HEALTH

simple practice routines

THROUGH

and a guide to the ancient teachings

YOGA

by

MIRA MEHTA

author of *Yoga: the Iyengar Way*

Thorsons

Thorsons
An Imprint of HarperCollins*Publishers*
77–85 Fulham Palace Road
Hammersmith, London W6 8JB

The Thorsons website is www.thorsons.com

™
and *Thorsons*
are trademarks of HarperCollins*Publishers*

Published by Thorsons 2002

1 3 5 7 9 10 8 6 4 2

Studio photography: Guy Hearn
Text illustrations: PCA Creative

A catalogue record for this book is
available from the British Library

ISBN 0-00-711620-9

Printed and bound in Great Britain by
Scotprint, Haddington, East Lothian

Dedication

This book is dedicated to the memory of my mother. A key figure in the spread of Yoga in this country, she was a fount of inspiration to hundreds of teachers and generations of students, myself included. Her disciplined and structured teaching methods, based on a thoughtful practice and wide reading, were set within an immense love for her students and for Yoga. She spared no pains to help each person and she sacrificed personal comfort to fulfil demands for a teacher in distant localities. In this subject of her choice her multi-faceted brilliance was honed, surely, by the agony she daily suffered from a spinal injury, to make her an exemplar of perceptiveness, compassion and indomitable spirit.

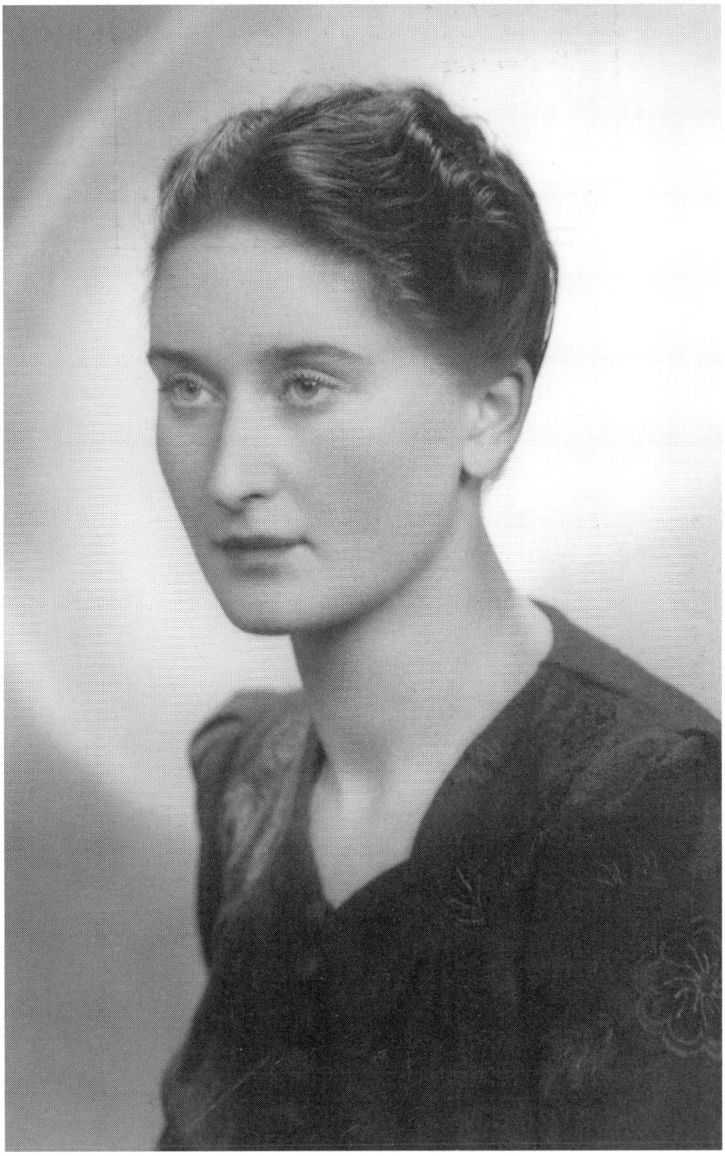

SILVA MEHTA
1926–1994

Acknowledgements

In the preparation of this book I am indebted to the following:

Prashant S. Iyengar for his support and encouragement and for going through the Yoga theory portions to ensure that no point was missed;

Professor Krishna S. Arjunwadkar, formerly of Bombay University, for his insistence that a book dealing with Yoga for health must include philosophy for health of the mind and for correcting my translations from the Sanskrit to ensure their accuracy;

Dr Mrunalini Kulkarni BAMS of the Tilak Maharashtra University, Pune for helping me to organize the Āyurveda section and for checking statements and references;

Dr L. Mahadevan BAMS, MD of Sarada Ayurvedic Hospital, Kanya Kumari for his timely and lively overview of Āyurveda while I was writing and for acting as a sounding board regarding the links between Āyurveda and Yoga;

Dr Tirun L. Gopal MD, DAy of Allentown, P.A. for answering some of my questions and for making corrections to the Āyurveda section;

Shyam Mehta for being the male model and for reading and testing the Yoga programmes for omissions and improvements;

Dr John Harrison PhD, FRCPath of King's College Hospital, London for explaining the disadvantages of chairs and for checking the paragraphs introducing the Yoga programmes;

Robert McLoughlin DO for scrutinizing the diagrams of the vital sites of the body so as to ensure that the arrows pointed to exactly the right spot;

Paul Heyda for his avuncular willingness to read the whole work in draft and for his gentle but pertinent suggestions;

Sallie Sullivan for supervising the photo sessions;

The Arsha Vidya Gurukulam in Saylorsburg, Pennsylvania for allowing me to enjoy the peace and beauty of their ashram while I wrote and for providing me with a computer;

Sarah Drake for her idea for the costume;

Gandolfi for making the costume;

Guy Hearn for the photography;

Michael Alcock for his always sensible agential advice;

Belinda Budge for her enthusiasm for this book, leading her to commission it;

Susan Berry for her keen editorial eyes and judgement;

Kate Latham for her excellent ideas and meticulous efficiency in overseeing the project;

Jacqui Caulton for her expertise in transforming bald text and bare photos into gorgeously designed pages.

Contents

Preface

This book arose out of my desire to understand more precisely how Yoga works. In pursuit of that desire I undertook formal studies in Āyurveda and in Yoga philosophy, refreshing my knowledge of Sanskrit in the process. For nearly three years I was a student at the Āyurveda Department of the Tilak Maharashtra Vidyapeeth (University) in Pune, India. For five years I also enjoyed one-to-one tutoring on the *Yoga Sūtras* and other Yoga texts by a retired Professor schooled in the ancient tradition of Sanskrit learning, Krishna S. Arjunwadkar. My practical studies have always been with the Iyengar family of Yogins and, above all, with my mother.

I have been fortunate in having many exceptional teachers, and in being able to consult the source works in the original language. I have tried to present the subject faithfully, but my efforts are of course limited by my own understanding. To the extent that I have succeeded I owe thanks to all those who have turned their minds to Yoga and Āyurveda before me, from the ancient thinkers on. Where I have failed, the misinterpretations are my own.

As a teacher myself, I am always conscious of the interaction between teacher and pupil. My own students in many countries have helped me to develop and refine my teaching methods. Their bodies and their questions have made me constantly search for ways of teaching which quicken the process of understanding. I have tried to be concise in my explanations, setting down not more yet not less than necessary. At the same time I have tried to convey my own passion for Yoga, in the hope that others will find in it the same deep satisfaction. To the extent that I have succeeded in this I owe thanks to my students.

Finally, as a poet I care about language. Words are the tools of communication. In teaching they can clarify or obscure; they can inspire or bore. I have tried to clothe my meanings neatly and aesthetically with clear syntax and fitting expression. To the extent that I have succeeded I owe thanks to my Muse.

In offering for consideration Yoga as a means to health it is both courteous to the reader and instructive to give some personal background. Except for a lucky few who are born with excellent constitutions and pass through life without experiencing accidents or the ravages of stress, everyone has minor or major health concerns. It is a condition of living.

Mine have been the following: At the age of eleven I realized that I had a severe curvature of the back (kyphosis). Ever since then my Yoga practice has been a constant struggle to conquer and reverse the natural progression of this curvature into rigidity and hunchback. Missing even a few days causes backache, neck pain and early fatigue from exertion to reappear. Fourteen years ago I suffered a whiplash injury where one of my cervical vertebrae dislocated. I immediately applied the countermeasure of plenty of spinal twists and standing poses. After that I developed chronic fatigue syndrome and was virtually bed-ridden for many months. The cause was diagnosed by chance some years later: amoebiosis, which I had had unknowingly for six years and which by that time had wreaked havoc with my digestion. The amoebae were eliminated by antibiotics, but for several years my practice was restorative, to rebuild strength. By chance again, I discovered I was hosting two other aggressive invaders which had been with me since childhood:

the Epstein Barr virus and an amoebic infection of the lungs. They were both treated with homeopathic medicine. As soon as the lung parasite had gone my back ceased to feel like concrete: the parasite must have indirectly caused the kyphosis. As I continued Yoga practice throughout, I am now enjoying robustness and energy rather than coping with a body debilitated by structural and systemic damage. My back is straight, my neck is strong, and my chest and lungs open well. I look forward to a trouble-free digestion, if not to the ability to consume poison, claimed for the Yogins of old (through the practice of *Mayūrāsana*, the Peacock Pose – HYP 1.31).

My brother Shyam, who demonstrates the postures along with me, has had since childhood the unusual combination of strength and suppleness. Blessed with a strong constitution too, he seems to manage with ease a high-pressure job in the world of finance involving regular travel abroad as well as Yoga teaching and family commitments. But in late 1998, through a medical examination required for a new job, he was diagnosed as having a hereditary genetic disorder involving a serious malfunction of the thyroid. He was told that the disease operated to a biological clock, that it would start within a few months and that he would need daily medication. Choosing instead to try to keep the disease at bay by Āyurvedic medicine and careful Yoga practice, he has so far succeeded: he is symptom-free.

Our mother Silva sustained a spinal fracture in her twenties and was told she would be in a wheelchair by the age of fifty. She was advised to take up Yoga, and, being in India at the time, did so. As a result she was mobile for the rest of her life, though she was never free of pain. Later she developed Graves disease, and swung between hypothyroidism and hyperthyroidism until she was given the right balance of medication. Her strong will carried her through this, and she taught a Yoga class the evening before she died.

Our stories are not unique. There are countless people who could testify to the healing power of Yoga. In my own teaching career I have seen amelioration of all types of conditions affecting the body's structure and functioning: sprained and torn muscles and ligaments, backache, scoliosis, arthritis, asthma, constipation, irregular menses, amenorrhea, cystitis, chronic fatigue, migraine, depression and hypertension. The list is endless, as is a list of ailments.

Yoga is not a panacea, even though it can sometimes substitute for medicine or surgery. It is, after all, primarily a path enjoining mental control for the sake of spiritual emancipation and the health benefits it bestows can be regarded almost as side effects. It has, however, two particular strengths. The first is that it works on the body through the body itself. Thus it has a direct contact with nature without any intermediary. What is direct is uniquely powerful. The second is its optimistic outlook, imbuing the mind with positive energy. A fundamental tenet of its philosophy is that "future pain is to be avoided" (PYS 2.16). The practice of Yoga is given as the way this can be achieved, for the individual's ultimate good.

Mira Mehta
April 2001

Introduction

The path of Yoga has as its goal the harnessing and transcendence of the mind in order to restore the experience of spiritual integrity. A pure spiritual nature is considered the birthright of all human beings, but one which is lost in the overlay of mundane activities. In pursuit of this goal it advocates practices which systematically train body, mind and senses, breaking habitual and instinctual behaviour and cultivating one-pointed awareness of the inner being. Stripped of the mass of thoughts and reflexes which surround and obscure the pure centre of consciousness which is the soul, that core shines out in its true nature.

There are five aids to Yoga which act as steps to this summit of experience, a profound absorption (*samādhi*) undisturbed by the sense of individual identity and other externals. These aids are ethical principles (*yama*), personal disciplines (*niyama*), mastery of the body through posture (*āsana*), mastery of the breath (*prāṇāyāma*), and withdrawal of the senses from their stimuli (*pratyāhāra*). The portal to this supreme experience is mental focus (*dhāraṇā*) on the desired object which deepens into meditation (*dhyāna*). From *yama* to *samādhi* there are thus eight parts to Yoga, metaphorically called limbs. The whole subject was systematically expounded more than two thousand years ago by Patañjali in his "Aphorisms on Yoga" (*Yoga Sūtra*).

Aside from their role in spiritual training, Yogic postures and breathing techniques have long been praised for their health benefits. A 15th century manual of practice, the *Haṭha Yoga Pradīpikā* of *Svātmārāma*, states that as a result of *āsana* practice "there is sturdiness, absence of disease and lightness" (HYP 1.17). In describing various *āsanas* it also details their effects: for example, through *Paścimottānāsana*, the seated forward bend (see page 104), the digestive power increases, the abdomen reduces and the practitioner becomes free of disease (HPY1.29). *Prāṇāyāma* practice is repeatedly said to eradicate diseases. Each *prāṇāyāma* has specific benefits: for example, *Ujjāyi* (see page 167) destroys disorders of *kapha* in the throat, increases the digestive power and cures dropsy and disorders of the channels and tissues of the body (HYP 2.52-53).

A major reason for the contemporary popularity of Yoga practice is its prophylactic and curative value. Another powerful attraction is its philosophy of tranquillity. These two together make Yoga a peerless tool for coping with the stresses of life, both physical and mental.

While the efficacy of Yoga as a health-bestowing practice is well attested, the reasons why it works are not elucidated in detail in the traditional texts. To discover the science behind the practice it is necessary to turn to its sister subject Āyurveda, traditional Indian medical science. Literally "the science of life", Āyurveda comes from the same matrix of philosophical thought as Yoga. Its sphere of enquiry is the body-mind complex, from the point of view of the maintenance of health and the treatment of diseases. Its explanations of the workings of the body, its interaction with the universe, its care and healthy living greatly illuminate Yoga practice.

Āyurveda and Yoga share a common heritage of Vedic culture. This refers to the civilization which produced a body of literature known as the *Vedas* (sciences or sources of knowledge). There are three principal *Vedas*: the *Ṛg* (prayer) *-Veda*, the *Yajur* (ritualistic formula) *-Veda* and the *Sāma* (chant) -*Veda*. The *Ṛg-Veda* is the oldest and is broadly a collection of prayers to deities. It is entirely in metrical form, consisting of over 10,000 couplets. It displays poetic genius of a high order and is occasionally marked by lofty philosophical musings. The *Yajur-Veda* is the oldest prose writing; it interprets the *Ṛg-Vedic* prayers as incantations for use in rituals and sacrifices. The *Sāma-Veda* is musical version of the ninth book of the *Ṛg-Veda*, refashioned for employment in rituals. A fourth *Veda*, the *Atharva-Veda*, contains mainly spells for magical rites and health cures, many of which involve the use of medicinal plants. It is assigned to the same period as the *Ṛg-Veda* and is also mostly metrical in form. This *Veda* is said to represent the religion of the "masses", while the *Ṛg-Veda* represents that of the "classes". The date of the *Vedas* is not known with certainty: a conservative estimate is 2,000–1,500 BC, but 3,000 BC is also suggested.

The composers of the Vedic hymns are by tradition regarded as seers who experienced mystic revelations of eternal truth. The culmination of Vedic thought is in the *Upaniṣads*, which contain, amongst other matters, teachings of deep spiritual import. It is here that Yoga is clearly mentioned, for example, in the *Kaṭha* and *Śvetāśvatara Upaniṣads*. The *Bhagavad-Gītā*, another ancient work on spiritual life, contains a whole chapter on Yoga practice and philosophy as well as many scattered passages relating to it. It describes itself as a Yoga treatise, although it employs the term Yoga in a wider sense of "a spiritual means". It is from this body of literature and also, undoubtedly, from knowledge of contemporary practices passed down from guru to disciple that Patañjali summarized the fundamental elements of the Yoga science. His epitome of Yoga (*Yoga Sūtra*) cannot have been the first work of its kind, but because of its excellence it superseded previous works and still stands today as the supreme authority.

The seeds of Indian medical science are traced to the *Atharva-Veda*. Among its magico-religious spells are included herbal remedies for ailments together with their methods of administration. The exegetical literature of the *Atharva-Veda* collects these together; however, at this stage they do not form a systematic medical science. Caraka's Compendium (*Caraka Saṁhitā*) is the earliest extant work of this nature, and it claims to be a redaction of an earlier work. As with Patañjali's treatise, its excellence eclipsed earlier works and it remains a sourcebook of authority.

Works on Yoga and Āyurveda are naturally concerned with the details of their own subjects. They take for granted the philosophical and cultural axioms of the society from which they spring. For the modern reader this background of ideas needs to be brought to the fore. The readings in the final section of this book present at first hand aspects of the world-view which nurtured the two sciences. For example, the important doctrine of the three intertwining strands of nature – light, energy and darkness or inertia (*sattva*, *rajas*, *tamas*) – is dealt with at length in the *Bhagavad-Gītā* and the *Sāṁkhya* philosophical school. Similarly, the doctrine of transmigration finds an explanation in the *Upaniṣads*. These texts also discuss the nature of the human being and the world, the existence of an Ultimate Reality as the ground of the universe, the experience of living as the experience of suffering, the path of Yoga as the means of spiritual release, and the distinction between mundane knowledge and knowledge of the transcendent reality. All these doctrines form the bedrock of thought on which both Āyurveda and Yoga are based.

This book is in three parts: the first part, *How Yoga Works*, gives a synopsis of the main principles of Āyurveda. On the criterion of relevance to Yoga, it does not deal with Āyurvedic clinical medicine and materia medica. It then applies the theory of Āyurveda to explain Yoga practice. The second part, *Practice Routines for Longevity*, gives sequences of Yoga *āsanas* and *prāṇāyāma* for maintaining health. The third part, *Readings for Serenity*, introduces Yoga philosophy for the health of the mind. The passages, chosen from ancient works, illustrate the Yogic approach to life situations and problems.

The intention of the book is threefold: first, to be a practical guide to the Yogic way of thinking; secondly, to introduce the wisdom of Āyurveda regarding health and healthy living; and thirdly, to link the two subjects so as to throw light on the theory behind Yoga practice. Wherever possible the presentation of ideas follows closely those of the original ancient texts. The source references are given so as to enable the interested reader to navigate the subject independently. A guide to the pronunciation of Sanskrit words and a list of abbreviations used are given at the back of the book.

Although Yoga is a discipline with eight spheres of operation, known as limbs, it is pre-eminently the third and fourth ones involving postures (*āsana*) and breath-control (*prāṇāyāma*) which lend themselves to detailed analysis in terms of the teachings of Āyurveda. The first two limbs comprise ethics and personal disciplines and mainly relate to the incorporeal, and the final limbs dealing with meditation go beyond normal states of body and mind. The method of *āsana* and *prāṇāyāma* practice followed in this book is that of B.K.S. Iyengar, who is recognized as a leading authority on Yoga and whose books (*Light on Yoga* and *Light on Prāṇāyāma*) are regarded as modern classics. His guru was T. Krishnamacharya, a renowned scholar of many branches of traditional Sanskrit learning as well as a Yogin, who ran a Yoga school at the palace of the Maharaja of Mysore. Krishnamacharya's guru was Ram Mohan Brahmachari, a Yogin recluse living in Nepal.

Summary of Major Conclusions

In applying the principles of Āyurveda to Yoga practice it became clear that these principles were powerful explanatory tools. The major conclusions are summarized below:

Anatomy

- The Āyurvedic enumeration of the vital sites of the body (*marmasthānas*) correlates to the actions needed in these areas in order to perfect the performance of the *āsanas*.

Physiology

- The existence of three distinct functional energies (*doṣas* – *vāta*, *pitta* and *kapha*) as governing physiology and psychology provides an explanation of how the *āsanas* produce their effects: they alter the balance of the *doṣas*.

- In particular, the division of each *doṣa* into five according to location and function enables a detailed explanation of how each individual posture and *prāṇāyāma* works and why different ones have different effects.

Psychology

- The Āyurvedic explanation of psychological health based on the right use of the senses and mind helps to understand the Yogic approach where mind and senses are quieted and purified in order to achieve mental peace.

Rejuvenation

- Āyurveda emphasizes the constant care of the body and its rejuvenation by tonics and special treatments. Yoga has a similar philosophy, and its practice has a rejuvenating effect.

Energy Management

- The Āyurvedic classification of constitution, temperament and stages of life according to the predominance of *doṣas* provides a guide to individual practice in terms of energy management and suitable postures.

- The Āyurvedic explanation of the stages of life and the menstrual cycle in terms of *doṣas* provides a basis on which to understand the special Yoga programmes needed by women during menstruation and pregnancy and by growing children.

- Āyurvedic guidelines on exercise are useful for understanding the limits of exertion in Yoga practice.

Pain Management

- The Āyurvedic explanation of the process of disease can be used to understand the management of pain through Yoga practice. This applies to mental as well as physical pain.

Healthy Lifestyle

- Āyurvedic guidelines on diet and a healthy daily routine provide a framework for Yoga practice which is conducive to physical and mental well-being.

- Āyurveda prescribes periodic cleansing procedures to rid the body of toxins. Yoga techniques also have this effect.

- Āyurveda stresses the importance of healthy progeny and has a special branch dealing with sexual potency. This highlights the importance of the health of the pelvic organs, which is improved by Yoga practice.

Therapeutics

- The Āyurvedic division of treatment into purifying and pacifying provides a theoretical basis on which to understand the therapeutic application of *āsanas*.
- Similarly, its analysis of the disease process is useful in understanding the evolution and counteracting of pain. This is of help in understanding the method of alleviating pain through Yoga *āsanas*.

THE SOURCE WORKS ON ĀYURVEDA

For Āyurveda the source works used are those known as the "Great Three":

The *Caraka Saṁhitā*, "Caraka's Compendium", an exhaustive compilation of all the branches of Āyurveda, particularly internal medicine. Its date is variously given as 1000 BCE or the 3rd or 2nd centuries BCE.
The *Suśruta Saṁhitā* "Suśruta's Compendium", another encyclopaedia of Āyurveda, whose specialty is surgery. It date is thought to be approximately 600 BCE.
Vāgbhaṭa's *Aṣṭāṅga Hṛydaya* "The Heart of the Eightfold [Science of Health]" a succinct presentation of the whole of Āyurveda which draws on the former two works. Opinions on the date of this work are divided between the 5th century CE and 600 CE.

THE SOURCE WORKS ON YOGA

For Yoga the main source works used are the following:

Selected *Upaniṣads*, "Sitting-Close Meetings", ancient philosophical treatises on the nature of life and the universe containing the seeds of ideas developed by later thinkers. The *Upaniṣads* are considered to be the end or culmination of the Vedas (*Vedānta*). The date of these works cannot be estimated with certainty. The Vedic literature is much earlier than the *Mahābharata* (see below), being dated variously between 3,000 BC and 1,500 BC.
The *Bhagavad-Gītā*, "The Song of the Lord", an immensely popular poetic discourse on spiritual life and liberation, forming part of the epic *Mahābhārata*. The composition of this epic took place from 400 BCE to 400 CE, according to the Critical Edition by the Bhandarkar Oriental Research Institute. Some scholars place the *Bhagavad-Gītā* a little before that, in the 5th century BCE.
Patañjali's *Yoga Sūtra*, "Aphorisms on Yoga", a systematic exposition of Yoga philosophy. It is thought to date from the 2nd century BCE.
Vyāsa's *Bhāṣya*, "Commentary", an important elucidation of Patañjali's *Yoga Sūtra* composed in the 4th century CE.
Svātmārāma's *Haṭha Yoga Pradīpikā,* "Light on the Yoga of Force", a manual of *āsanas* and *prāṇāyāmas* as well as esoteric practices written in the 15th century CE.

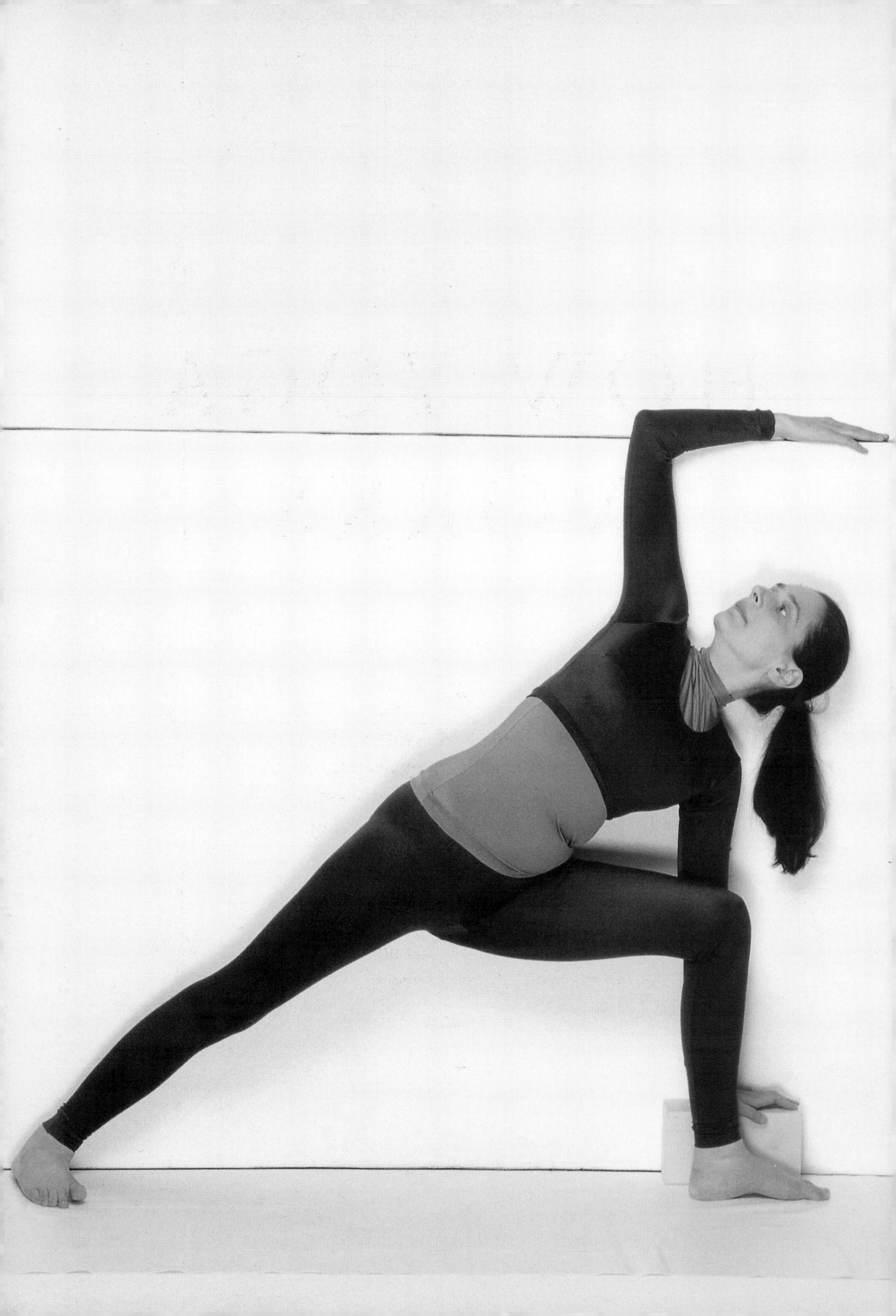

HOW YOGA WORKS

Indeed, the aim of Āyurveda is,
For those afflicted by disease,
Complete freedom from disease,
And for the healthy, safeguarding.

(SS-Sū 1.14)

One should know that unyoking
From the yoke of pain is designated Yoga.

(BG 6.23)

Introducing Āyurveda

When I began the study of Āyurveda I was fortunate in having some knowledge of Sanskrit and Indian philosophy to ease me into the ocean of concepts that differed vastly from modern Western ones. However, they are not so far removed from ancient Greek and mediaeval ideas, which are also becoming more and more alien to the contemporary mind. As I learned to swim in this ocean, as it were, certain features of Āyurveda showed themselves distinctly.

The first is a theoretical framework that views the human being and all nature as interconnected. Everything emanates from nature and consists of three principles: light, energy and inertia and five elements: space, air, fire, water and earth. Bodies have different shapes and qualities according to the combination and proportion of these elements; the senses of living creatures are designed to interact with these elements. Everything in the world can be classified according to its properties: hot or cold, liquid or solid, rough or smooth, and so on. Everything has a use.

This theoretical framework is anthropocentric. The rationale of classification is utility to human life and endeavour. This can be seen in the listing of foods and their properties so that their benefit or otherwise to different constitutions can be ascertained. It is even more evident in the taxonomy of Āyurvedic *materia medica*. The properties of plants, animals and minerals are schematized so that they can easily be identified and used to remedy deficiencies and imbalances in human tissues. The calculation is almost like a mathematical equation.

Within this sophisticated and systematic world view, Āyurveda sets its special subject of study: life and longevity. It has a common-sense approach to life and health. To withstand wear and tear, the body needs regular maintenance: a good diet, a daily health regimen and periodic internal cleansing. Not only does Āyurveda recognize the importance of a sensible life-style and diet, it lists exhaustively the activities and attitudes which promote or endanger health. Most of these resemble good parental advice, such as washing before eating and avoiding walking at night. However, a few are striking. To give a thought-provoking example, sitting on a hard seat of knee height is said to be injurious to health. Western medicine recognizes that pressure for long periods on the veins at the back of the thigh, together with immobility of the legs and dangling feet, leads to stagnation of blood and possible deep-vein thrombosis in the calf. This drives home the disadvantages of using chairs as opposed to sitting cross-legged on the floor. In this more natural position, the feet are level with the hips and support the legs, which also support each other. The legs are firm, not flaccid, so blood does not pool in the lower legs, and the possibility of thrombosis is avoided. Some other Āyurvedic recommendations, such as to avoid associating with lunatics, do not accord with modern thinking.

Āyurveda is considered to have been handed down from ancient savants, who were instructed by the gods themselves. Whatever its history, it is certainly remarkable that its theories, as well as many of its medicinal recipes, have enjoyed continuous currency for centuries, for the very good reason that they work. Subsequent doctors and medical authors have added their contributions within this time-tested framework and have not overturned it. The theory of three *doṣas*, embodying the principles of motion, heat and cohesion, as the operating principles of the body accounts for the variety of constitutional types, for different physiological processes and for the states of health and disease. In the field of anatomy, Āyurveda's contribution is the identification of numerous vital, vulnerable sites in the body: *marmas*.

If Āyurveda can provide a logical explanation of how the body works, it follows that it must be able to explain how Yoga postures and breath control work, as their province is the body, mind and breath. This was the premise I started with and, in working out a detailed analysis based on the effects of different postures and breath controls, I was delighted, though not surprised, to find that this premise was correct. My analyses corroborated the brief statements given in early Yoga texts.

On the specific topic of the link between Āyurveda and Yoga, there is no authoritative body of texts which can be consulted. The Yoga literature provides only hints. What I have set down is thus largely interpretative, in the sense not of creative speculation but of the application of the principles of Āyurveda to a particular set of data.

This section is in two parts. The first part sets out the world view and fundamental tenets of Āyurveda. They are divided into four major topics: life, the conceptual framework of Āyurveda, the body and health. The second part is concerned with understanding Yoga through Āyurveda. The topics covered are anatomy, physiology and psychology, the management of energy and pain, cleansing routines and special therapies.

Life

Life is defined as the union of body, senses, mind and soul. It is described as the support which does not let the body decay, the holder of the vital force constantly passing away and getting bound.

Health is the root which promotes longevity and sustains the achievement of all purposes of life. Indian thought, from which Āyurveda springs, recognizes four purposes: the performance of social and religious duties, the acquisition of wealth, the pursuit of pleasure and happiness, and finally, the striving for spiritual enlightenment. It is said that those wishing to enjoy a long life should follow the teachings of Āyurveda. Diseases create impediments to all activities.

Āyurveda is the science which gives knowledge (*veda*) about life (*āyus*). It defines life and states that there are four grades of life: good, not good, happy and unhappy. It further speaks of the span of life, which can be prolonged or shortened according as one follows or ignores health-promoting rules. It therefore explains in detail what is good or wholesome for life, and what is not good.

A life is considered happy when there are no physical or psychological diseases and when there is youth, strength, energy, success, capability, courage, spiritual and worldly knowledge, strong sense organs and body qualities, such as complexion, voice, smell, taste, touch, sight, wealth, enjoyments, achievement of undertakings, and freedom of movement. An unhappy life is the opposite of this.

A life is considered good when one wishes others well, speaks the truth, is calm, acts with circumspection and is level-headed. One follows the purposes of life without conflict, honours worthy people, has spiritual and worldly knowledge, is serene and serves the elderly. One controls the emotions of passion, anger, envy, mania and pride. One is always generous and is devoted to ascetic practices, knowledge and peace. One has knowledge about the soul and is concerned both with this world and the next. One has a good memory and intellect. A life is not considered good when these qualities are lacking.

Certain features of a new-born baby are held to indicate longevity such as the quality of hair, skin and eyes. The texts also list signs and portents of imminent death, such as sudden changes in complexion and voice and in other physical and mental characteristics. Signs and symptoms indicating that diseases are progressing towards death are also noted.

The span of life is to a certain extent determined by individual constitution. *Kapha*-predominant people tend to live long lives; *vāta*-predominant people tend to have a short life span and *pitta* people a medium life span.

The span of human life is taken to be 100 years, but it is recognized that death can be timely or untimely. The parallel is given of the axle of a cart which can get destroyed quickly if the cart is overloaded, if the road is rough, if there is no road, if a wheel breaks, if the driver is careless, if the bolt comes loose, and so on. In the same way, life span can be reduced by over-exertion, by a mismatch between food consumed and digestive power, by erratic eating habits, awkward postural habits, too much sex, resorting to falsehood, controlling physical urges, failure to control emotions that should be controlled, by possession by evil spirits, by poison, by turbulent winds, by fire, by accidents, by not eating and by failing to take remedial measures. For these reasons it is necessary to know and follow what is healthful for life. This is explained in Āyurveda.

The Conceptual Framework of Āyurveda

Everything in this universe, including the human body, is formed from the five elements, earth (*pṛthvī*), water (*āp*), fire (*agni*), air (*vāyu*) and space (*akāśa*). The body is understood in terms of functional units, tissues and waste products (*doṣa, dhātu, mala*). Similarly the substances in the universe are understood with respect to the effect they have on the body. They are described in terms of taste (*rasa*), potency (*vīrya*), post-digestion taste (*vipāka*), qualities (*guṇa*) and a special property (*prabhava*).

THE FIVE ELEMENTS

There are five elements in the universe which combine to form the perceptible substances of earth, water, air, fire and space. For example, water consists of all the five elements with the water element predominant. Different substances are formed from a combination of these five elements. Earth consolidates, water lubricates, air produces movement, multiplicity and separation, fire is responsible for metabolism and space accommodates. These five elements combine in different proportions to produce the multiplicity of substances in the world, both within and outside the body.

The elements have a hierarchical order from the subtle to the gross: that is, from space to earth. Each element has a main property: space has sound; wind has touch; fire has form-and-colour;

Role of Elements in Body Parts

ELEMENT	BODY COMPONENT DERIVED FROM ELEMENT
Earth (*pṛthvī*)	Smell Organ of smell Weight Stability Hardness / Solidity Bones
Water (*jala*)	Tastes Organ of taste Coolness Softness Unctuousness Moisture
Fire (*agni*)	Colour Sight Digestion Body heat Perception / Brightness
Air (*vāyu*)	Sense of touch Organ of touch + Dryness + Energy + Breathing Activities of body Organization of constituents (*dhātus*) Respiration
Space (*ākāśa*)	Sound Organ of hearing Lightness Minuteness Division Hollowness, Orifices

water has taste and earth has smell. Each also possesses the properties of the elements preceding it. Thus, for example, in addition to smell, earth has taste, form-and-colour, touch and sound.

The predominant element present in a substance can be recognized by the qualities of that substance. A substance is said to be earth-predominant when it is heavy, gross, stable and characterized by smell. It produces these qualities in the body, as well as bulk and hardness. A substance is water-predominant when it is cold, heavy, oily, slow-acting, semi-liquid and characterized by taste. It produces oiliness, secretions, wetness, satisfaction from nourishment and binding in the body. A substance is fire-predominant when it is dry, sharp, hot, cleansing, minute and characterized by form-and-colour. In the body it produces a burning sensation, lustre, colour, sight and digestion. A substance is wind-predominant when it is a dry, cleansing, light and characterized by touch. It produces dryness, lightness, cleanness, movements and loss of energy. A substance is space-predominant when it is minute, cleansing, light and characterized by sound. It produces porosity and lightness in the body.

Parts of the body, their actions, qualities and functions are all classified according to the five elements. Space correlates to the ears, the voice and empty spaces. Wind correlates to the sense of touch, the skin, the breath, impetus, the organization of tissues and body movements. Fire is associated with form-and-colour, the eyes, the power of sight, digestion and heat. Water relates to taste, the tongue, coldness, softness, oiliness and wetness. Earth governs smell, the nose, heaviness, stability and shape. The correlation of body parts and elements is given in the table on page 4. There is a correlation between the *doṣas* and the elements. *Vāta* is formed predominantly from wind and space. *Pitta* is formed predominantly from fire. *Kapha* is formed predominantly from water and earth.There is similarly a correlation between the senses and the elements: space with the ears, air with the skin, fire with the eyes, water with the tongue, and earth with the nose.

PROPERTIES AND TASTES

Substances in the world are understood in terms of how their properties act on the human body. There are twenty main properties, divided into ten pairs of opposites. The table overleaf gives the effect of each property on the body.

Substances are also classified according to their basic taste, their post-digestion taste, their potency and their special property.

There are six tastes (*rasa*): sweet, sour, salty, bitter, pungent and astringent. Each taste is formed predominantly from two elements (*mahābhūta*):

Tastes and their Associated Elements

TASTE	ELEMENTS
Sweet	Earth and Water
Sour	Fire and Earth
Salty	Water and Fire
Pungent	Fire and Wind
Bitter	Space and Wind
Astringent	Earth and Wind

The first three tastes (sweet, sour and salty) decrease *vāta* and increase *kapha*. The last three (bitter, pungent and astringent) decrease *kapha* and increase *vāta*. Astringent, bitter and sweet tastes decrease *pitta*. The remaining three (sour, salty and pungent) increase *pitta*. The first taste (sweet) gives the maximum strength to the body, while the last (astringent) gives the least.The specific taste that is produced at the end of digestion as a result of the contact of substances with the digestive fire is called *vipāka*. Generally substances that are sweet and salty have a sweet *vipāka*. Sour substances have a sour *vipāka*. Bitter, astringent and pungent substances have a pungent *vipāka*.

Over and above the basic taste and post-digestion taste, a substance is considered to have a potency (*vīrya*) that is hot or cold in its effect. In a general sense, *vīrya* is also the term for the strongest acting quality of any substance.

The special property of a substance, other than the properties of taste, post-digestion taste and potency, is called *prabhava*. This property is unique to the substance and is unexpected or unpredictable. An example of this is ghee (clarified butter), which, despite having a cold potency like milk, increases the digestive fire.

The 20 Properties and their Effects

PROPERTY	EFFECT ON BODY	PROPERTY	EFFECT ON BODY
Cold (*śīta*)	Produces cheerfulness, obstruction; overcomes fainting, thirst, sweating and burning sensation	**Hot** (*uṣṇa*)	Opposite in effect to cold; aids digestion
Unctuous (*snigdha*)	Gives oiliness, softness, strength and good complexion	**Dry** (*rūkṣa*)	Opposite in effect to oily; produces rigidity and roughness
Slimy (*picchila*)	Nourishes life; gives strength; unites fractures; increases kapha; is heavy	**Clean** (*viśada*)	Opposite in effect to Slimy; is cleansing; heals wounds
Sharp (*tīkṣṇa*)	Produces burning sensation; aids digestion; causes secretions	**Mild** (*mṛdu*)	Opposite in effect to Sharp
Heavy (*guru*)	Causes loss of body vigour; increases waste products; gives strength; nourishes; increases bulk	**Light** (*laghu*)	Opposite in effect to Heavy; produces slimness; aids slimness; aids healing of wounds
Liquid (*drava*)	Causes moisture	**Viscous** (*sāndra*)	Is gross and non-permeating; builds up (the body)
Smooth (*slakṣṇa*)	Similar to Slimy	**Rough** (*karkaśa*)	Similar to Clean
Motile (*sara*)	Initiates actions and processes	**Sluggish** (*manda*)	Constipating
Pervasive (*vyavāyin*)	Pervades body before digestion	**Expanding** (*vikāsin*)	Releases elements (*dhātus*) as it extends
Speedy (*āśukārin*)	Moves fast like oil in water	**Subtle** (*sūkṣma*)	Operates in tiny channels

SIMILARITY AND DISSIMILARITY

A basic principle of Āyurveda, on which all treatment is based, is that similarity is always responsible for increase, while dissimilarity is responsible for decrease. The equilibrium and disequilibrium of body tissues occurs because of the operation of similarity and dissimilarity. The exclusive and excessive use of substances and actions similar to a particular body tissue will cause imbalance by increasing that tissue. The exclusive and excessive use of substances and actions dissimilar to particular body tissue will decrease it, leading to imbalance. However, if similar and dissimilar things are both used together at the same time, the balance of body tissues is maintained.

Tissues are increased by food and actions having the same qualities and are decreased when food and actions have the opposite qualities. There are three types of similarity and dissimilarity: of substance (*dravya*), of property (*guṇa*) and of action (*karma*). As an example of the first kind, flesh gets increased by eating flesh (similarity of substance), while *vāta doṣa* gets decreased (dissimilarity of substance). As an example of the second, milk increases regenerative tissue and semen (similarity of property); cold water reduces the sensation of burning (dissimilarity of property). As to the third, sleep increases *kapha doṣa* (similarity of action), while exercise decreases it (dissimilarity of action).

CORRESPONDENCE OF MANKIND AND THE UNIVERSE

The union of the five elements with the soul (*ātmā*) brings about the existence of each individual being, known as *puruṣa*. The individual being is conceived as the microcosmic counterpart of the universe. Within the individual are to be found as many entities as are present in the universe, and vice versa. These include various deities, heavenly bodies, principles and ages of creation. Some main points of correspondence between the body and the universe are given below.

This knowledge of the universe in the self and the self in the universe produces true knowledge. The individual recognizes that he or she alone is the cause of happiness and sorrow lies in one's inclination to worldly things. With this knowledge the individual rises towards emancipation.

Main Correspondences between Microcosm and Macrocosm

HUMAN BEING	UNIVERSE
Soul	Universal consciousness
Mind	The Creator
Ego	The Lord of gods
Intake of food and water	The sun
Anger	The deity of destruction
Nourishment	The moon
Happiness	The group of eight gods called *Vasus*
Lustre	The gods of medicine
Vigour	The wind god
All senses & their objects	The group of gods called *Viśvadeva*
Delusion	Darkness
Knowledge	Light
Creation of the foetus	Divine worlds, heaven, and so on
Childhood	The first age marked by perfect *dharma*, the supporting principle
Youth	The decadent second age marked by the rise of theft
Old age	The decadent third age marked by the rise of falsehood
Disease	The decadent last age marked by the rise of conceit
Death	End of ages

The Body

The body is stated to be the seat of consciousness and derived from the five elements. The Sanskrit word for body, *śarīra*, is derived from a verbal root meaning to wear out or decay. Hence the body is taken to be "that which degenerates every moment".

The body is considered to be pervaded by three principle, or energies, called *doṣas*: *vāta*, *pitta* and *kapha*: concerned respectivly (roughly speaking) with movement, metabolism and cohesion. Physically, the body consists of seven tissues (*dhātus*): plasma, blood, flesh, fat, bone, marrow and regenerative tissues. There are three main waste products (*malas*): urine, faeces and sweat. *Doṣas*, tissues and wastes are the root substances of the body, which are present from its formation to its disintegration. Their role is likened to the root of a tree, which is responsible for its development, maintenance and destruction. In equilibrium they maintain the health of the body; unbalanced, they lead to disease.

FUNCTIONAL ENERGIES (*DOṢAS*)

The *doṣas* control all the functions of the body. The word comes from the verbal root "*duṣ*" meaning to spoil or become spoiled. The *doṣas* become disturbed and lose equilibrium as a result of imappropriate food and behaviour; they also disturb the other bodily substances, the tissues (*dhātus*) and waste products (*malas*). The inherent tendency of the *doṣas* to become disturbed, as well as their capacity to disturb, has given them their name, "spoilers".

There are three *doṣas*: *vāta*, *pitta* and *kapha* The word *vāta* is derived from "*va*", which indicates motion. *Pitta* is derived from "*tapa*", which indicates heat. That which gets increased by water is *kapha*. (An alternative name for *kapha* is *śleṣma*, which comes from "*śliṣ*", to embrace or to hold together.) Thus the names *vāta*, *pitta* and *kapha* themselves indicate their functions in the body. *Vāta* is mainly responsible for motion, *pitta* for heat and conversion and *kapha* for cohesiveness and for growth.

Though the *doṣas* are present throughout the body, each has a specific area of operation. *Kapha* is located predominantly above the heart. The site of *pitta* is between the heart and navel. *Vāta* is located below the navel. The *doṣas* are formed in the digestive tract. Each one is associated with particular tissues (*dhātus*). *Vāta* resides in the

Sites and Functions of the *Doṣas*

DOṢA	SEATS	FUNCTIONS
Vāta	Large Intestine (*pakvāśaya*) [major seat] Pelvis (*kati*) Thighs (*sakthi*) Ears (*śrotra*) Bones (*asthi*) Skin (*sparśanendriya*)	Vigour, Freshness Exhalation Inhalation Movements Producing urges Maintenance and motion of tissues Maintenance of activities of organs
Pitta	Navel (*nābhi*) [major seat] Sweat (*sveda*) Serum (*lasika*) Blood (*rudhira*) Plasma (*rasa*) Eyes (*dṛṣṭi*) Skin (*sparśana*)	Digestion Maintenance of body temperature Sight Hunger Thirst Taste, liking Glow of complexion Intellectual retentive power Analytical intelligence Strength Slenderness and softness of body
Kapha	Chest (*uras*) [major seat] Throat (*kaṇṭha*) Head (*śiras*) Right lung (*kloma*) Finger joints (*parva*) Stomach (*āmāśaya*) Plasma (*rasa*) Fat (*medas*) Nose (*ghrāṇa*) Tongue (*jihvā*)	Sturdiness of body Oiliness Holding joints together Tolerance

bones; *pitta* in the blood and sweat and *kapha* in all the other tissues.

The table opposite gives the sites and functions of the three *doṣas*.

BODY TISSUES (*DHĀTUS*)

Those substances that support the body are called *dhātu*. The *doṣas* reside in the body with the support of the *dhātus*, the body tissues. In their normal quantity and quality, they support the body. When they are disturbed by the *doṣas*, they lead to diseases. The *dhātus* are also termed "*duṣya*": "spoilable": that which gets disturbed or vitiated. *Dhātu* comes from the verbal root *dhṛ*, meaning "to hold". The tissues hold the body in the sense that they form the base of body. They are the cause of the existence of the body and form its structure.

There are seven *dhātus*: plasma (*rasa*) – an approximate equivalent as the functions of *rasa* are not identical with those of plasma; blood (*rakta*); flesh (*māṁsa*); fat (*meda*); bone (*asthi*); marrow (*majjā*); and semen and regenerative tissue (*śukra*). Their functions are given in the table below:

Functions of *Dhātus*

TISSUES	FUNCTIONS
Plasma (*rasa*)	Nourishment of other *dhātus*, particularly of blood; contentment
Blood (*rakta*)	Complexion; nourishment of flesh; life support
Flesh (*māṁsa*)	Nourishment of body and fat; plastering of body
Fat (*meda*)	Oiliness of body; sweat; sturdiness; nourishment of bones
Bone (*asthi*)	Formation of supporting structure of the body; nourishment of bone marrow
Bone marrow (*majjā*)	Filling of bones, nourishment of regenerative tissue; strength, oiliness; affection
Semen and regenerative tissue (*śukra*)	Courage, motility, attraction (to and for the opposite sex), body strength, sexual excitement, reproduction

The quintessence of all the seven tissues is called *ojas*. It is responsible for resistance, vitality and balance of mind. Though it is present throughout the body, its site is the heart and it is responsible for the continuance of the body; without it life is destroyed. *Ojas* is oily, cool and reddish-yellow in colour. It gets decreased as a result of anger, hunger, obsession, grief and overexertion. The signs of decreased *ojas* are: fear, loss of strength, constant worry, impairment of the senses, loss of the glow of health, loss of mental vigour, and dryness and emaciation. When *ojas* increases, happiness, growth and body strength also increase.

WASTES (*MALA*)

Substances which make the body unclean if they remain in it for a long time are called impurities (*mala*). These waste products also have certain functions in the body. However, if they are retained for too long, they disturb its normal functioning. The three main *malas* produced in the body are stools, urine and sweat.

Functions of Body Wastes

WASTE	FUNCTIONS
Stool (*purīṣa*)	Supports the body; supports *vāta* and digestive power. A decrease of stool inside the body leads to weakness
Urine (*mūtra*)	Fills the bladder; maintains water balance
Sweat (*sveda*)	Keeps the skin moist and delicate

There are two types of waste products: those produced as a result of the main digestive process, (stools and urine) and those produced during tissue metabolism. The most important of these is sweat. Other tissue wastes are: *kapha*, produced during the conversion of plasma into body tissue; *pitta*, produced during the formation of blood; earwax and sticky secretions of the mouth and nose, produced during the formation of flesh; sweat, produced during the formation of fatty tissue; nails and body hair, produced during the formation of bones; oily secretions of the eyes and skin, produced during the formation of bone marrow.

DIGESTIVE FIRE (*AGNI*)

The manifestation of the element of fire in the body is called *agni*. This is the power of metabolism. *Pitta* is the manifestation of *agni*. The normal functioning of the *doṣas*, *dhātus* and *malas* depends on the normal functioning of *agni*. *Agni* is present everywhere but its specific location is the stomach. It is also present in each body tissue.

Metabolic fire can be disturbed by diet, activities or stress. Impairment occurs in three ways: it can be slow, hyperactive or erratic. Impaired *agni* is the cause of all metabolic diseases, as a weak metabolism leads to improperly digested food material (*āma*), a main cause of all diseases.

The Āyurvedic explanation of digestion, assimilation and formation of body tissues is as follows. Food is brought by *vāta* into the digestive tract. The *kapha* situated in the stomach mixes with this food and separates the particles from each other, thus making the food ready for the action of the digestive power (*agni*). The digestive fire is fanned by *vāta* present in the abdomen. The stomach is the site of *kapha*, and the sweet taste is predominantly present in it. Therefore the food becomes sweet and *kapha* is produced.

Food taken on to the small intestine is partly digested and becomes sour, because that is the site of *pitta,* where the sour taste predominates, and where *pitta* is produced. Subsequently, in the large intestine, food is separated into nutrient and waste. It becomes pungent in taste, since the large intestine is site of *vāta* and the pungent taste is present. *Vāta* is produced here. Later the five metabolic fires (*agnis*) of the five elements transform this digested food so that it can nourish the properties of each element in the body. The properties of each element are present in food and nourish their respective elements in body substances. For example, heaviness – a property of earth – nourishes the earth element in the body.

Later still "subtle" digestion takes place, during which the metabolic fires (*agnis*) of the seven body tissues (*dhātus*) act on this digested food and nourish their respective tissue. From the seven tissues certain subsidiary tissues are produced. Breast milk is produced from plasma (*rasa*); menstrual blood from plasma and blood (*rasa* and *rakta*); large muscles, tendons and blood vessels are produced from blood (*rakta*); the six skin layers from flesh (*māṁsa*); and muscles from fat (*meda*).

CONSTITUTION *(PRAKṚTI)*

Āyurveda groups people into seven constitutional types, depending on the predominance of *doṣas*. A person's constitution is decided by the predominance of *doṣas* in the semen and ovum of the parents at the time of conception. When all the three *doṣas* are equal, this is known as a balanced constitution, and is supposed to be the best, giving good health. When one *doṣas* is predominant, this results in a mid-quality constitution. A constitution with two *doṣas* predominant is the least desirable, because the precarious balance of the *doṣas* often causes illness.

All three *doṣas* are present in every body. A person with a *vāta*-predominant constitution will also show some qualities of *kapha* and *pitta*. Similarly, *pitta*- and *kapha*-predominant constitutions also have some qualities of the other *doṣas*. In addition to the *doṣas*, mental constitution (*manasprakṛti*) and the quality of body tissues also determine physical structure and temperament. The following tables list the characteristics of the three main constitutional types.

CHARACTERISTICS OF *VĀTA* CONSTITUTION

Having broken, dull (greyish) hair and limbs
Hating cold
Having unstable mind, memory, intellect, actions, friendship, eyes and gait
Being excessively talkative
Having little wealth, strength, life span and sleep
Having a feeble, mumbling, rapid, cracking voice
Non-believing
Gluttonous
Indulging in lavish living
Fond of music, laughter, hunting and quarrelling
Habituated to and desiring sweet, sour, pungent and hot foods
Not robust
Lacking control over senses
Ignoble
Not liked by the other sex
Having few children
Having rough, dull, round unattractive eyes like those of a dead man, half-open during sleep and seeking in dreams mountains, trees and the sky
Mean
Filled with jealousy
Thieving
With excessively bulging calves
Resembling in nature a dog, jackal, camel, vulture, rat and crow

CHARACTERISTICS OF *PITTA* CONSTITUTION

Having intense hunger and thirst
Being fair and hot in body
Having red palms, soles and face
Being brave
Being proud
Having brown or reddish hair and scanty body hair
Having a good character
Being kind to dependants
Being wealthy
Being adventurous
Being intelligent
Being strong
Offering help even to foes in the event of dangers
Endowed with retentive power
Having loose joints and muscles
Not liked by the other sex
Having little semen and libido
The abode of white hair, wrinkles and veins
Eats sweet, astringent, bitter and cold foods
Hates heat
Sweaty
Malodorous
Extreme in speech, anger, drinking food and envy
In dreams sees red and yellow blossoms, burning surroundings, shooting stars, lightning, the sun and fire
Having reddish / brown, unsteady eyes* with scanty, thin lashes, fond of coolness and quickly reddening with anger, alcohol and sunlight
Having a medium life span and medium strength
Learned
Averse to physical stress
Resembling in nature a tiger, bear, monkey and cat.

(*In the case of coloured eyes, brightness or oiliness is the constitutional marker.)

CHARACTERISTICS OF *KAPHA* CONSTITUTION

- Gentle
- Having deep set, adipose and well-knit joints, bones and muscles
- Not troubled by hunger, thirst, pain, stress and heat
- Endowed with superior intelligence and goodness, and true to his or her word
- Having a complexion [fresh] like creepers and grasses, [bright] like a weapon, yellowish, [pink] like a lotus
- Long-armed
- Having a broad and plump chest
- Having a large forehead
- Having thick, dark hair
- Soft-limbed
- Having a charming, well-proportioned and well-defined body
- Having plenty of vitality, sex, nutritive body tissue *(rasa)*, semen, sons and dependants
- Pious
- Soft spoken
- Harbouring enmity covertly, steadfastly and for a long time
- Having a gait like a majestic elephant in rut
- Having a voice like that of a thunder cloud, the sea or a drum
- Having a good memory
- Persevering
- Well-bred
- Not much given to crying or greediness even in childhood
- Eating little, bitter, astringent, pungent, hot and dry food, yet maintaining strength
- Having eyes with thick lashes and red outer corners, deeply affectionate, large, long, distinct, with white cornea and dark iris
- Habituated to little speech, anger, drinking and eating,
- Having a long life-span and immense wealth
- Far sighted
- Eloquent
- Having faith
- Serious
- Munificent
- Forgiving
- Noble
- Prone to sleep
- Unhurried
- Grateful
- Straightforward
- Learned
- Popular
- Devoted to his or her elders
- Stable in friendship
- In dreams sees lakes with lotuses, flocks of birds and rain clouds
- Resembling in nature *Brahmā* (god of creation), *Rudra* (god of destruction), *Indra* (overlord of the gods), *Varuṇa* (god of waters), the eagle, swan, lordly elephant, lion, horse and bull

TEMPERAMENT

Āyurveda classifies temperaments according to the predominance of the *guṇas*, *sattva*, *rajas* and *tamas*. The table below shows the mental qualities associated with each *guṇa*.

There are seven types of *sattvic* temperament, six types of *rajasic* temperament and three types of *tamasic* temperament. There is a correlation between *guṇas* and *doṣas* as follows: *vāta - rajas, pitta - sattva, kapha - tamas.*

The following tables, showing the different temperaments, are arranged according to their correlation with the *doṣas*.

GUṆAS AND MENTAL QUALITIES

GUṆA	MENTAL QUALITY
Sattva (Light)	Kindness Sharing nature Tolerance Truthfulness Righteousness Belief in morality leading to divine life Knowledge Discrimination Retentive faculty Memory Courage Non-attachment
Rajas (Activity)	Predominance of suffering Unsettledness Unsteady nature Pride Falseness Unkindness Hypocrisy Vanity Excitement Lust Anger
Tamas (Darkness, ignorance)	Despondency Lack of belief in morality leading to divine life Unrighteousness Stunted intelligence Ignorance Perverted mind Lethargy Sleepiness

Rajasic Temperaments

TEMPERAMENT	CHARACTERISTICS
Demonic-type	Brave Wrathful Envious Wealthy Deceitful Terrifying Ruthless Self-praising
Ogre-type	Intolerant Habitually angry Striking at weak points Cruel Gluttonous Liking meat excessively Sleeping excessively Prone to excessive exertion Envious
Ghost-type	Eating a lot Uxorious Desiring to be alone with women Dirty Hating the clean Cowardly Terrifying Having unnatural diet and behaviour
Snake-type	Brave when angry Timid when not angry Acerbic Prone to excessive exertion Amenable to charms or diplomacy Given to eating and loitering
Evil Spirit-type	Gluttonous Causing distress by own behaviour and treatment of others Envious Not sharing with others Excessively greedy Idle
Bird-type	Perpetually desiring sex Constantly eating and moving about Unsteady Intolerant Disinclined to save

Sattvic Temperaments

TEMPERAMENT	CHARACTERISTICS
***Brahmā*-type** (Creator of World)	Pure Adherent of truth Self-controlled Sharing nature Having intellectual and experiential knowledge Skilled in debate Having a good memory Free from passion, anger, greed, ego, delusion, envy, joy, intolerance Equal in behaviour towards all beings
Sage-type	Devoted to ritual, study, religious vows, offerings and celibacy Hospitable Has subdued mania, ego, passion, hatred, delusion, greed and rage Endowed with genius, eloquence and expertise Having power of retention
***Indra*-type** (Overlord of the gods)	Lordly Authoritative Devoted to ritual Brave Vigorous Brilliant Not indulging in mean acts Far-sighted Devoted to piety, wealth and pleasures (the three worldly goals)
***Yama*-type** (God of Death – the justice giver)	Following the letter of the law Acting in keeping with propriety Invincible Alert Having a good memory Asserting authority Free from attachment, envy, hatred and delusion
***Varuṇa*-type** (God of Waters)	Brave Steadfast Pure Disliking impurity Devoted to ritual Fond of sporting in water Not indulging in mean acts Manifesting anger and pleasure in the proper context
***Kubera*-type** (Treasurer of the gods)	Possessing status, honour, luxuries and retinue Devoted to piety, wealth and pleasures (as goals of life) Pure Moving about comfortably Manifesting anger and pleasure
Divine Musician-type	Fond of dancing, singing, musical instruments and conversation Expert in panegyric, narrations, histories and legends Given to perfumes, flowers, unguents and clothes Taking pleasure in dalliance with women Not envious

Tamasic Temperaments

TEMPERAMENT	CHARACTERISTICS
Bestial-type	Repudiating Badly dressed Having disgusting food habits and behaviour Addicted to sex Prone to sleep
Fish-type	Timid Indiscrete Greedy for food Unsteady Addicted to anger and passion Ever-moving Desirous of water
Vegetable-type	Lazy Solely interested in food Deficient in all aspects of intelligence

THE SOUL *(ĀTMĀ)*

In order to understand the Āyurvedic concept of the soul, it is necessary to understand the theory of the universe posited by another ancient school dealing with metaphysics, *Sāṁkhya*. According to this school, there are two eternal principles, nature or matter (*prakṛti*) and spirit (*puruṣa*). *Puruṣa* is inactive and is the principle of consciousness. *Prakṛti* is active but insentient. It has three qualities (*guṇa*), light (*sattva*), motion (*rajas*) and darkness (*tamas*).

At the time of evolution nature (*prakṛti*) and spirit (*puruṣa*) come together. The light (*sattva*) property of nature becomes prominent and the cosmic principle of intelligence (*mahat*) is produced. Then the motion (*rajas*) property becomes prominent and ego (*ahaṁkāra*) or the principle of individualization evolves.

Sattva, with the aid of *rajas*, produces the five senses (seeing, smelling, perceiving touch, hearing and tasting), the five organs of action (grasping, speaking, moving, procreating and excreting) and the eleventh power (the mind). The mind is called the inner organ and it has the power both of sensing and acting.

Separately from the ego-principle, *ahaṁkara*, the darkness (*tamas*) property, becomes prominent with the help of motion (*rajas*), and the five subtle elements (*tanmātra*) are produced. These are the subtle principles from which the five elements (*mahābhūtas*) of space, wind, fire, water and earth evolve, in progressive order of heaviness.

The three qualities of nature (*guṇas*) correlate with the five elements as follows:

CORRELATION BETWEEN ELEMENTS AND *GUṆAS*

ELEMENTS	*GUṆA*
Space	*Sattva*
Air	*Rajas*
Fire	*Sattva* and *rajas*
Water	*Sattva* and *tamas*
Earth	*Tamas*

Evolution

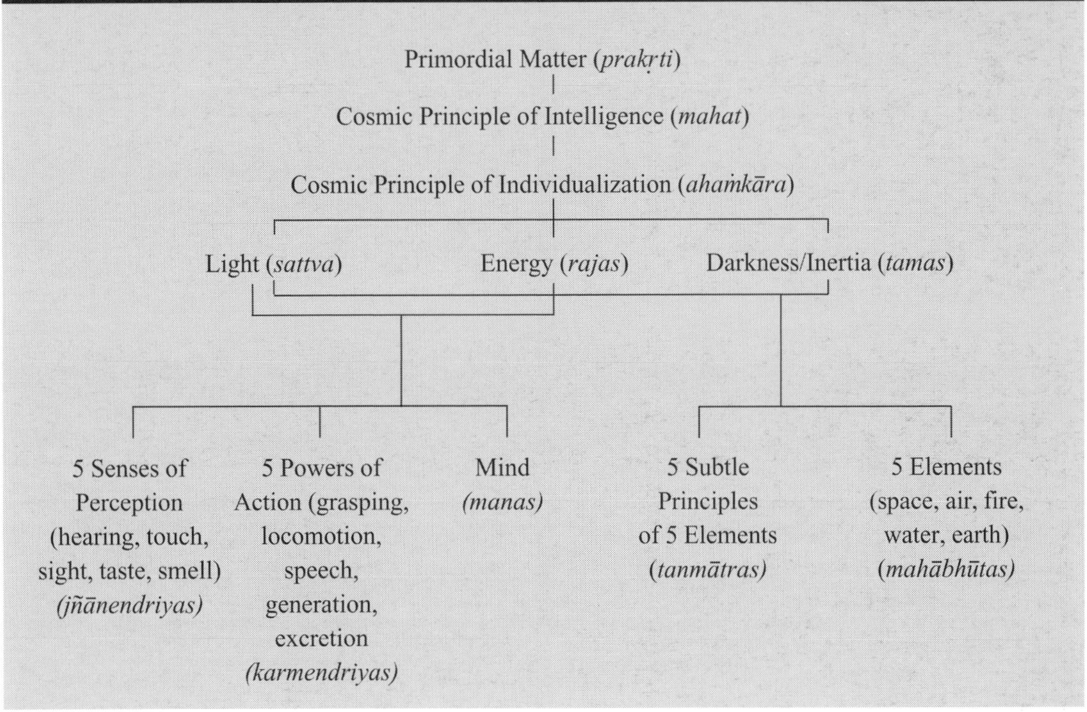

Āyurveda speaks of two eternal souls or selves: the higher self (*paramātmā*) which is eternal and is devoid of diseases and abnormalities, and the lower self (*ātmā*) which is subject to birth and death. This lower self, when conjoined with the mind, the properties of the five basic elements (sound, touch, form-and-colour, taste and smell), and the senses, is responsible for consciousness. It is a mere observer of actions. It does not have emotions like anger, hatred, happiness or sorrow.

The self has knowledge. Knowledge manifests when the self is united with the mind and senses. When it is not in contact with the mind and senses; or if the mind and senses are impaired, there is no knowledge. When the control of the mind over itself or over one of the senses is lost, perception and the thinking process are impaired and so, ultimately, is knowledge. Just as one cannot see in a dirty mirror or water, similarly, it is said, one cannot see when the senses are masked.

The higher self (*paramātmā*), being eternal, has no original cause. However, the entity known as *puruṣa*, person, uniting self (soul), mind and senses, has its origin in faulty intellect, which leads to desire and aversion. These in turn impel the individual *puruṣa* to act, thereby getting enmeshed in the cycle of birth and death.

At the time of dissolution or death the soul or self becomes separated from the elements. At the time of evolution or embodiment the soul is associated with *rajas* and *tamas* and manifests itself from nature. This becomes the living body, made up of the five elements and the soul, which is perceivable to the senses. At the time of death, the body of six constituents (five elements and the soul) dissolves again. This cycle of birth and death continues for those who are strongly attached to *rajas* and *tamas* in the form of actions and pleasures and who are ego-centred. Those who have overcome *rajas* and *tamas* and are not ego-centred are freed from the round of birth and death; they have attained liberation (*mokṣa*).

The indications or signs of the soul are: breathing, flickering and movements of the eyes, life, movement of the mind, movement of the mind from one sense to another, initiation of action and controlling of the mind itself, movement of the mind in different places in sleep, the knowledge of death, the identical perception of things by both eyes, desire, hatred, happiness and sorrow, effort, consciousness, and firmness of mind, intellect, memory and ego.

THE MIND *(MANAS)*

The mind is active but not conscious, while the soul is inactive but gives consciousness. The mind in association with the soul acts; when not in association with it, it does not act. Since the soul is conscious, it is held responsible for all actions, while the mind, though active, is not considered responsible because it is not conscious.

The mind is indicated by the presence/absence of knowledge.When the mind associates itself with the senses, the chain of soul-mind-sense-object is complete, producing knowledge. This infers that the mind is subtle and only one. Without the mind/senses association, there is no knowledge even if the senses, their objects and the soul are present.

The mind cannot be perceived by the senses. Its actions are dependent on its objects and on the soul. These actions include the perception of happiness, unhappiness, thinking, and associating the senses to their objects. The soul, the seat of consciousness, is behind any efforts to perceive objects.

Anything that can be known by the mind is considered to be an object of the mind. Control over the senses and over itself are actions of the mind. The objects of the mind are:

- Thinking (*cintya*) – in terms of what should or should not be done
- Analysis (*vicarya*) – in terms of good or bad, proper or improper
- Inferring (*ūhya*) – exposed to reasoning
- Focusing (*dhyeya*) – that which is constantly thought of
- Determination (*saṅkalpya*) – after evaluating in terms of good and bad points

VITAL SITES (*MARMASTHĀNAS*)

Āyurveda lists 107 critical points of the body (*marmasthānas*). These are sites beneath which the physical structures of the body intersect. They are classified according to the structures involved (muscles, blood vessels, tendons and ligaments, bones, joints), location, consequences of injury (instant death, death after some delay, death upon the removal of an object penetrating the spot, disability and severe pain). There are 22 *marmas* in the arms and hands, 22 in the legs and feet, 12 in the abdominal and chest region, 14 in the back, and 37 in the neck and head. Their size is measured in finger-widths (*anguli*).

The table opposite lists the *marmas*.

MARMA	NAME	LOCATION	SIZE IN FINGER-WIDTHS	NO.	TISSUE
1	*Tālahṛdaya*	Centre of palms and soles	½	4	Muscle
2	*Kṣipra*	Between thumb and forefinger and big toe and second toe	½	4	Tendon
3	*Kūrca*	Mound of thumb and big toes	4	4	Tendon
4	*Kūrcaśira*	Below wrist and below ankle	1	4	Tendon
5	*Maṇibandha*	Wrist	2	2	Joint
6	*Gulpha*	Ankle	2	2	Joint
7	*Indrabasti*	Bulge of forearm and calf	½	4	Muscle
8	*Kurpara*	Elbow	3	2	Joint
9	*Jānu*	Knee	3	2	Joint
10	*Aṇi*	Just above elbow and knee	½	4	Tendon
11	*Urvi*	Just above middle of biceps and quadriceps	1	4	Blood vessel
12	*Lohitākṣa*	Front of armpit and centre of groin	½	4	Blood vessel
13	*Kaśadhāra*	Centre armpit	1	2	Tendon
14	*Viṭapa*	Lower groin	1	2	Tendon
15	*Guḍa*	Anus	4	1	Muscle
16	*Basti*	Bladder	4	1	Muscle & ligament
17	*Nabhi*	Navel	4	1	Blood vesel
18	*Hṛdaya*	Heart	4	1	Blood vessel
19	*Stanamūla*	Bottom of breast (mammary artery)	2	2	Blood vessel
20	*Stanarohita*	Areola	½	2	Muscle
21	*Apastamba*	Just below middle of collar bone (apex of lungs)	½	2	Blood vessel
22	*Apālāpa*	Pectoral fold (insertion of pectoral muscle in humerus)	½	2	Blood vessel
23	*Kaṭikataruṇa*	Lumbo-sacral joint	½	2	Bone
24	*Kukundara*	Sacro-iliac joint	½	2	Joint
25	*Nitamba*	Iliac crest	½	2	Bone
26	*Parśvasandhi*	Kidneys	½	2	Blood vessel
27	*Aṁsaphalaka*	Shoulder blade	½	2	Bone
28	*Bṛhatī*	Thorax inside shoulder blades	½	2	Blood vessel
29	*Aṁsa*	Shoulder ligaments	½	2	Muscle & ligament
30	*Manya*	Carotid artery	4	2	Blood vessel
31	*Nīla*	Side of throat	4	1	Blood vessel
32	*Sirā Mātṛkā*	Jugular vein	4	8	Blood vessel
33	*Kṛkātikā*	Junction of head and neck (atlanto-occipital joint)	½	2	Joint
34	*Vidhura*	Depression at base of ears	½	2	Tendon
35	*Phaṇa*	Sides of nose (maxillary sinus)	½	2	Blood vessel
36	*Apāṅga*	Outer corners of eyes	½	2	Blood vessel
37	*Āvarta*	Towards outer eyebrow	½	2	Joint
38	*Śaṅkha*	Temple	2	2	Bone
39	*Utkṣepa*	Above temple (Frontal and parietal joint)	½	2	Ligament
40	*Sthapani*	Between eyebrows (Corresponds to pituitary)	½	1	Blood vessel
41	*Śṛṅgātaka*	Inside mouth, behind uvula	4	4	Blood vessel
42	*Sīmanta*	Along cranial sutures	_	5	Joint
43	*Adhipati*	Centre of back of head	½	1	Joint

Health

Āyurveda has a concept of positive health. Well-being, without any disease, is said to be the state of health in which one exists in one's own natural state.

A person is said to be healthy when the following conditions are met: when the *doṣas* are in equilibrium; when the digestive fire is also in equilibrium; when the body tissues and wastes are in the right amount and performing their functions properly; and when the soul, mind and senses are contented.

Āyurveda has a twofold objective: the maintenance of health and the treatment of disease. In both, its concern is the equilibrium of the body constituents; in the first aspect it prevents disequilibrium, and, in the second, it restores equilibrium. A diseased condition is considered to be an imbalance of this equilibrium. Disease is also defined as sorrow, and health is considered equal to happiness.

In its teaching regarding the maintenance of health, Āyurveda gives guidelines on how to prevent the imbalance of body constituents. These guidelines cover three broad areas: healthy routines to follow on a daily basis, those to follow on a seasonal basis, and rules to follow in order to safeguard against diseases.

DAILY REGIMEN

Information is given about each aspect of the daily regimen: sleep, hygiene, the care of the body, exercise, diet, behaviour and sexual conduct. A health-promoting daily regimen is shown on the right. Diet, sleep, exercise, and good conduct will be considered in detail as they are of relevance to yoga practice.

Diet

Food is considered to be the vital breath of living beings. On it depend complexion, cheerfulness, good voice, life, power of imagination, happiness, contentment, good physique, strength and understanding. Fire is said to be the internal manifestation of God, and eating is a fire sacrifice.

Wholesome food should be taken at the proper time. It should be hot and oily rather than dry. It should be an appropriate amount, which can be easily

Recommended Daily Regimen

Rising: Rise early (4 am to 6 am). Attend to the calls of nature.

Oral hygiene: Clean the teeth. Massage the gums. Scrape the tongue. Gargle with water and oil.

Eye-care: Splash the eyes with cold water. Apply collyrium to the eyes to enhance vision. Apply a herbal ointment once a week.

Nose-care: Apply oil drops in nostrils to give strength to shoulder muscles, prevent sinusitis and spondylosis, promote clarity of the senses, strong hair growth and a good voice.

Massage: Do oil massage (including head, ears and feet) to mitigate *vāta* and promote strength, sleep and growth, except when indisposed by coughs, colds, fever, or diarrhoea, for example. *Kapha* people should do dry massage.

Exercise: Exercise to produce lightness of the body, to reduce fat, to make the body firm and to be fit for work.

Bath: Take a bath. Bathing improves appetite and vigour, and removes fatigue.

Eating: Eat in a quiet, clean place. Do not engage in unnecessary conversation or argument while eating. Chew food thoroughly before swallowing. Do not exert yourself after eating.

Take betel leaves (pan), as they are good for the heart and digestion, except in diseases related to *pitta* and blood.

Profession: Follow a profession that is noble, well-respected, and beneficial to society and self.

Duties and Conduct: Spend time in the company of good people and follow the scriptures; be humble, charitable and enthusiastic; perform religious rites.

Ethics: Avoid sinful behaviour, such as cruelty, stealing, unlawful sex, backbiting, telling lies, harsh speech, jealousy and impiety. Recollect the events of the day. Adopt what is the best in life and avoid improper conduct. A person who is at odds with duty and right conduct (*dharma*) cannot be happy and contented. It is believed that the actions (*karmas*) of this life can affect not only this life but even future lives.

digested. Solid food should fill half the stomach, liquids one quarter, and the remaining quarter should be left free for the action of digestion. Food should be taken only after the previous intake of it is completely digested. Incompatible foods (such as milk and sour fruits) should be avoided. Food should be taken in pleasant surroundings and should not be eaten very quickly or very slowly, or while conversing or laughing. One should concentrate while eating and think about the suitability of the food.

All the six tastes should be present in every meal since this is most likely to create balance, but the sweet taste should predominate as it gives nourishment. However, each *doṣa* is compatible with specific tastes that originate from the same elements. There should be variations in the tastes according to the season.

When one is worried, grieved, afraid, angry, unhappy, or when one sleeps too much or too little, food is not properly digested and does not give its full benefit.

Certain foods are wholesome for all constitutions on a daily basis. These include rice, wheat, mung beans, bown lentils, milk, ghee, rock salt, pomegranates, amla fruits (rich in Vitamin C) and certain light meats. Beef and pork are recommended only in certain conditions, such as weakness, hyperactive digestion and diseases causes by *vāta*.

Certain foods aggravate or alleviate each *doṣa* according to their preponderance of taste. The table below gives the effects of different tastes on the *doṣas*.

While food provides nourishment for the body tissues, *ojas*, strength and good complexion, it is the digestive power (*agni*) which is the effective agent. The body tissues cannot develop from undigested food. The digestive fire is the root cause of life, colour, strength, health, enthusiasm, plumpness, lustre, vitality (*ojas*), heat (*tejas*), metabolic powers and breath energies. When it is extinguished one dies; with its proper maintenance one lives long and healthily. When it is impaired one becomes ill.

The digestive fire becomes vitiated through not eating, eating before digestion is complete, over-eating and irregular eating; through eating unwholesome, heavy, chilled, very dry and spoiled food; and some other causes. An impaired digestive fire cannot digest even light food. This undigested food becomes acidic and toxic.

When the digestive fire and the amount of food eaten are as they should be, digestion is smooth and the body tissues remain in equilibrium.

Sleep

Sleep is said to be the wet-nurse of the earth. Happiness or unhappiness, a well-developed or a thin body, strength or weakness, sexual potency or impotence, knowledge or ignorance, and life itself or death are dependent on sleep.

When the mind and senses are fatigued and turn away from objects, a person sleeps. The ideal time for rising is in the early hours of the morning just before sunrise. At this time the mind is alert. It is the period of *vāta* (wind), which is conducive to the voiding of stools and urine. (Note: One should sleep with the head to the east or south.)

Going to sleep late at night increases *vāta*; sleeping during the day increases *kapha* and *pitta*. Neither is advisable.

Exercise

Exercise is prescribed as a daily activity. It is defined as those actions of the body that are regarded as good, that are expected to produce stability of the body, and that improve the strength of the body. They should be performed in the proper amount.

Effect of Foods on *Doṣas*

DOṢA	AGGRAVATING FOODS	ALLEVIATING FOODS
Vāta	Pungent, bitter and astringent	Sweet, sour and salty
Pitta	Pungent, sour and salty	Sweet, bitter and astringent
Kapha	Sweet, sour and salty	Pungent, bitter and astringent

Exercise refers only to bodily actions; mental actions are not included. These actions should be good or approved. Physical exertion, such as carrying heavy loads, is not included in exercise. Walking is included, however, as are traditional forms of physical training, such as wrestling and martial arts.

Exercise is said to bring lightness to the body, the capacity to work hard, a strong digestion, and reduction of fat. It develops the physique. In addition, it gives stability and the capacity to tolerate sorrow and stress. It decreases excess *kapha doṣa*, which in normal conditions is responsible for growth but in excess can produce heaviness, obesity and poor digestion. Exercise increases the power of digestion, enhancing metabolism. It enables one to endure hunger, thirst, cold and heat, and prevents laziness. It is cleansing for the body and promotes good health and a good complexion.

It is said that there is nothing like exercise to reduce obesity. When one exercises regularly one fears nobody, thanks to one's physical strength. One's muscles become firm. One wards off old age, and diseases stay away from one, as small animals from a lion. One looks good even if one is not young, handsome and attractive. One can digest any food without any bad effect, even if it is incompatible or improperly cooked.

For those who are strong and who also eat oily food, exercise is always the right path. During the cold season and in spring it is particularly beneficial. In winter and spring, one should perform exercises to half one's strength, less in the other seasons. Before performing exercise, one should consider factors such as age, strength, physique, habitat and climatic conditions, season and diet, as ignoring these factors could invite disease.

There are certain physical indications which mean that one should stop exercising: sweating, heavy breathing, a feeling of lightness in the body, and a feeling of an obstruction at the heart. When one starts breathing through the mouth, it indicates that one has used half one's strength. Other indications of this are excessive sweat at the armpits, forehead, nose, palms, soles of feet and joints, and dryness in the mouth. Over-exertion can kill. Take the example of the lion and elephant fighting: the lion may be the victor, but the exertion will kill it.

Exercise beyond one's capacity can produce exhaustion, fatigue of mind and senses, the degeneration of body tissue, bleeding though the body orifices (ears, nose, eyes, mouth, anus and so on) and broken capillaries on the skin. It can even cause severe breathing disorders with symptoms akin to asthma and bronchitis. It can also cause coughs, fever and vomiting.

Certain people should avoid exercise: those who have become emaciated; those who have to endure physical strains, such as carrying heavy loads and walking long distances; and those who are under the sway of anger, grief or fear. Exercise is not suitable for young children, elderly people, *vāta*-predominant people, those who have to use their voice a lot, and those who are hungry or thirsty.

Good Conduct

Āyurveda recognizes the importance of good conduct in maintaining the health of the mind, senses and body. Good conduct includes physical acts and ethical behaviour and positive actions, as well as those to be avoided. The advice given resembles sensible parental guidance, leaving nothing to doubt and standing good throughout life.

Āyurveda recommends that one should pay respect to those worthy of it, perform prescribed rituals, maintain body cleanliness, regularly cut their hair and nails, wear good clothes, be cheerful, and apply oil to the head, ears, nostrils and feet. One should act with kindness to those in adversity, honour guests, perform obsequies, speak considered, helpful and sweet words, be self-controlled, dutiful, ambitious for the means not the end, careful, fearless, modest, wise, enthusiastic, skilful, forbearing, virtuous, religious-minded and devoted to spiritually enlightened teachers. One should use an umbrella, stick, head-covering and shoes, avoid places with rags, bones, thorns, refuse, hair, and so on. One should stop exercising before exhaustion. One should be friendly towards all creatures, conciliatory towards the angry, heartening towards the frightened and helpful to the wretched. One should be truthful, of equable nature, tolerant of the harsh words of others, and of patient and peaceful disposition. One should eradicate the roots of attachment and aversion.

One should not tell lies, appropriate what belongs to another, covet another's wife or goods, indulge in enmity or evil, do evil even to someone wicked, speak of another's faults, pass on another's secrets, or associate with unprincipled people, enemies, lunatics, low people, abortionists, mean and bad people.

Āyurveda lists a number of actions which should be avoided. They include actions that could result in physical harm, such as riding in or on unsound vehicles, sitting on hard seats of knee-height, sleeping without a pillow, approaching snakes and animals with teeth and horns, eating and drinking to excess, provoking quarrels, among others. There are prohibitions regarding food, such as eating without washing first, with a disturbed mind or in the presence of hungry people. Food should not be dirty, served by inimical people or stale.

With regard to habits and urges, one should not sneeze, eat or sleep in a prone position, or attend to other work while under the pressure of a natural urge. Cautions regarding sex include not having intercourse with a menstruating or unwilling woman, or in a public place, in water, after fasting or overeating, or after exertion or exercise. Certain times are noted as unsuitable for study, such as during storms and important festivals.

In general, deviation from the normal code of conduct is not advised. Thus walking at night or in an inappropriate place, making unsuitable friends, drinking, gambling, prostitution, insults, arrogance, backbiting, harsh speech to the elderly and the distancing of family and helpers is disapproved of. So is impatience or foolhardiness, neglect of servants, lack of trust in close kin, solitary enjoyment, over-dependence on others or over-suspiciousness.

Procrastination, unconsidered actions, domination by the senses, fickleness of mind, over-burdening of the intellect and senses, dilatoriness, subservience to anger or elation, dwelling on grief, pride in success and despair at failure should all be avoided. Instead, one should constantly remember one's own nature and the inevitable power of a cause to initiate an effect. In fine, one should be intent on chastity, knowledge, charity, friendship, compassion, joy, detachment and peace.

SEASONAL REGIMENS

Seasonal Regimen (*ṛtucarya*) denotes the regimen to be followed by people during different seasons to maintain health. It is said that time is divine and has no beginning or end. It denotes change. The changes in the atmosphere are called seasons; they follow a definite order and this transformation affects the body. As the human being is an integral part of the universe and both have the basic elements in common, any change in the latter, the macrocosm, is reflected in the former, the microcosm.

Āyurveda divides the year into six seasons beginning in mid-January: late winter, spring, summer, rains, autumn and early winter (snows). For the first half of the year, as the sun increases in power, people have less strength and herbs less potency. As the power of the sun decreases in the second half of the year, people and herbs have more strength. In the extremely cold, warm and hot seasons, bitter, astringent and pungent tastes are increased progressively. In the wet, cool-night, and cold seasons, sour, salty and sweet, tastes are increased. The following table gives the correlation of the seasons with their properties. They apply to temperate as well as tropical climates.

Properties of the Seasons

SEASON	CLIMATE	TASTE
Late Winter	Extreme cold	Bitter
Spring	Warm	Astringent
Summer	Hot	Pungent
Rainy	Wet	Sour
Autumn	Cool nights	Salty
Early Winter	Cold	Sweet

Each *doṣa* accumulates, aggravates and becomes normal in different seasons. It is recommended that the excess *doṣa* are eliminated in order to prevent the occurrence of diseases associated with seasonal changes. The table overleaf summarizes the cyclical changes.

As each season has different properties, different diets and regimens are recommended to balance these. They are shown in the subsequent table.

Doṣas and Seasons

DOṢA	SEASON OF ACCUMULATION	SEASON OF AGGRAVATION	SEASON OF PACIFICATION	METHOD OF ELIMINATION
Kapha	Winter	Spring	Summer	Emesis
Pitta	Rainy Season	Autumn	Winter	Purgation
Vāta	Summer	Rainy season	Autumn	Enema

Recommended Seasonal Regimens

SEASON	PROPERTY	COMMENT	SUITABLE DIET AND REGIMEN
Winter (early and late)	Cold Unctuous Promoting good digestive fire	Health and digestive power are good	Strength-promoting foods: sweet, sour and oily Oil massage Vigorous exercise
Spring	Hot	Digestive disorders are common as a result of the accumulation of *kapha* in winter which liquefies due to the warmth of spring	Light dry foods which do not tax the digestion Exercise is essential
Summer	Hot Dry	Dryness is due to the loss of *kapha* and accumulation of *vāta*	Light, liquid, oily and sweet food Minimum exercise
Rainy	Cold Dry from previous heat	The digestive power is disturbed, reducing strength	Oily, hot, sweet, sour and salty foods (to counteract *vāta*)
Autumn	Hot Sharp		Sweet, bitter, astringent and cool foods (to counteract *pitta*)

SAFEGUARDS AGAINST DISEASES

The disequilibrium of bodily factors (*doṣas* and *dhātus*) is called disease. It is always expressed as pain or suffering.

There are three types of diseases: endogenous, produced internally by the three factors above (*doṣas*, body tissues and waste products); exogenous, produced by external agents like trauma, poison and fire; and, lastly, mental, produced by emotional factors. Another classification is as follows: traumatic, such as accidents, insect bites, and weapon injury; fated (being the effects of past deeds, which are brought on by seasonal influences, planetary disposition and natural events like old age and death); and, lastly. idiosyncratic, denoting hereditary and congenital conditions and acquired *doṣic* imbalance.

There are three causes of disease: relating to

the senses, actions and time. Regarding actions and the senses, there can be misuse, overuse or under-use. Time concerns the seasons and unseasonable weather.

Listening to very loud sounds, such as thunder, drums or screaming, overburdens the auditory sense; not listening to sounds at all is deemed under-use. Listening to harsh words, those indicating loss or bereavement, frightening words, bad language, or words which convey calamity is deemed misuse.

With regard to tactile sense, lack of touch, as in bathing, massage or the application of creams and so on, is under-use. Overuse is an excess of these. Misuse is the touch of spirits, poison and winds and the touch of oily, cold and hot objects at the wrong time.

Looking at very bright objects to excess leads to loss of vision. Looking at minute objects or not using vision at all also leads to loss of sight. Looking at hateful, frightening, immense, horrific, distant and very close objects is misuse of the eyes.

Enjoying a taste to excess is overuse of the gustatory sense. Omitting a taste or eating it minimally is under-use. Taking unaccustomed, improperly processed food or incompatible combinations of food is misuse of the taste organs.

Inhaling very faint or very strong or sharp smells, or not inhaling any smells at all impairs the olfactory sense. Inhaling putrid, abhorrent smells, those which decrease the intellect, damp and poisonous fumes is misuse of the nose.

The excessive use, under-use or lack of use of speech, mind and body causes disease. Misuse of the body includes controlling or forcing the various natural urges, falling awkwardly, walking unevenly, the awkward disposition of the limbs, being struck or twisted and other actions which cause pain.

Misuse of speech includes making sly hints, lying, speaking at the wrong time, quarrelling and disagreeable, irrelevant and harsh speech.

Misuse of the mind includes fear, grief, anger, greed, delusion, pride, envy and false ideas.

The seasons are associated with particular climates such as hot, cold and rainy. Excessive, low or unseasonable heat, cold and rain produce disease.

The root cause of all diseases is said to be the failure of intelligence, willpower and memory. This is termed the "crime of the intellect". It is said that diseases inflicted by external factors like spirits, poison, wind, storms, fire, accidents and so on are also caused by faulty intellect. The emotional states mentioned above like envy, grief, fear, anger, egoistic pride and hatred are considered to be mental abnormalities caused by offences against the intellect, stemming from lack of knowledge or improper knowledge. The same applies to the abuse of the senses.

The thirteen physical urges of passing wind, faeces, and urine, sneezing, thirst, hunger, sleep, coughing, panting, yawning, crying, vomiting and ejaculation should never be suppressed. *Vāta* is responsible for all these urges; if suppressed it becomes vitiated and causes various diseases.

There are various actions of the mind, speech and body that are not recommended and should be controlled. Undesirable mental impulses are: greed, sorrow, fear, anger, pride, impudence, envy, excessive desire, and malice. With regard to speech, the urge to speak harshly, to talk too much, to denigrate others, to tell lies, and to speak irrelevantly, should be controlled. In respect of actions, those which harm or cause pain to others, such as sex with another's wife, stealing, violence, should be controlled.

Diseases caused by external factors can be prevented by the avoidance of "crimes of the intellect", the pacification of the senses, the recollection of things that could be harmful or were harmful previously, knowledge of place and time and knowledge of the soul, and following the directives of good behaviour.

In addition various purificatory treatments are prescribed, such as emesis, purgation, enema and nasal cleansing.

Understanding Yoga through Āyurveda

In order to use Āyurveda to understand Yoga it is necessary to examine what is written in the Yoga literature regarding practice. As full details were transmitted orally from guru to disciple, the texts give clues, not comprehensive explanations. From these the logic behind Yoga practice can be deduced, with the help of the knowledge of Āyurveda.

However, over and above the physical body and the mind, Yoga also deals with the esoteric body and mind-transcending experiences. As Āyurveda has nothing to offer in these spheres, the esoteric aspects of Yoga are not considered in this book. The most important Yoga text giving information about practice is the *Haṭha Yoga Pradīpikā*. Relevant passages from this work will be presented wherever possible.

The knowledge given in Āyurveda informs Yoga practice in several ways. First, Āyurvedic anatomy and physiology provide a theoretical basis for understanding the way in which Yoga *āsanas* and *prāṇāyāma* work. Secondly, Āyurveda teaches the general principles of energy management. These principles are as valid in Yoga practice as elsewhere. Thirdly, it recommends various daily and periodic health-care routines for the preservation and strengthening of the body. Understanding the necessity for these brings the understanding of how Yoga can provide an alternative to them, without recourse to doctors and medication. Fourthly, an overview of its approach in other specializations gives a perspective of the extent to which Yoga can provide alternative or supplementary methods of treatment.

The above points outline the overlap between Yoga and Āyurveda, showing how Yoga can also be prophylactic and curative. While Yoga is not a medical science, it is outstandingly efficacious in maintaining health and preventing disease. It can alleviate or cure structural defects and physiological dysfunction. It can help in the management of illnesses which require medication, and in rehabilitation after surgery or accidents. It has a methodology of health for the mind. In these respects it parallels medical science.

Medical science has as its purpose the relief of suffering. Yoga, too, has this aim, but it seeks a permanent end to suffering by aspiring to a state of being which pain cannot touch. Thus the two sciences have fundamentally different spheres. The commonality and distinction between medical science and Yoga are pithily summed up in the commentary of the *Yoga Sūtras* of Patañjali. Vyāsa, the commentator, takes the scheme of Āyurveda as a model for Yoga (VB II.15):

> Just as medical science has four divisions: disease, the cause of disease, the cure (health) and therapeutics, so Yogic science has four divisions: the problem (suffering), the cause of suffering (ignorance), the cure (liberation) and the means (the eightfold Yoga).
>
> (In fact, Āyurveda (CS-Sū 1) classifies knowledge of health and disease under three heads: causes, symptoms and treatment; Vyāsa's fourth category spells out its aim.)

The two distinct spheres of Yoga and Āyurveda make them complementary. The scope of Āyurveda is the maintenance and restoration of health and in this regard it recognizes the importance of mental and emotional factors. Its pharmacopoia and treatments are aimed at bringing about physical and psychological normalcy.

For Yoga, however, physical and psychological well-being is the starting point. Western medicine has treatments for many ills of body and mind, but it has no remedy for life's sorrows. This is where Yoga comes into its own. Its practice and philosophy aim to replace egocentric considerations, agitation of mind, insecurity and spiritual ignorance with a large-hearted perspective, serenity, self-assurance and self-knowledge.

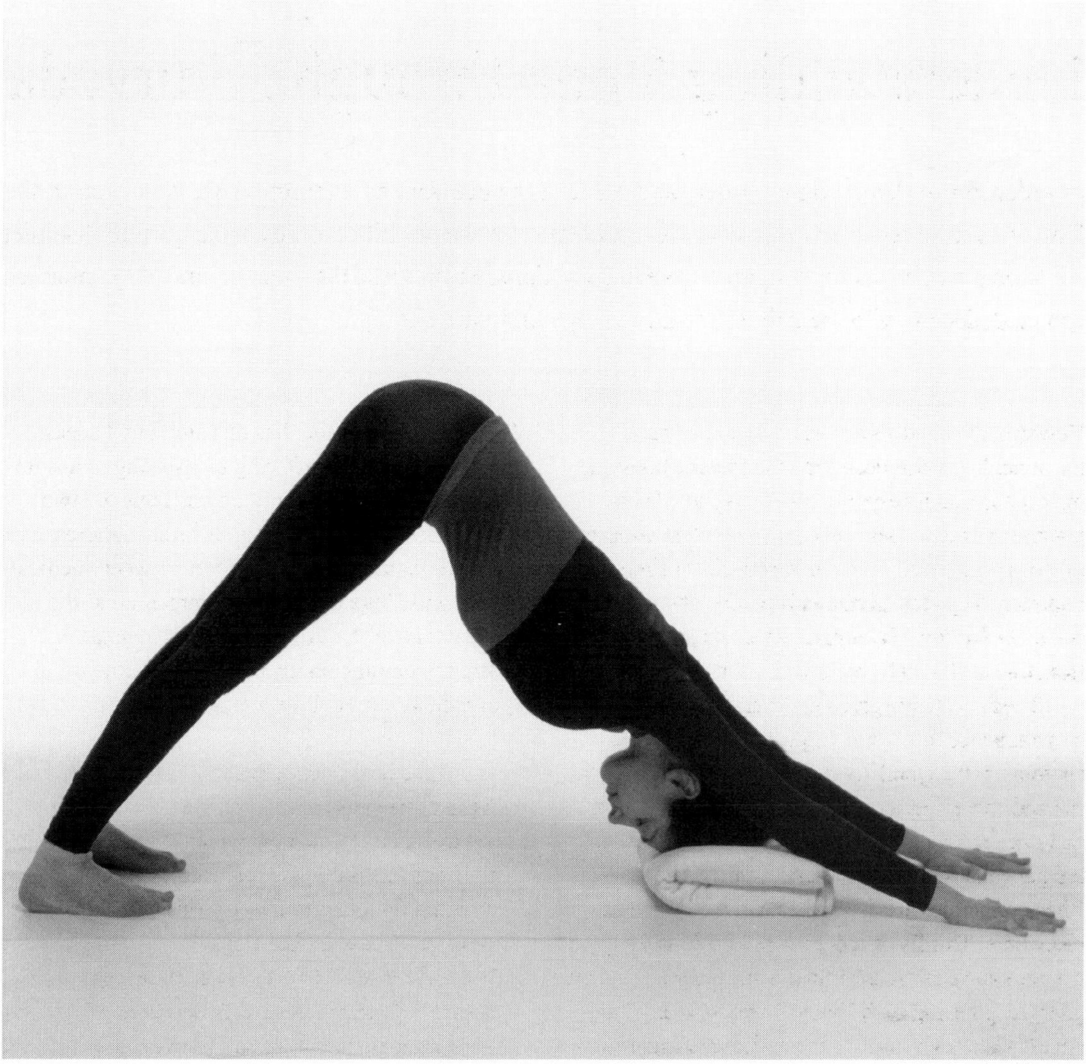

Dog Pose Head Down: a simultaneous stretch and relaxation

Anatomy: Vital Sites and *Āsanas*

In Yoga practice concentration on the vital sites first prevents the dissipation of energy and then maintains and increases it. In this way strength and resilience are maximized. Maintaining awareness at these points simultaneously in the *āsanas* results in a dynamic body and relaxed mind.

There is no written source for linking the *marmasthānas* to *āsana* practice. The knowledge of *marmas* was developed for warfare and for surgical purposes. Most of the sites can be verified by consulting modern anatomy books as sites of important nerves, arteries or junctures where the body structure is delicate and therefore vulnerable. This being the case, it is a matter of logic to apply this knowledge to *āsanas*, which are concerned with strengthening the body and maximizing energy.

For example, in the pose illustrated above, the knees and elbows – individual *marma* sites – need to be kept firm while the head – containing several *marma* sites – needs to be relaxed.

The diagrams overleaf show the sites of the *marmas* and the table indicates the action required in the *āsanas*.

Marmas and their Locations

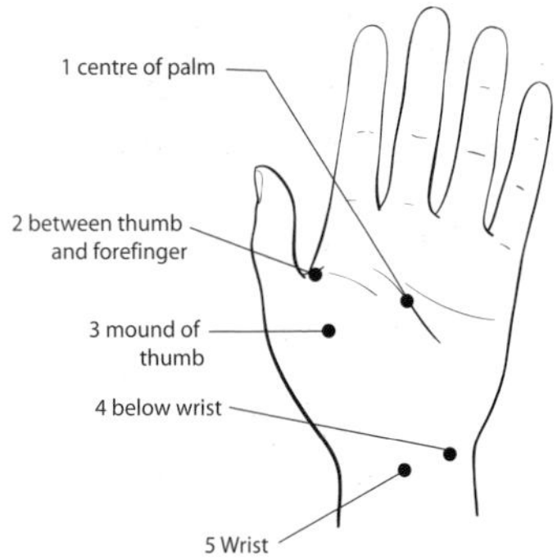
1 centre of palm
2 between thumb and forefinger
3 mound of thumb
4 below wrist
5 Wrist

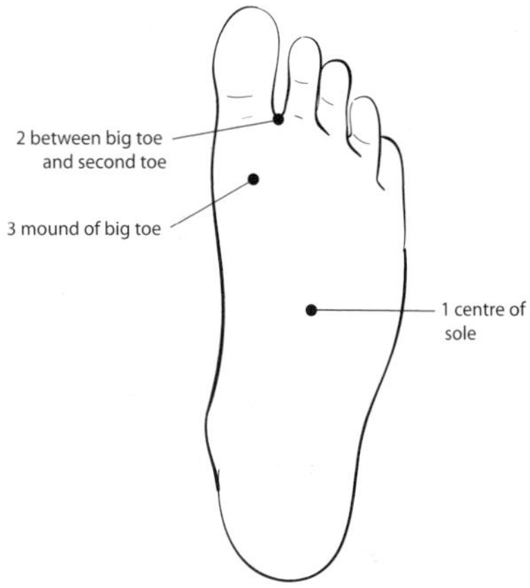
2 between big toe and second toe
3 mound of big toe
1 centre of sole

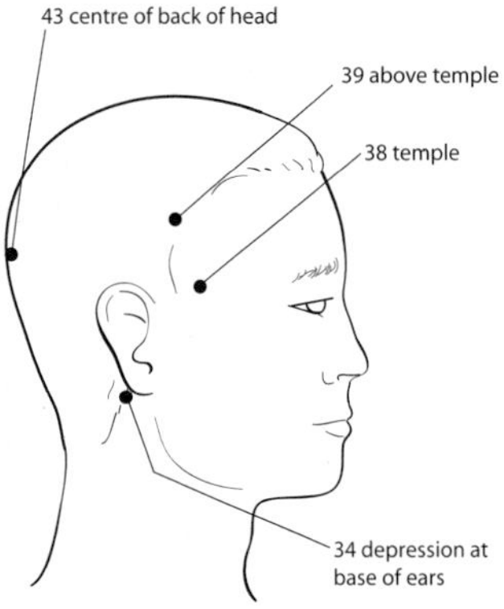
43 centre of back of head
39 above temple
38 temple
34 depression at base of ears

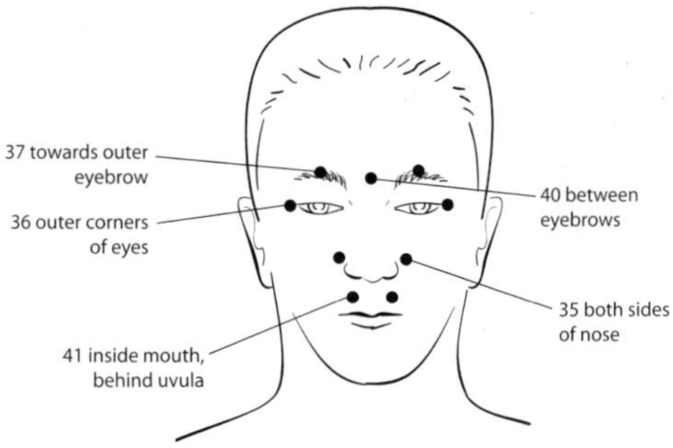
37 towards outer eyebrow
36 outer corners of eyes
41 inside mouth, behind uvula
40 between eyebrows
35 both sides of nose

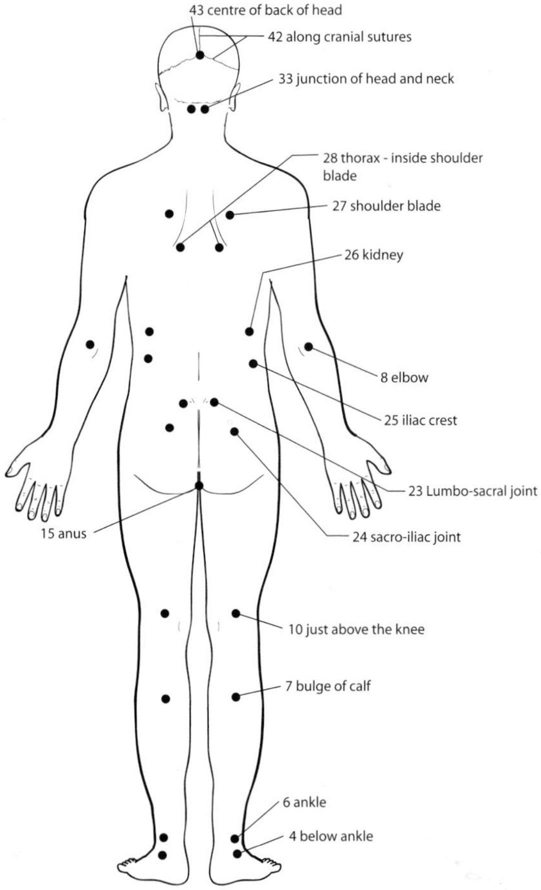
43 centre of back of head
42 along cranial sutures
33 junction of head and neck
28 thorax - inside shoulder blade
27 shoulder blade
26 kidney
8 elbow
25 iliac crest
23 Lumbo-sacral joint
15 anus
24 sacro-iliac joint
10 just above the knee
7 bulge of calf
6 ankle
4 below ankle

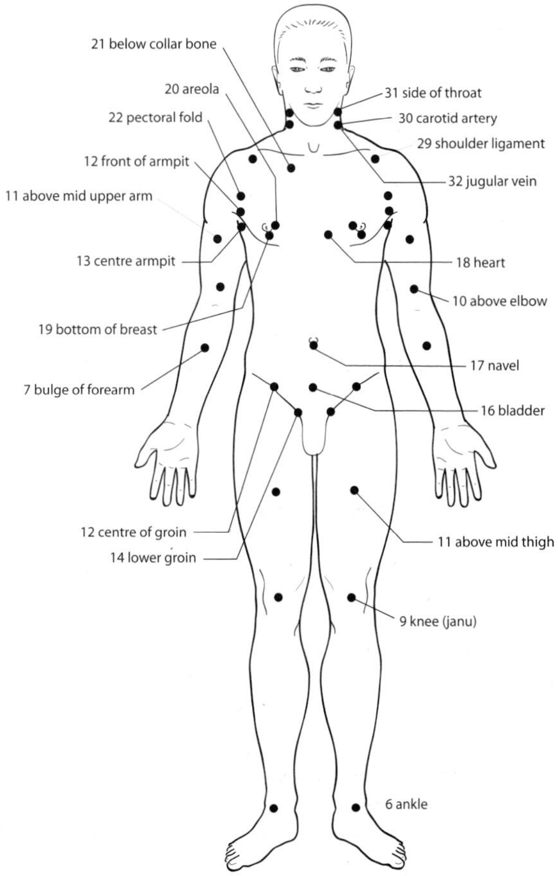
21 below collar bone
20 areola
22 pectoral fold
12 front of armpit
11 above mid upper arm
13 centre armpit
19 bottom of breast
7 bulge of forearm
31 side of throat
30 carotid artery
29 shoulder ligament
32 jugular vein
18 heart
10 above elbow
17 navel
16 bladder
12 centre of groin
14 lower groin
11 above mid thigh
9 knee (janu)
6 ankle

KEY NO.	MARMA NAME	LOCATION	NO.	YOGA ACTION
1	*Tālahṛdaya*	Centre of palms and soles	4	Stretch; Increase height of foot arch; during relaxation deepen hollow.
2	*Kṣipra*	Between thumb and forefinger and big toe and second toe	4	Keep closed when hands in air; stretch when hands on floor; maintain space between big toe and second toe.
3	*Kūrca*	Mounds of thumb and big toes	4	Press towards floor to maintain stability.
4	*Kūrcaśira*	Below wrist and below ankle	4	Increase depression to maintain space between the wrist and hand and ankle and foot.
5	*Maṇibandha*	Wrist	2	Rotate outer wrist towards it to maintain alignment and strength.
6	*Gulpha*	Ankle	2	Extend and make firm.
7	*Indrabasti*	Bulge of forearm and calf	4	Stretch; divide stretch from this point towards upper and lower and lower muscle insertions.
8	*Kurpara*	Elbow	2	Stretch and make firm.
9	*Jānu*	Knee	2	Stretch and make firm.
10	*Aṇi*	Just above elbow and knee	4	Stretch.
11	*Urvi*	Just above middle of upper arm and thigh	4	Stretch; tie thighs together at this point.
12	*Lohitākṣa*	Front of armpit and centre of groin	4	Soften to increase depth when armpit and groin are closed; extend when armpit and groin are exposed.
13	*Kaśadhāra*	Centre of armpit	2	Soften to increase depth when armpit is closed; extend when armpit is exposed.
14	*Viṭapa*	Lower groin	2	Soften and draw in when groin is closed; extend when groin is open.
15	*Guḍa*	Anus	1	Tighten and draw buttocks together when legs are together.
16	*Basti*	Bladder	1	Draw back and lift.
17	*Nabhi*	Navel	1	Draw back and lift.
18	*Hṛdaya*	Heart	1	Lift and project.
19	*Stanamūla*	Bottom of breast (mammary artery)	2	Lift and project.
20	*Stanarohita*	Areola	2	Lift, project and open outwards.
21	*Apastamba*	Just below middle of collar bone (apex of lungs)	2	Lift and project.
22	*Apālāpa*	Pectoral fold (insertion of pectoral muscle in humerus)	2	Open outwards by drawing shoulders back.
23	*Kaṭikataruṇa*	Lumbo-sacral joint	2	Lengthen overlying muscles towards legs. Initiate outward rotation of leg from here.
24	*Kukundara*	Sacro-iliac joint	2	Press into body to move coccyx in.
25	*Nitamba*	Iliac crest	2	(see 4 as it arcs) Contract overlying muscles to keep erect.
26	*Parśvasandhi*	Kidneys	2	Press in (to stimulate kidneys).
27	*Aṁsaphalaka*	Shoulder blade	2	Press towards rib cage (to give firm support to chest).
28	*Bṛhatī*	Thorax inside shoulder blades	2	Press in (to make thoracic spine concave).
29	*Aṁsa*	Shoulder ligaments	2	Draw downwards and press in.
30	*Manya*	Carotid artery	2	Lengthen.
31	*Nīla*	Side of throat	2	Relax; draw towards back of neck.
32	*Sirā Mātṛkā*	Jugular vein	8	Stretch.
33	*Kṛkātikā*	Junction of head and neck (atlanto-occipital joint)	2	Stretch; press forward to maintain curvature of neck.
34	*Vidhura*	Depression at base of ears	2	Lengthen and draw back to maintain erect position of head/skull.
35	*Phaṇa*	Both sides of nose (maxillary sinus)	2	Relax and increase depression of skin.
36	*Apāṅga*	Outer corners of eyes	2	Relax and draw outwards.
37	*Vartaa*	Towards outer eyebrow	2	Draw back and keep level.
38	*Śaṅkha*	Temple	2	Relax.
39	*Utkṣepa*	Above temple (frontal and parietal joint)	2	Relax.
40	*Sthapani*	Between eyebrows (Corresponds to pituitary)	1	Relax and widen area.
41	*Śṛṅgātaka*	Inside mouth, behind uvula	4	Relax.
42	*Sīmanta*	Along cranial sutures	5	Relax.
43	*Adhipati*	Centre of the back of the head (Medulla)	1	Relax.

Physiology: *Āsanas* and *Doṣas*

In order to understand how *āsanas* work it is necessary to look at the clues given in the historical texts on Yoga. These form the basis from which a more detailed explanation can be made, using the information of Āyurveda.

Mediaeval works on Yoga are the first to record the physiological effects of certain *āsanas*. Before that, in the commentaries on the *Yoga Sūtras*, the *āsanas* are merely named and a brief description given. The *Haṭha Yoga Pradīpikā* often gives results as well as instructions. It uses the terminology of Āyurveda: *doṣas*, body tissues, digestive fire and so on. The following is a sample:

Matsyendrāsana (a spinal twist)

The right foot is placed at the root of the left thigh, the left foot twisted outside the [right] knee. Maintaining this arrangement, one should stay with the body turned...
Matsendra's pose intensifies the digestive [fire] and is a weapon that shatters a host of powerful diseases.
Through practice it awakens Kuṇḍalinī *and blocks the 'Moon' [left nostril,* Idā *channel] in men.*
(HYP 1.26–27)

Paścimottānāsana (a forward bend)

Stretching the legs on the ground like a staff, and grasping the two tops of the feet [toes] with the arms,
One should stay in that position with the forehead placed on the knees...
Paścimottānāsana, *the foremost of the postures, makes the air [in the stomach] flow to the back;*
It boosts the gastric fire, slims the stomach and brings health to men.
(HYP 1.28–9)

Mayūrāsana (a balance on palms and upper arms)

Holding the ground with both palms, then resting the sides of the navel on the elbows, Poised high, one should elevate [the body] like a staff...
The exalted Mayūrāsana *quickly cures all diseases such as tumours and dropsy and overcomes [imbalance of] the doṣas.*
It consumes completely bad foods eaten in large quantities, stimulates the gastric fire and destroys [even] deadly poison.
(HYP 1.30–31)

Śavāsana (relaxation)

Lying stretched out on the ground like a corpse is Śavāsana.
Śavāsana *removes tiredness and gives rest to the mind, the physiological effects of certain.*
(HYP 1.32)

To understand how *āsanas* and *prāṇāyāma* bring balance back to the *doṣas,* it is necessary first to know the symptoms of *doṣic* imbalance. The three *doṣas* lose of equilibrium as a result of unsuitable diet and activities, as well as external or genetic factors. They either increase or decrease, producing various symptoms in the body by which their abnormality can be recognized. The table opposite gives a summary of these symptoms.

Yoga *āsanas* affect the *doṣas* in the body and therefore its structure and functioning. It was seen earlier that the *doṣas* correlate to the five elements as follows: *vāta* to space and air, *pitta* to fire, and *kapha* to water and earth. All *āsanas* increase the space aspect of *vāta* because they lengthen muscles, open out compacted joints and decompress the soft parts of the body. Therefore for the purpose of analysing *āsanas* in terms of their action on the *doṣas* only the air aspect of *vāta* needs to be considered. The space aspect of *vāta* becomes pre-eminent in *Śavāsana*, the Corpse Pose, which is not concerned with any of the other elements.

The *āsanas* affect the *doṣas* in accordance with the principle of similarity and dissimilarity. In general they balance *vāta*, regulate *kapha* and maintain *pitta. Kapha* and *pitta* are both inactive; *vāta* impels them to increase or decrease. The table overleaf gives the *doṣic* effect of the pose types.

Symptoms of Imbalance of *Doṣas*

DOṢA	SYMPTOMS OF INCREASE	SYMPTOMS OF DECREASE
Vāta	Thinness Blackness Desire for hot things Tremors Accumulation of stools (and flatus) Constipation Loss of Strength Loss of Sleep Impairment of functions of senses Irrelevant talk Vertigo Helplessness	Loss of energy Reduction or loss of speech and action Impairment of perception Symptoms of increased *kapha*
Pitta	Yellow stool, urine, eyes and skin Hunger Thirst Little sleep	Weak digestive power Cold Dull complexion
Kapha	Weak digestive power Excess salivation Laziness Heaviness Whiteness Coldness Laxness of body Difficulty in breathing Cough Excessive sleep	Vertigo Dryness at sites of *kapha* Palpitations Looseness of joints

The Effect of *Āsanas* on the *Doṣas*

POSE TYPE	*DOṢIC* EFFECT	BENEFITS TO BODY AND MIND
Standing Poses	*Kapha* +	Muscles are built up and strengthened; joints are made firm.
	Pitta +	Digestive energy is enhanced and blood circulation improved by stretching; laxness of joints is reduced; fat is converted into muscle (metabolism).
	Vāta balanced	Natural mobility is restored.
Supine Poses	*Kapha* +	Immobility and calmness are induced.
	Pitta +	The digestive fire is enhanced by the abdominal stretch.
	Vāta balanced	*Prāṇa* and *udāna* circulate well; there is steadiness of mind; agitation of *pitta* does not occur as *vāta* does not fan it.
Fast Sequences and Jumpings; Salute to the Sun	*Kapha* -	Inertia is reduced.
	Pitta +	The digestive fire is fanned by increased *vāta*; circulation improves as all the *vātas* are increased, enhancing all the metabolic fires.
	Vāta +	Speed of movement and lightness are increased.
Twists	*Kapha* -	Stiffness is decreased.
	Pitta +	Metabolism, especially that of elimination, is increased.
	Vāta +	The mobility of the spine (joints) is increased.
Backbends	*Kapha* -	Laziness and slowness are reduced.
	Pitta +	The digestive fire improves because of the abdominal stretch; circulation and all *pittas* improve.
	Vāta +	The mobility of the spine increases.
Forward Bends	*Kapha* +	Absence of activity brings coolness and slowness to the body and head.
	Pitta +	*Apāna* is encouraged to move in its proper direction so that it does not disturb the gastric fire, which increases (i.e. *apāna* and *samāna* are regulated).
	Vāta -	Stillness of body and mind is induced.
Inverted Poses	*Kapha* -	Congestion in the chest lessens and brain power increases because *prāṇa* circulates well as the block caused by *kapha* is reduced.
	Pitta +	Digestion is enhanced; metabolism and hormonal balance are regulated.
	Vāta balanced	*Prāṇa* and *udāna* circulate well.

In order to manage the *doṣas* and to counteract their increase and decrease, a regular practice of all types of *āsanas* needs to be maintained. The practice should be balanced and should consist of effective sequences.

In order to understand the *āsanas* more precisely it is necessary to examine the functions of *vāta*, *pitta* and *kapha* in detail. Āyurveda gives each of these principles five designations according to location and function. These designations are ancient, being found in the *Upaniṣads* and other ancient writings on Yoga. They are helpful in understanding the therapeutics of *āsanas*. *Vāta* as the principle responsible for movement is particularly important. The divisions of the *doṣas* are noted in the tables on the following page.

Location of the Five *Vātas*

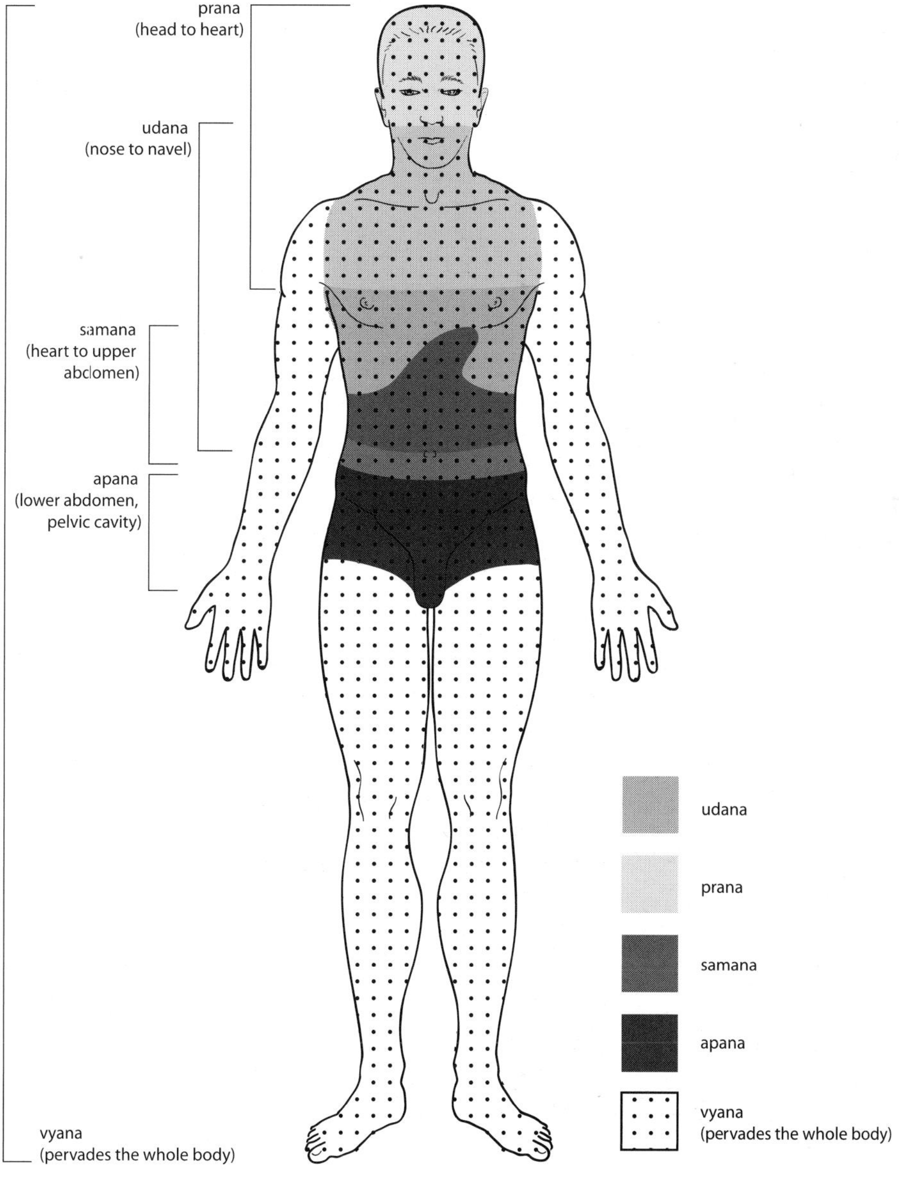

The Five Divisions of *Vāta*

SUBSIDIARY *VĀTA*	LOCATION	FUNCTION
Prāṇa	Main site: brain Area of action: throat and chest	It supports intelligence, heart, organs and mind. It causes the operations of spitting, sneezing, belching, exhalation and the swallowing of food.
Udāna	Chest, moving to the throat, nose and umbilicus	It causes the operations of speech, volition, life-process, stamina, complexion and memory.
Vyāna	Main site: heart It moves all over the body	It is fast moving and is the ultimate cause of almost all actions of creatures such as walking, throwing down and up, and closing and opening of the eyes.
Samāna	Near fire (*agni*), i.e. digestive system It moves in the stomach and intestines	It absorbs and digests food, separates nutrients and expels waste products.
Apāna	Abdomen It moves in the region of the waist, bladder, genitals and thighs	It causes expulsion of semen, female discharge, faeces, urine and the foetus.

The Five Divisions of *Pitta*

SUBSIDIARY *PITTA*	LOCATION	FUNCTION
***Pācaka Pitta* or *jaṭharāgni*, the digestive fire**	Small intestine	Its function is digestion, assimilation and separation of essentials and wastes. It aids the other *pittas*.
Rañjaka	Stomach	It imparts colour to plasma.
Sādhaka	Heart	It helps to achieve the aims of life, and is responsible for intelligence, retentive power and pride and enthusiasm.
Ālocaka	Eyes	It governs vision.
Bhrājaka	Skin	It gives colour and lustre to the complexion.

The Five Divisions of *Kapha*

SUBSIDIARY *KAPHA*	LOCATION	FUNCTION
Avalambaka	Chest	It supports the lower part of the spine by itself, the heart by food essence and the other *kaphas* by moisture.
Kledaka	Stomach	It moistens food.
Bodhaka	Tongue	The perception of tastes is attributed to it.
Tarpaka	Head	It nourishes the sense organs.
Śleṣaka	Joints	It lubricates the joints.

The analysis of *āsanas* in tems of the five *vātas*, five *pittas* and five *kaphas* greatly aids understanding of their mechanics.

Standing Poses and Twists

Standing poses and twists enhance the mobility of the joints and the extension of the muscles. Standing poses also improve the firmness of the joints. The physiology of these poses in Āyurvedic terms is as follows:

In the poses, the joints are made to flex or tighten. Joints are the seat of *kapha*. Making them firm increases the *śleṣaka kapha* in the joints. Bending them to make them more mobile channels *vāta* into its proper direction so that it does not go astray, vitiating *kapha* and causing pain.

The muscles are also the site of *kapha*. Stretching them increases *kapha*, making the muscles stronger. The thighs are the seat of *vāta*, as they are concerned with locomotion. Pulling up the thigh muscles (quadriceps) increases *kapha* and, hence, the strength of the thighs, preventing the dissipation of *vāta*.

The lateral rotation of the spine releases trapped *vāta* so that it can flow in its proper direction. Trapped *vāta* disturbs the *kapha* in the joints and causes pain. Free-flowing *vāta* enables supple movements. Lateral rotation of the lumbo-sacral vertebrae also acts on *apāna*, the abdominal air, improving its functioning. Lateral rotation of the thoracic vertebrae acts on *prāṇa* and *udāna* in the chest area, stimulating movement and preventing stagnation. This brings a feeling of freshness and alertness. Lateral rotation of the cervical vertebrae also acts on *prāṇa* and *udāna* in the throat region, easing tension in the head, neck and throat.

Forward Bends

These poses involve a prone position of the head and trunk. The weight of the back and the back of the head fall onto the front. The effect is as follows:

The head is the site of *kapha*. Gravity increases *kapha*, and brings it to bear on the *pitta* in the eyes (*alocaka*), cooling them. This brings relaxation. It also quietens *prāṇa* which is active in the brain. *Udāna* in the throat region is stilled by the increase of *kapha* due to gravitational weight, bringing relaxation. The voice box becomes passive.

The chest is the site of *kapha*, and also of *prāṇa* and *udāna vātas*. The prone position improves the functioning of *prāṇa* by encouraging respiration into the back of the lungs. At the same time, *udāna*, which controls speech, is quietened. The chest is also the site of *vyāna vāta*, which controls cardiac function as well as the opening and closing of the eyelids, yawning, sweating and motility. In this position *vyāna* is slowed down: the heart gets rested, the limbs become immobile, the eyes tend to close and coolness pervades the body.

The abdomen is the site of *pacaka pitta*, the digestive fire, and *samāna* and *apāna*. The prone position, which increases *kapha,* soothes the *pacaka pitta* and relieves acidity. *Kledaka kapha* increases. The increased *kapha* pushes *apāna* along the intestinal tract, thus helping to expels gas. The abdominal organs become soft.

Inverted Poses

On account of the numerous physiological and psychological effects of inverted poses they are of paramount importance. The physiology of inverted poses is as follows:

Gravity increases *kapha* in the head, making it quiet and passive. *Tarpaka kapha* which nourishes the sense organs is itself nourished and reinforced.

In *Śirṣāsana* (Head-Balance) the shoulders and chest have to lift against gravity. *Vāta* introduced into the shoulders by the action of lifting refreshes *avalambaka kapha*,which supports and balances the body systems. In *Sarvāṅgāsana* (Shoulder-Balance) the lift of the chest away from the shoulders continues to reinforce the actions of *avalambaka kapha*. In all inverted poses, the circulation of *prāṇa* and *udāna* in the upper trunk increases, improving respiratory efficiency and the qualities they control: cortical/brain function, perception, heart functioning (*prāṇa*); and vocal power, memory, insight, courage, discrimination and alertness (*udāna*).

The inversion of the abdominal and pelvic organs moves *samāna vāta* and *apāna vāta*, refreshing them. *Samāna vāta* fans the gastric fire (*pācaka pitta*) so that digestion is enhanced. *Apāna vāta* moves freely in its proper direction in the excretory and reproductive systems, bringing health.

The inversion of legs and trunk alters the gravitational pull on *vyāna vāta*, responsible for cardiac function and circulation. This gives rest to the heart and stimulates circulation. *Sādhaka pitta*, located in the heart, is fanned; its functions of intelligence, pride, enthusiasm and achievement of goals are enhanced.

Supine Poses

In these poses the front of the body is stretched. As space is created in and around the abdominal and pelvic organs *samāna* and *apāna* move freely. *Samāna* fans the gastric fire, *pācaka pitta* and also *rañjaka pitta* in the stomach, liver and spleen, enhancing digestion. Through the proper movement of *apāna* elimination and the working of the reproductive system are enhanced. When the rib cage is raised on a bolster, *prāṇa* and *udāna* move freely, improving respiration. The heart is supported, slowing down *vyāna vāta*. This produces restfulness with its accompanying characteristics: the tendency to close the eyes, coolness and the absence of movement. At the same time *sādhaka pitta* is increased, imbuing the mind with positive energy. Located in the heart, it controls intelligence, pride, enthusiasm and achievement of goals.

Fast Sequences/Jumpings

In this method of performing postures at speed the fast forward and backward movements of the body activate all the *vātas*. The head and chest are flushed with *prāṇa* and *udāna*, and the rate of respiration increases. *Vāta* increases in the legs, giving them speed and lightness. *Vyāna vāta* is stirred, increasing the heart rate and the pulse and range of circulation. It reaches and fans *bhrājaka pitta*, which is located in the skin and heightens its colour. *Samāna vāta* is increased, fanning *pācaka pitta* (the gastric fire) and speeding up metabolism. *Apāna vāta* is shaken up and is able to move past blockages or remove them. Thus the excretory and reproductive systems get toned.

Backbends

In these poses the backward arching of the spine gives a strong extension to the front of the body. This again increases all the *vātas*. However, because *avalambaka kapha* supports the chest it maintains the stability of the *vātas*. The psychological as well as the physiological functions of the *vātas* become enhanced. As the heart is in a lifted position, *sādhaka pitta* is also strongly enhanced, increasing confidence and positive energy.

Relaxation

In lying flat on the floor the body succumbs to the force of gravity and *kapha* is increased. *Vāta* becomes quiet, and the body still. This enables the body and mind to relax.

Psychology: *Doṣas* and *Prāṇāyāma*

Just as the results of *āsana* practice were noted, the effects of *prāṇāyāma* were recorded. On this subject the *Haṭha Yoga Pradīpikā* begins with a caution:

> *Just as lions, elephants and tigers should be tamed by slow degrees,*
> *So should breath be, otherwise it will kill the practitioner.*
> *Through proper [practice of]* prāṇāyāma *etc, all diseases are eradicated;*
> *Through improper practice all diseases are generated.*
> *Hiccups, asthma, coughs, headache, pains in the head, ears and eyes:*
> *Various diseases occur through disturbance of the breath.*
> *(HYP 2.15–16)*

Specific *prāṇāyāmas* are said to have specific effects. To give some examples (HYP 2.48–53, 57–58): Alternate nostril breathing *(Sūrya Bhedana Prāṇāyāma)* purifies the cranium, destroys [diseases of] *vāta doṣa* and eradicates worms. The Conquest-Helping Breath (*Ujjayi Prāṇāyāma*) destroys disorders of *kapha doṣa* in the throat and increases the fire of the body [digestive fire]. It destroys disorders of the channels, dropsy and body tissues (*dhātus*). The Cooling Breath (*Śītali Prāṇāyāma*) nullifies tumours, enlarged spleen and so on, fever, bile, hunger thirst and poisons.

It is said that the nose is the gateway to the head (VA Sū 20.1). Āyurveda attributes to *prāṇa vāta* and *udāna vāta* the functions of the brain and mind. The brain is a seat of *vāta* (see page 32). *Sādhaka pitta* and *tarpaka kapha* are also involved as the former governs intelligence and the latter nourishes the senses. Although they have these functions ultimately they are controlled by *vāta*, which is responsible for all actions in the body. The *vāta* used in respiration is *prāṇa*. From the functions of *prāṇa* it can be seen that it is closely associated with the senses and nervous system. This explains the risks attending the incorrect practice of *prāṇāyāma*, and how *prāṇāyāma* brings health by balancing *vāta doṣa*.

The regulation of *vāta* in *prāṇāyāma* is achieved with the aid of three important physical "locks" (*bandhas*). One is the chinlock (*jālandhara bandha*) which controls *prāṇa* and *vyāna* in the thorax and throat. The second is the diaphragmatic grip (*uddiyāna bandha*) which controls the movement of *samāna* in the gastric region. The third is the clenching of the anus (*mūlādhara bandha*), which controls *apāna* by retaining it in its seat, the lower abdomen.

However, *prāṇāyāma* goes beyond respiration as it is primarily concerned with the management of the life force. This is also called *prāṇa*, and should be distinguished from *prāṇa vāta*, which is a functional aspect of *vāta doṣa*. Thus in *prāṇāyāma*, as opposed to ordinary respiration, exhalation is the operation of *prāṇa* while inhalation is the operation of *apāna*. *Prāṇa* and *apāna* here are not *doṣas* but cosmic forces. The aim of Yoga is their control: to reverse the downward flow of *apāna* so that it rises to meet *prāṇa* and the two then unite, leading to the awakening of spiritual energy.

Prāṇāyāma is not concerned only with *vāta doṣa*. When this *doṣa* is balanced, it goes beyond the doṣas entirely and is concerned with the *guṇas* (*sattva*, *rajas*, *tamas*, as applied to the mind. A peaceful, intelligent mind is predominantly *sattva*. Under the influence of *rajas*, it initiates activities and becomes disturbed by emotions. Under the influence of *tamas,* it becomes dull and despairing. In *prāṇāyāma,* the mind is trained to turn away from activity to concentrate on the breath. This diminishes its *rajasic* quality. By exploring the subtle inner world of breath the faculty of intelligence is honed. This diminishes its *tamasic* quality.

There is a definite correlation between the breath on the one hand and the mind and emotions on the other. Each emotion is associated with a specific type of breath. For example, when someone is angry, the breath comes out in short gusts; when they are sad, they sigh, and so on. Similarly, when breathing is made even and slow, the mind follows suit and becomes quiet and serene. Brain activity also become slow and finally ceases altogether, resulting in an all-pervading sense of peace. The autonomic nervous system, which is usually overactive, becomes quiet, thus slowing the pulse and bringing down the blood pressure. The *Haṭha Yoga Pradīpikā* explains the relationship between mind and breath as follows:

> *The mind has two stimulants, instincts and breath.*
> *Of these, when one is destroyed the two also are destroyed.*
> *Where the mind dissolves, there breath dissolves;*
> *Where breath is dissolved the mind is dissolved.*
> *Mind and breath are blended like milk and water,*
> *And both are alike in their operation.*
> *Where there is breath there is operation of mind;*
> *Where there is mind there is operation of breath.*
> *Hence, through the destruction of one there is the destruction of the other;*
> *Through the operation of one there is the operation of the other.*
> *As long as they are not destroyed the senses operate;*
> *When they are destroyed the state of liberation is achieved.*
> *(HYP 4.22–25)*

Vāta as concerned with higher mental functions is correlated to *rajas*, the principle of activity. The fundamental nature of the mind, however, according to Yoga and *Sāṁkhya*, is not *rajas* but *sattva*, the principle of intelligence. It is heavily affected by *rajas* only when it is full of desires and emotions. Āyurveda considers *sattva* as the property of the mind and *rajas* and *tamas* as defects (*doṣas*), which create mental disorders. However, although it speaks of liberation, Āyurveda is more concerned with the mind as manifest in the body in this life; Yoga is concerned with the metaphysical mind and the return of a clouded and sullied mind to its pristine purity.

Energy Management

Āyurveda delineates the parameters of constitution, age, strength, climate, season, and so on, according to which activities should be carried out in order to maintain health throughout life. This amounts to the sensible management of energy, having the whole life-span in view.

A second general principle regarding the optimization of energy is that, for any object or activity, there can be right use, overuse, under-use and misuse. Right use maintains health; the others undermine it. This applies to use of the senses, eating, exercise, mental activity, and so on. It applies equally to Yoga practice.

Yoga, however, has a bolder objective than just the maintenance of health: nothing less than conquering and transcending the forces of nature. Setting out with this aim, its techniques for tapping into and harnessing the energies of the body and mind are incomparable. It channels, dams and directs these energies in the most efficient way, cutting through blockages and preventing dissipation. This gives it the power not merely to maintain health, but to maximize it and, ultimately, to transcend all health considerations.

The ground rules for Yoga practice, based on the common-sense teachings of Āyurveda, are set out below. They are intended for people living life in the world, with full work, family and social commitments. Incorporating Yoga into daily life as a support and spiritual practice is different from having Yoga as an exclusive aim. The latter case applies to recluses who have renounced mundane activities and who follow their own rules of spiritual discipline, as exemplified in the various Yoga texts.

Constitution

A person in normal health should do all the various postures, so as to have a rounded balance of practice. However, individual constitution should also be taken into account by placing emphasis on those poses that balance it. The Āyurvedic classification of constitutional types into *vāta-*, *pitta-* and *kapha-*predominant is useful for evaluating the suitability of *āsanas* for each individual.

CONSTITUTION	SUITABLE *ĀSANA* PRACTICE
Kapha	Someone who is heavy but strong and tireless should do vigorous postures, and postures vigorously, to counterbalance the tendency towards lethargy. This applies to *kapha*-predominant people, but also to others during periods of strong health, stable life circumstances and freedom from stresses. Someone who is heavy but strong and tireless should do vigorous postures, and postures vigorously, to counterbalance the tendency towards lethargy. This applies to *kapha*-predominant people, but also to others during periods of strong health, stable life circumstances and freedom from stresses.
Pitta	Someone who is mentally hyperactive or emotionally agitated should do postures that soothe the mind. This applies to *pitta*-predominant people, but also to others during periods of intense intellectual activity and emotional strain.
Vāta	In broad terms, someone who is thin, erratic in activity, and gets easily tired should do plenty of restorative postures. Staying quietly in these builds up energy and stability. This applies both to people of *vāta*-predominant constitution, but also to others at critical periods of change, insecurity and debility due to illness, stress and so on.

Age

Āyurveda notes childhood as a time when *kapha* is predominant, the middle years of adulthood as *pitta*, and old age as *vāta*. These natural stages of life require different approaches to Yoga practice. To match their exuberant power, children and young people should do fast, energetic practice. Adults should do postures to maintain physical strength and firmness, and as a buttress against mental and emotional pressures. The elderly should do postures that maximize their intake of oxygen and safeguard them against fragility and debility.

The *Haṭha Yoga Pradīpikā* has no bars to practice, declaring that it can be done by everyone, irrespective of age, ill health or weakness.

Illness, Stress and Trauma

Āyurveda has a methodology of treatment. The first step is to treat the disease by curative medicines and to bring back the body to normalcy. The second step is to strengthen the body by the use of tonics.

Similarly in Yoga there are two stages of therapy. The first is to give relief from pain, as with a painkiller, or to apply measures to effect a return to normalcy. The second is to build up the tissues to a superior degree. This can be compared to rejuvenation. During the period of convalescence, a gentle routine of recuperative practice should be adopted. This should be intensified only gradually, commensurate with the recovery of strength and stamina.

Time of Day

Āyurveda divides the day into periods of four hours, governed in turn by *kapha, pitta and vāta.* The first part of the day and night are governed by *kapha*, the middle part by *pitta* and the last part by *vāta.* There is a gradual overlap of *doṣas* at the junction of the periods.

Cycle of *Doṣas*

DOṢA	DAY	NIGHT
Kapha	6–10 am	6–10 pm
Pitta	10 am–2 pm	10 pm–2 am
Vāta	2–6 pm	2–6 pm

The different qualities of these periods affect Yoga practice. In the morning and evening when *kapha* is strong, dynamic practice is possible. In the afternoon, under the influence of *vāta*, restful postures alone are suitable. (Āyurveda itself recommends that exercise be done in the morning.) The *Haṭha Yoga Pradīpikā* does not indicate any particular time for *āsana* practice. For *prāṇāyāma* , it gives four times: early morning, mid-day, evening and midnight. For people not devoting their lives exclusively to Yoga, the most practical times are early morning and evening.

Climate and Season

Āyurveda recognizes that seasonal and climatic alteration should be reflected by changes in a person' s diet and activities. What is appropriate for hot weather is not so for cold weather, and so on. Similarly, Yoga practice needs to be adapted to the seasons, as shown in the table overleaf.

Diet

Āyurveda notes that food and drink, if taken in the proper manner, promote growth, life, intelligence and health. Food is the fuel for the internal fire, *agni*, which is the chief protector of the body. There are seven factors to be considered when selecting and eating food. These are its natural properties, such as heavy or light, healthful or incompatible combinations, the processing it has undergone, its quantity, its provenance in relation to the eater, its seasonality and time of consumption, and the manner in which it is consumed. With regard to quantity, it is said that half the stomach should be filled with solid food, one quarter with liquids, and the last quarter should be left unfilled, for air (and the operation of digestion).

The *Haṭha Yoga Pradīpikā* advocates moderation in food and prescribes and prohibits certain items for the Yogin. Its recommendations are in accord with Āyurvedic principles. Basically, such a diet increases *kapha* and reduces *vāta* and *pitta*. *Kapha* is responsible for stability and placidity. It is strengthened by milk, ghee, grains and fruits. *Vāta* is characterized by instability, a quality increased by dry, stale foods. *Pitta* is characterized by desires and activity. Pungent, salty, sour foods and meat increase these. This is why a vegetarian diet is recommended for Yogins. Light, fresh foods

SEASON	SUITABLE YOGA PRACTICE
Cold (Winter) (Two seasons)	Poses which generate heat by vigorous movements and strong stretches. Standing poses, twists, inverted poses, jumps and backbends effectively promote circulation, warm the body and overcome stiffness.
Post-Winter Cool (Spring)	Poses which regularize digestion and rid the body of coughs and colds. Standing poses, forward bends, twists, supine poses, inverted poses and backbends are beneficial. Inverted poses in particular clear congestion and boost the immune system.
Hot (Summer)	Poses which cool the body and involve passive rather than active stretches. Supine poses, supported forward bends and supported inverted poses keep the body flexible without exertion. Staying in these poses for a length of time helps to throw off body heat.
Wet (Rains)	Poses which enhance digestion and make the body warm. Standing poses, twists, forward bends, backbends, inverted poses and supine poses with stretching are all helpful.
Post-Summer Warmth (Autumn)	Poses which cool and soothe the body. Forward bends, supine poses, inverted poses and supported backbends all have this effect.

also promote the *sattvic* qualities of the mind. Milk and ghee are advised in the initial stages for those undertaking *prāṇāyāma*. *Prāṇāyāma* is concerned with the element of air and *vāta doṣa*, whose characteristics are dryness and lightness. Milk and ghee have the opposite qualities of heaviness and oiliness. Their consumption balances the drying effect of *prāṇāyāma*, thus preserving health.

Overall, the postures increase metabolic efficiency and certain one, such as inverted poses, forward bends and supine poses enhance the power of digestion and eliminate wind (*apāna*). In this way they help to preserve a good digestion throughout life. Even if sensible food habits are not adhered to, Yoga can help counter the negative effects so that the energy of body and mind is maintained. *Prāṇāyāma* regulates the actions of the five *vātas* and thus also enhances metabolism. Yoga practice highlights the effects of different foods on the body and mind, and gives a keen understanding of what is healthful and what is harmful. Its enhancement of well-being and sensitivity encourages the rejection of what is deleterious to health.

Pain Management

Pain is always due to *vāta*. *Vāta* resides in all the cavities of the body, in the bones, the feet and thighs (the source of locomotion), the skin, ears and the brain in its functional aspect. In addition, in its five functions it pervades the entire body and is the catalyst for all the body processes. As an air, or principle of motion, it needs to move freely in its proper channels in order to perform its functions properly.

Āyurveda provides a paradigm for the development of pain in its analysis of the stages of a disease. These stages are as follows:

(1) Accumulation of the *doṣa* in its seat
(2) Aggravation
(3) Spreading
(4) Localization
(5) Manifestation
(6) Particular symptoms

Taking the general pattern of disease as the model, it is possible to understand the process of pain. When *vāta* is blocked or increased, it accumulates (stage 1) and becomes agitated (stage 2). It finds other routes and moves where it should not (stage 3). It settles in its new (unauthorized) location (stage 4) and manifests as pain or disease (stage 5). In this location it may also be associated with the other *doṣas*, producing specific symptoms (stage 6).

Āyurveda notes the different types of pain that manifest in different diseases, such as dislocating, dilating, pricking, throbbing pain, cramps, pain with numbness, myalgia, severe pain, splitting pain, constricting pain, pain as if the whole body is constricting and hypersensitivity. These pains are sharp or dull, according to *doṣic* predominance. A dull pain is correlated to *kapha*, a sharp pain to *vāta* or *pitta*. When *pitta* and *kapha* are involved together with *vāta* there may be inflammation or itching.

From the point of view of Yoga practice it is important to differentiate between the harmful pain symptomatic of a problem and the beneficial pain of stretching. When a muscle extends or a joint opens, *vāta*, which is associated with movement and space, is increased. If the muscle is habitually contracted and the joint compressed, this extension may be accompanied by pain. Such pain is to be expected in this training process, as in any new activity. As the action becomes habitual, pain decreases or disappears. *Vāta* is balanced when it fulfils its proper potential for space and movement within the body structure. In this case there is no pain at all in the flexion, extension and rotation of the limbs and the pain involved in bringing *vāta* to this ideal state is not harmful.

As *vāta* is mobile and unpredictable, the extension of muscles and joints should always be executed smoothly, with full mental awareness. By this means *vāta* is channelled and does not run zigzag and out of control. If *vāta* is increased suddenly or is introduced in the wrong place, it produces pain, indicating wrong movement. This warning pain should not be ignored: over-stretching and misalignment can lead to the tearing of muscles and ligaments, dislocation, and sprains.

Yoga is effective in relieving pain. As pain is due to *vāta*, it is the balancing of *vāta* and increase of *kapha* that gives relief. The postures remove obstructions to the flow of *vāta* in the joints and increase *kapha* by making them more stable. Similarly they increase space in the organs and soft tissues. When there is no obstruction to the flow of *vāta* in the body, there is no pain.

When inflammation occurs, the affected part should be rested. Doing postures with support is a constructive way of giving rest. For example, in the case of inflammation of the knee, doing inverted poses where the legs are supported is more soothing than merely being inactive, as the weight is taken off the legs completely. While rest quietens *vāta*, the removal of pressure on the legs reduces the irritation due to aggravated *pitta*.

To relieve itching, the skin needs to stretch. Again, this should done in supported poses as these reduce the agitation of *vāta*, which is the root cause of pain. Stretching the skin reduces the sensation of congestion caused by aggravated *kapha*, in a similar manner to the natural response of scratching.

Mental pains, such as grief, anxiety and fear, have somatic consequences that manifest themselves immediately or after a period of time. The process is akin to physical pain: the energy of the mind does not flow unhampered in creative pursuits but is either caught in painful reflections or diverted to avoid these. In the normal course of events, it takes a long time for the mind to return to cheerfulness. Yoga practice helps the speedy return to a healthy frame of mind. This is achieved by supported backbends and supported inverted poses. By energizing the body and preventing the collapse of the chest region, these poses convert *tamas*, characterized by dullness and inertia, to *sattva*, characterized by lightness and fresh intelligence. At the same time they quieten agitation, the characteristic of *rajas* and also of *vāta doṣa*.

Cleansing Treatments

In the normal course of life impurities and toxins accumulate in the body. Āyurveda considers that it needs to be regularly cleansed of these in order to maintain good health. Cleansing procedures must be undertaken under the supervision of a doctor.

Āyurveda divides treatment into two types, purification (*śodhana*) and pacification (*śamana*). The former is that which removes *doṣas* from the body, and the latter restores them to normalcy. There are five types of purification, involving procedures that rid the body of accumulated toxins and rejuvenate it. These are to be undertaken periodically, according to the season, and when suffering from particular ailments. The purpose of these procedures is to rebalance the *doṣas* and the keep the five *vātas* in their sites, for the sake of optimal physiological functioning.

The main procedures are always preceded by pre-operative procedures. Here the principle is to bring the *doṣas* from other parts of the body to the gastro-intestinal tract so that it is easy to cleanse away the excess toxins. The two preliminary procedures are oleation and sudation:

The first step is the application and ingestion of medicated oils (oleation). This is especially for *vāta* problems. Oil massage can be done regularly at home and is followed by a warm bath. Another separate procedure is the streaming of liquid, particularly oil and ghee, onto the head (*śirodhāra*). This is done for ailments above the shoulders and for psychological problems.

After oleation, heat therapy (sudation) is carried out. This involves the application of dry heat, hot liquid or medicated steam to induce sweating.

The five principal cleansing methods *(pañcakarmas)* are emesis, purgation, enema, nasal medication and bloodletting.

Emesis is done to cleanse the upper part of the body. Excess *kapha* is brought to the stomach by means of oleation and sudation and expelled by medicines to induce controlled vomiting.

Purgation effects the downward expulsion of *doṣas*, particularly *pitta*.

Enema is the treatment for *vāta* in its own seat. Medicated oils or herbal decoctions are used.

Nasal medication is used for diseases of *vāta*, *pitta* and *kapha* above the shoulders. It can be done daily as a preventive measure. Medicated drops are instilled in each nostril.

Bloodletting is used to purify the blood. It is done by the application of leeches, and was previously also done by venesection.

After the main cleansing rest is advised. There is a gradual return to normal food.

A parallel may be drawn between the "Five Procedures" (*pañcakarma*) or Āyurveda and the "Six Procedures" (*ṣatkarma*) of Haṭha Yoga. These cleansing techniques are advised only when fat or *kapha* is excessive. Others in whom the *doṣas* are balanced should not do them. According to the *Haṭha Yoga Pradipikā*, the purpose of these cleansing procedures is to rid the body of excess *doṣas* so that *prāṇāyāma* can be practised successfully. However, it also notes that according to some teachers *prāṇāyāma* itself removes impurities and they do not recommend the *ṣatkarma*. As it is not safe to attempt these procedures without the guidance of a teacher they are mentioned only briefly. The six principal techniques are: internal cleansing, enema, nasal cleansing, concentrated gazing, abdominal massaging and frontal-brain cleansing.

The importance of the regular cleansing and palliation of *doṣas* to maintain the health of the

Comparison of Cleansing Procedures in Āyurveda

CLEANSING NEEDED	ĀYURVEDIC PROCEDURE	YOGIC PROCEDURE THROUGH *ĀSANAS* AND *PRĀṆĀYĀMA*
***Kapha* Excess**	Emesis	Inverted poses and backbends help to expel excess *kapha* from the upper body and prevent it from accumulating.
***Pitta* Excess**	Purgation	Inverted poses, supine poses, forward bends and twists help to regulate excess *pitta*.
***Vāta* Excess**	Enemas	Inverted poses, supine poses and forward bends help to regulate excess *vāta*.
Blood	Bloodletting	Vigorous movements, standing poses and inverted poses help to purify the blood.
Head Congestion	Nasal medication	Inverted poses and *prāṇāyāma* relieve tension and congestion in the head.

body is recognized in Yoga. The systematic practice of *āsanas* and *prāṇāyāma* performs these cleansing, rejuvenating and balancing functions.

Other treatments also have their equivalents in Yoga. Regular massage with oils is recommended in Āyurveda in order to keep the muscles and joints pliable, to nourish the body tissues and to reduce fatigue and increased *vāta*. It is said to improve eyesight and induce good sleep. Yoga practice performs these same functions. The nourishment comes internally from a blood supply made more efficient by the stretching of muscles, rather than externally from oil applied by stroking. Because of their similarity in action, and because both may cause fatigue, massage and *āsana* practice should be done at separate times. After each the body needs time to assimilate what it has received. If a time gap is kept, the two can enhance each other: massage will be more effective because the body tissues are already soft and receptive, and the oil lubricates the tissues so that the body can stretch and flex better.

For calming the mind Āyurveda gives a treatment wherein medicated oil is streamed slowly onto the forehead for a period of time. In Yogic *prāṇāyāma* exhalations perform a similar function by rhythmically dispelling tension from the forehead and therefore the brain.

Corresponding with Āyurveda, in Yoga vigorous standing poses, jumps and Salute to the Sun done in a warm temperature produce sweating.

Any Yoga programme includes and normally ends with inverted poses which are restful and bring balance back to the body and mind. The principle is the same as that governing the post-operative procedures in Āyurveda.

Other Specializations

Āyurveda classically has eight branches: internal medicine, including psychiatry, the diseases of the head and neck, surgery, toxicology, possession by spirits, paediatrics (including obstetrics and gynaecology), rejuvenation therapy and aphrodisiacs and reproductive diseases. In several of these Yoga can provide alternative or complementary treatments.

MENTAL HEALTH

Āyurveda does not treat psychiatry as a separate branch of medicine. It considers the psychological causes of all diseases: for example, fear or grief giving rise to diarrhoea or desire or grief producing fever. Insanity and epilepsy are dealt with under internal medicine.

The misuse of intelligence and the increase of *rajas* and *tamas* are considered to be important origins of mental diseases. They may have external or internal causes. Psychoses and neuroses are caused by the vitiation of all the three *doṣas* and are classified according to the dominance of *vāta*, *pitta* and *kapha*. Phobia, neurosis, delusion, hallucination, obsession and mania vary according to their *doṣic* predominance. Sitting immobile, and excess salivation are symptoms of *kapha* predominance. Excessive movement and moodiness are symptoms of *vāta* predominance. Anger is a symptom of *pitta* predominance. Aggression could be a symptom of *pitta* or *vāta*. The treatment for these disorders consists of medicated ghees, cleansing procedures, oil streamed onto the head, rejuvenating tonics and sedatives. Head massage and medication administered through the nose are also given as well as counselling, advice on ethics and spiritual remedies.

The Yogic approach to psychological disorders is likewise to soothe or stimulate the mind, as appropriate, and to nourish and strengthen the nervous system. Inverted poses done with support are effective in achieving this. For *vāta*- and *pitta*-dominant conditions forward bends with the head resting on a support are calming, particularly if a bandage is wrapped round the forehead. Similarly, concentrating on the exhalations in *prāṇāyāma* induces mental relaxation. In the case of depression supported backbends are powerful mood lifters. Concentrating on the inhalations in *prāṇāyāma* induces confidence. In all postures and *prāṇāyāma* support is necessary so that there is no strain on the nerves. In addition to physical measures, Yoga has a whole literature concerning peace of mind. Once some degree of mental balance is restored through other means, reading its philosophy can help to give a perspective which allays personal anguish.

Āyurveda uses two principles of treatment: pacification (*śamana*) and purification (*śodhana*). Yoga applies these principles to mental disturbance, ranging from what is considered normal to pathological conditions. In common with Āyurveda it recognizes "enemies" of the mind which destroy equanimity. Āyurveda enumerates these as greed, grief, fear, anger, pride, shamelessness, envy, desire and covetousness (CS.Sū 7.27), and the Yoga list is similar. Mental disturbance in the form of stress, anxiety, frustration, and so on, can occur in any of three areas: the thought or ego centre, located in the brain and throat, the emotional centre, located in the heart and chest and the sensual centre, located in the pelvis. Yoga techniques of *āsana* and *prāṇāyāma* are effective in calming and purifying these centres.

CHILDREN

Āyurveda considers that a child spends one year inside the womb and seven years outside. The eighth year is the time for starting studies. Childhood is the time of *kapha*, promoting growth and strength. Childhood is considered to continue till the age of sixteen.

In childhood *kapha* predominates, in the middle years *pitta* predominates and in the last years of life, *vāta*. Puberty is the transition from *kapha* to *pitta*. In women menopause is the stage when *pitta* diminishes and gives way to *vāta*.

AGE	*DOṢA*
Childhood	*Kapha*
Adulthood	*Pitta*
Old Age	*Vāta*

Yoga practice may be started at the age of seven or eight, when the child is old enough to understand what is required. It aims at nurturing physical and mental development and at inculcating good habits for life. It is as suitable for the slower, less fit child as it is for the physically adept. In keeping with the bursting *kapha* strength of childhood, the *āsanas* should be done energetically and fast. In this way they train the body to be light and agile and the mind to be co-ordinated and concentrated. Mental energy is harnessed by the inverted poses, further developing concentration and willpower and laying the basis of emotional balance. This last is needed during the turmoil of puberty and adolescence. *Prāṇāyāma* is not suitable for children for the same reasons. While they are growing, their intellect and senses are exploring the outside world. It would be unnatural to force their still-expanding mental faculties to turn inwards. *Prāṇāyāma* can be attempted when the period of growth has stabilized at the end of adolescence.

WOMEN'S HEALTH

Āyurveda classifies the epochs of a woman's life according to age and body changes. These are summarized in the following table.

AGE	CHANGES IN THE BODY
Childhood	
10	General development
10–12	Development of secondary sex characteristics
12–16	Menstruation
Adulthood	
16–40	Maximum reproductive capacity
40–50	Pre-menopausal symptoms
Old Age	
After 50 or 55	Menopausal and after

The menstrual cycle is likewise understood in terms of *doṣic* predominance.

SPECIFIC STAGE	DURATION	DOMINANT *DOṢA*
Menstrual phase	3 days	*Vāta*
Optimum period for conception	12–16 days	*Kapha*
Post-ovulatory stage	9–13 days	*Pitta*

Taking into account the dominance of *vāta* during menstruation, Āyurveda advises the following balancing mode of living:

ACTIVITIES
Celibacy Avoidance of daytime sleep Cultivation of calmness and restful state of mind Thinking of good, auspicious things
FOOD
Eating *vāta*-reducing foods: milk, rice, barley, ghee Avoiding pungent, hot and salty foods (as they aggravate *pitta* and therefore increase bleeding) Eating less for easy digestion

Yoga practice helps women cope comfortably with the frequent physiological changes taking place in their bodies. The monthly cycle is respected, and the special routine advised at the time of menstruation (quiet supine poses and forward bends) is in harmony with nature. They reduce *vāta*. Pre-menstrual tension is minimized, and menstrual cramps and other discomforts alleviated. Irregular menses are regularized.

The general level of health improves, thus ensuring a sound base for pregnancy. Yoga can be safely done at this time; however, the supervision of an experienced teacher is necessary as the health of both mother-to-be and child must be monitored at each stage. Physical fitness and a calm attitude are of great value during delivery.

At the time of menopause troublesome symptoms such as hot flushes and mood swings can be controlled and relieved. Post-menopausal physical degeneration, as exemplified by osteoporosis, can be fought by maintaining a vigorous practice. This maintains heat in the body.

In the case of serious gynaecological conditions, Yoga practice can give relief from pain and can help to prevent the problem from worsening. Pain is the effect of *vāta* and the requisite postures all seek to balance *vāta*. If there are symptoms of aggravated *pitta*, such as excess bleeding, the postures indicated would be those that reduce heat, such as forward bends. If the condition indicates aggravated *kapha*, such as cysts, the postures would seek to improve the flow of *vāta* in the lower abdomen by creating space. Groin-opening poses and inverted poses are effective for this.

SEXUAL POTENCY

Another branch of Āyurveda deals with ways to increase sexual potency, for the sake of ensuring progeny. It is said that regulated sex is one of the three pillars of life and health, the other two being food and sleep. Āyurveda considers the ovum as *agni*, the fire principle, and the sperm as *soma*, the moon or cooling principle. The treatments to increase sexual potency consist of cleansing procedures such as purgation and enema followed by medicines and tonics to be taken internally.

In contradistinction to householders, celibacy was always enjoined on Yogins. It is one of the ethical vows (*yamas* – on which the practice rests. At the same time it was recognized that a life of celibacy increased sexual potency. The *Haṭha Yoga Pradīpikā* describes the alluring effect of a particular *prāṇāyāma*:

Sītkārī Prāṇāyāma (Hissing Breath)

> *One should make a hissing sound in the mouth [to inhale] and expel [air] only through the nose.*
> *By persistence in this, one becomes a second god of love.*
> *One is adored by the circle of yoginis and is able to create and destroy;*
> *Neither hunger nor thirst, nor sleep nor laziness arise.*
> (HYP 2.54–55)

It and other Tantric Yoga texts describe various practices by which to sublimate sexual energy into spiritual energy.

Using Yoga in a limited way as a means to maintain health, the practice of *āsanas* are a valuable adjunct to infertility treatments because they tone the pelvis and reproductive organs. In women, consistent practice of inverted poses, forward bends and groin-opening poses regularizes the menses and conduces to hormonal balance. Backbends invigorate the pelvic area. The body tissues remain well-nourished and supple. This optimizes uterine health. The same poses are beneficial for men.

REJUVENATION THERAPY

Rejuvenation therapy is called *rasāyana*, meaning the movement of *rasa*, the fundamental fluid of the body which nourishes the other tissues. As a therapy it recommends medicines and treatments which promote the excellence of *rasa*, thereby preventing illness and the symptoms of ageing and enhancing memory, intellect, youth, lustrous complexion and longevity. It also includes ethical conduct (*yama*) and life disciplines (*niyama*) that modify behaviour and create mental and physical health. The aim is regeneration of vitality, energy and stamina.

The body is inherently subject to degeneration. Apart from external factors such as accidents there are other causes of degeneration, related to food, activities and psychological stresses. With respect to diet, the causes are the consumption of excess salty, spicy, bitter, raw, non-nourishing and decayed foods, irregular dietary habits and alcohol abuse. Deleterious activities are excessive exercise, daytime sleeping and sexual activity, and the suppression of natural urges. Harmful psychological states are anger, violence, fright, sorrow, greed and dejection.

The first thing that occurs is the disturbance of the *doṣas*, which in turn vitiates the digestive fire (*agni*) and the seven body tissues (*dhātus*), beginning with *rasa*. This causes a diminution of the body's immunity (*ojas*) and thus degeneration. *Rasāyana* aims at restoring the balance of the *doṣas* and their proper interaction with the *dhātus*, thereby recovering vitality, the acuity of the sense organs, and digestive power, and removing fear, anxiety, depression and so on. It re-establishes the metabolism and enhances the zest for life and the capacity to work.

There are many benefits of *rasāyana*: increased life-span, memory, intelligence and overall vitality, the establishment of youthfulness, good colour and complexion, a good voice, clarity of the senses, good sleep and optimum health.

The practice of Yoga is recognized to be rejuvenative and to maintain the body at its peak. A Yogin is described as having physical and mental well-being, without disease, old age and pain. According to the *Haṭha Yoga Pradīpikā*:

> *Perfection of* Haṭha *Yoga is achieved when there is leanness of body, graciousness of face, manifestation of sound, clear eyes, absence of disease, control of semen, blazing [digestive] fire and purity of channels.*
> (HYP 2.78).

The benefits claimed for *rasāyana* can also be gained from Yoga practice. Instead of using procedures like purgation and enemas to expel toxins, and tonics and oil massage to nourish tissues, Yoga uses the body itself.

Memory and intelligence are sustained by inverted poses, which increase blood flow to the brain and the volume of air in the chest. Stale air is expelled efficiently.

Vitality, youthful grace and buoyancy are maintained by the various stretches, rotations and jumps, and by backbends. These enhance circulation to the joints, muscles and organs, which all become toned. Toxins are eliminated quickly and regularly. The skin becomes soft and the pores remain open. The spine and the nervous system are strengthened. All these features are characteristics of youth.

Clarity of voice and the senses is enhanced by inverted poses and forward bends. These quieten the mind and senses, and relax the throat.

Good sleep and emotional stability are promoted by mental and sensory relaxation in the *āsanas* and by the regulation of the breath. In this way health is maintained at its optimum.

Āyurveda recognizes that health depends not just on physical factors but on psychological harmony within the individual and with the world at large. Thus it enjoins ethical conduct and personal life disciplines. It is said that only those who are virtuous – defined as being truthful, free from anger, not addicted to alcohol and sex, non-violent, peaceful and pleasant in speech, stable, pious, compassionate, regular in their habits and consuming milk and ghee (*sattvic* food) – benefit from rejuvenation therapy. Those who are not free from mental and physical defects do not gain the effects.

In common with all spiritual paths and with Āyurveda, Yoga also lays down certain moral attitudes and life disciplines as fundamental to harmonious relationships and mental well-being. Its morals are the vows not to do violence, to speak the truth, not to steal, to be celibate or chaste, and not to accumulate possessions. Its disciplines are purity of body, mind and speech, contentment, ascetic practices, study of sacred texts and surrender to actions to God.

Āyurveda is the science of longevity. In Yoga, too, longevity is a serious aim. Following a long tradition asserting that breath control (*prāṇāyāma*) prolongs life the *Haṭha Yoga Pradīpikā* states:

> *As long as the breath remains in the body,*
> *that is called life.*
> *Death is when it leaves the body; hence one*
> *should retain the breath [in the body].*
> (HYP 2.3)

To achieve this control and channel the breath involves applying locks (*bandhas*) at various parts of the body. There are three main ones. The first is the rising or flying lock (*uddiyāna bandha*), which involves pulling back the abdomen in the region of the navel. The second is the root lock (*mūla bandha*), which involves pressing the perineum with the heel and contracting the anus and drawing the down-moving air (*apāna*) upwards so that it unites with the upper air (*prāṇa*). The third is the chin lock (*jālandhara bandha*), which involves contracting the throat and bringing the chin down onto the chest. All are said to transform an old person into a youth, and to destroy old age and death.

The locks (*bandhas*) occur in the *āsanas* themselves. The rising lock (*uddiyāna bandha*) occurs naturally in Head-Balance (*śirṣāsana*), where the abdomen is drawn towards the back and the navel moves towards the waist. The root (anal) lock (*mūla bandha*) occurs in Head-Balance (*śirṣāsana*) and Shoulder-Balance (*sarvāṅgāsana*) when the buttocks are tightened and drawn together. The chin lock (*jālandhara bandha*) occurs in the Shoulder-Balance (*sarvāṅgāsana*) and Plough pose (*halāsana*) when the chest is brought towards the chin. Thus the *āsanas* train the body for *prāṇāyāma*.

There are many other practices explained in the *Haṭha* Yoga tradition, which include those which are occult and which do not find favour with mainstream society. The main aim is to awaken the individual spiritual energy *Kuṇḍalinī* which lies coiled at the base of the spine and make it rise to the crown of the head where it unites with the universal energy. Beyond longevity, all these practices are said to confer immortality and the great teachers of the tradition are said to have conquered time (that is to say, death) to roam about the universe.

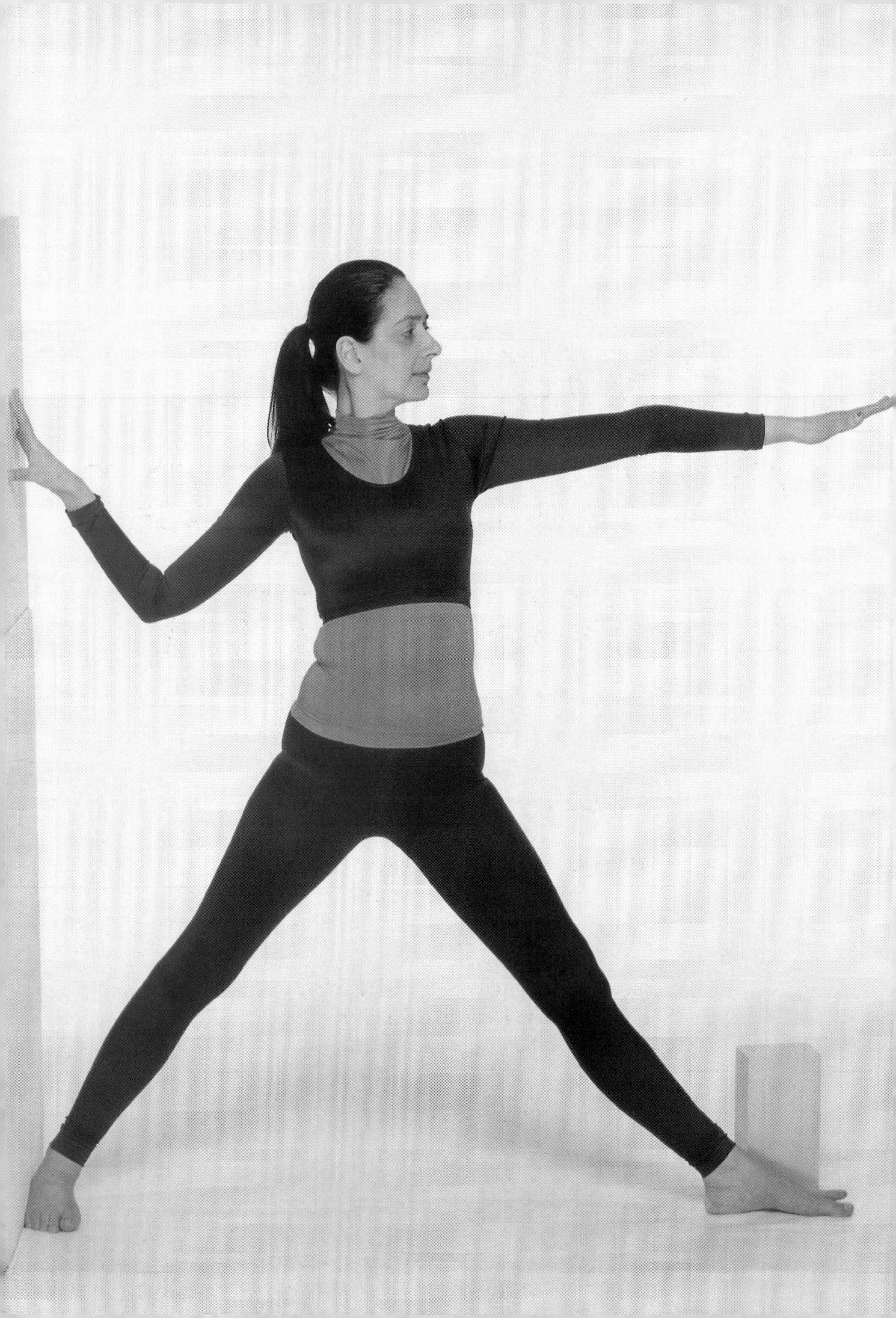

PRACTICE ROUTINES FOR LONGEVITY

Whether young, old, or very old,
Sick or feeble,
Through persistence the diligent achieve
Success in all the Yogas.

Success comes to one devoted to practice;
How can it come to the idler?
Merely by reading and teaching
Success in Yoga does not arise.

(HYP 1.64–65)

About the Practice Routines

These programmes address the various aspects of the body and mind: the skeleto-muscular system, the physiological systems and the psyche. They are designed progressively, with simple postures and methods introduced before more complex ones, and the body structure dealt with before its functions and before the mind. Taken together the programmes form a systematic course which can be followed from beginning to end.

In the ordinary course of events the postures are performed independently. However, with the aim of improving health it is helpful to make use of various supports. These enable the postures to be done efficaciously with confidence and without strain. They facilitate the alignment of the body and therefore the correct actions in the poses. Importantly also, they provide support for weak or injured areas. Common household items are used as props, such as walls, ledges, chairs, stools, benches, tables, blankets, bolsters or firm cushions, belts and bricks. In addition it is useful to have a foldable non-slip mat.

There is, in fact, a tradition of using aids for Yoga practice. The *Bhagavad-Gītā* (BG 6.11) describes the ancient equivalent to the modern mat and blanket: a deer skin covered with a soft cloth. *Vyāsa's* commentary on the *Yoga Sūtras* mentions a "supported posture" (PYS 2.46). In this a band is placed around the back and crossed legs while sitting for long periods. In more recent times an illustrated manuscript dating from the 19th century depicts Yoga postures done with the help of ropes hung from bars as well as the Yoga band (N.E. Sjoman – *The Yoga Tradition of the Mysore Palace*, Abhinav Publications, 1996). The systematic use of props for remedial purposes is, however, a hallmark of the Iyengar method.

Different props and methods are employed for the same postures. This variety in approach activates different parts of the body and gives a wide base of understanding. For example, doing standing poses with the back foot against the wall highlights and reinforces the action of the back leg, whereas doing them with the back against the wall supports the spine and removes the difficulty of independent balance. Little by little alignment, anchor points and the direction of stretches are learned and the body takes on the shape of the posture.

The cumulative effect of a series of postures is much greater than that of a single pose. A sequence of carefully graded poses builds a progression from mild to intense. It introduces different types of movements and actions. It maintains a balance between effort and rest: for example, stretching and relaxing. It allows time for assimilation of the work done. It ends with repose. As a result of Yoga practice there should be lightness of body and mind.

The postures are usually held for a period of time. By maintaining stretches in an unaccustomed configuration of limbs the joints and muscles gain pliability and strength. This is why there is often instant relief from aches and pains and in the long term even chronic pains are reduced in severity or disappear. Postures which have a powerful physiological effect, such as inversions, are usually held for a longer duration. Occasionally, to encourage litheness and liveliness, some postures are done as a series of quick movements linked by jumps.

Prāṇāyāma, control of the breath, has to be approached with care because breath is the life force. Traditionally *prāṇāyāma* is done while seated, although the *Haṭha Yoga Pradīpikā* states that *Ujjāyi* can also be done while moving about, standing or walking (HYP 2.53). For a beginner, however, sitting immobile in the required erect posture is strenuous. A non-fatiguing method is to practise while lying with the chest supported. The rib cage rests and broadens and the lungs expand effortlessly, facilitating deep breathing and relaxation.

For the sake of better understanding and consolidation of practice repeat each programme several times. Ultimately all of them should be practised regularly to maintain health. However, those who suffer from specific ailments will benefit by concentrating on the programme which relates to their condition.

Organization of the Routines

The practice routines are divided into those which develop anatomical strength, those which enhance physiological efficiency and those which promote mental and emotional well-being.

ANATOMICAL STRENGTH

The Feet and Legs
The Hips and Pelvis
The Back
The Neck, Shoulders, Arms and Hands

PHYSIOLOGICAL EFFICIENCY

The Abdominal Organs: Stomach, Liver and Intestines
The Abdominal Organs: Kidneys and Bladder
The Lungs and Heart
Circulation
The Female Organs
Body Immunity

MENTAL AND EMOTIONAL WELL-BEING

The Tension-Free Mind
The Affirmative Mind

GENERAL GUIDELINES FOR PRACTICE

Food
Yoga should be done on an empty stomach: 2–3 hours after a snack and 4–5 hours after a heavy meal. Food may be taken half an hour after practice, drink ten to fifteen minutes. This allows time for the body to switch gear from exercise to digestion.

Clothing
Clothing should be non-restrictive and the feet bare. This is necessary for effective stretches and for sensitivity.

Time
Any time of day can be suitable for practice. In the morning the body is stiff but the mind is fresh; in the evening the body is more supple but the mind is more tired.

Personal Hygiene
The bowels should be evacuated before a morning Yoga practice. A bath should be taken before or after practice.

Perspiration
In moderate temperatures Yoga practice does not make the body sweat excessively. Excessive perspiration is a sign of over-exertion or ill-health. Restorative poses should be done to recover lost energy. If heavy perspiration persists, the manner of practising should be changed and the advice of a teacher sought.

Breathing
Initially or when a new posture is learnt there is a tendency to hold the breath. This creates tension and should be avoided. When the mind is relaxed the rhythm of the breath synchronizes with the movements and extensions of the body.

Menstruation
Inverted poses should never be done during menstruation, as they inhibit the exit of body wastes. Vigorous Yoga practice is similarly inadvisable as it may put strain on the female organs. A gentle routine of supported supine poses and forward bends is suitable during this time of physiological change.

Medical Conditions
In the following circumstances supervision by an experienced teacher is essential: serious illness, chronic conditions requiring regular medication, recent accidents and surgery, and pregnancy. The programmes given in this book are general in nature and are not a substitute for individual guidance.

Children
All the postures can safely be done by children. For children who suffer from particular ailments (asthma, scoliosis, etc.) postures relevant to the area of their problem should be done. The support will need to be adapted and the length of time in the pose reduced. ***Prāṇāyāma* should not be taught to children.**

Anatomical Strength

The archetype of health is to remain composed in oneself, undisturbed by physical or physiological impairment or by mental stresses. This is the Āyurvedic concept of well-being. The purpose of sleep is to bring about this state after the exertions of the day.

The Āyurvedic doctrine of right use, overuse, underuse and misuse or abuse with regard to the senses can be usefully applied to physical as well as mental activities. The overuse of joints and muscles causes degeneration, while others stiffen or atrophy owing to lack of use. Wrong use causes pain or injury.

The right use of the body allows it to function optimally with minimum deterioration due to ageing. Through Yoga practice it is possible to transform deleterious postural habits into beneficial ones. Aches and pains, restricted movement and weakness can be eliminated or at least reduced. Instead, pain-free limbs and joints, ease of movement, strength and stamina can be enjoyed even when these did not exist before. Improvement occurs irrespective of age.

Ideally, muscles should be able to perform their functions of expansion and contraction without being impeded or restricted in the space allotted to them. Those which lie along a bone should be able to extend along the whole length of the bone. Those which move the bones and tendons at a joint should be able to give the maximum flexion, rotation or stability required. When all is working well there is good co-ordination and balance, bringing lightness and gracefulness.

There are several factors which diminish the natural grace of the body. First, the in-built cycle of growth and decay sets a life-span for all cells and organisms. The etymological explanation of the Sanskrit word for body in Āyurveda is "that which perishes". Part of the process of decay is a decreasingly efficient metabolism and the consequent reduction of nutrients to all tissues. This leads to frailty. Secondly, the body is always contending with the force of gravity which tends to compact whatever is above into what is below. This produces rigidity and stiffness. Another major factor is a life-style in which walking barefoot or with footwear that does not constrict the toes, sitting on the floor and squatting do not feature. There is no occasion for regularly stretching with a long reach or for bending low. This seriously erodes natural physical abilities, as is expressed by the adage, "Use it or lose it". Other reasons for less-than-optimum physical functioning are illness, accidents, recurrent stresses, traumas and inappropriate or inadequate diet.

Care and respect for the body as the vehicle by means of which we live our life and fulfil our desires is taught by both Yoga and Āyurveda. This is why Āyurveda enjoins a daily regimen which includes exercise, and why Yoga includes *āsana,* posture or postures, as one of its eight aspects. Physical discipline is seen as necessary both for health and as a step towards understanding and controlling the mind. In fact, the practice of postures can improve the performance of the body, maintain it at its peak for a long time and retard the ageing process. And as with the body, so with the mind.

The postures (*āsanas*) are effective for the following reasons:

CIRCULATION

The postures involve stretching, flexing, rotating and gripping the joints and muscles while the limbs, trunk and head are held in different directions – forward, backward, laterally and upside-down. This huge range of actions systematically improves the circulation of blood to all parts of the body. The blood vessels are exercised regularly. They contract in upright poses, an anti-gravitational action, and expand in inverted poses in harmony with gravity. They rest in supine and prone poses where there is negligible gravitational force. Thus the tissues are constantly replenished with nutrients and degeneration is prevented. Well-nourished tissues work efficiently and new cells which replace dead ones are of a high quality. They preserve the vigour of youth.

RESISTING GRAVITY

In the postures, emphasis is given to lengthening muscles and creating space in the joints by stretching. Extension should occur before any other action. In this way the compression and contraction of the skeleto-muscular system as well as of the organs is reversed. Inverted poses where the feet are higher than the head also powerfully counteract the effect of gravity on the body. Extensions and inversions help to maintain body height and chest expansion. This in turn maintains and then improves lung capacity. Plentiful reserves of oxygen and therefore energy are the boon of youth.

HEALTHY MOVEMENTS

Repeated practice of the postures makes the body regain and retain flexibility and steadiness. In old age the loss of independence and dignity because of the inability to perform everyday tasks is much feared. When there is minimum loss of movement that fear is replaced by the confidence of youth.

BREATHING

The multiplicity of postures matches the complexity of the body and helps to maintain the health of all its parts. Similarly there are different *prāṇāyāmas* through whose techniques the various states and moods of the mind can be controlled. Depression, dullness, poor concentration, emotional agitation and excess can be replaced by cheerfulness, intellectual vigour, focus and mental balance. Initially the capacity for *prāṇāyāma* is small; with time the lungs become more elastic and practice can be sustained for longer periods. This builds up good reserves of energy over time and prevents the shrinking of the rib cage and enfeebled lungs characteristic of old age. Instead, it preserves youthful lungs and a youthful mind.

OTHER FACTORS

The postures can bring about improvement in physical health and mobility even when there is debility as a result of illness, injury or faulty nutrition. In these cases the personal guidance of an experienced teacher is advisable, as the programme should be carefully designed to meet individual need. Dietary advice is also the province of specialists. Āyurveda has much to say regarding the relationship between diet and health. It classifies foods as wholesome or unwholesome and as suitable or unsuitable for a person's constitution and for particular seasons and climates. This principle of suitability with respect to constitution, health, age and life situation applies equally to Yoga practice. All these factors should be taken into account in order to derive the maximum benefit from it. Yoga practice should be a happy and satisfying time alone spent on self-improvement and self-exploration. In this way it becomes a harmonizing force in oneself and a support in times of stress.

The Feet and Legs

The Feet

The feet are the base of the body, designed to take its weight. The toes, heels and arches bear the body in its upright stance. Any misalignment, contraction or misplacement of weight, such as dropped arches, squashed toes or elevated heels, destroys the alignment of the body. As a result, the delicate balance of the skeleton, musculature, organs and systemic conduits is disturbed. Other parts compensate for the part which is not doing its job properly. For example, when the weight is placed on the toes instead of the heels, the body leans forward and the front of the body – the shins, knee-caps, front thighs (quadriceps) abdomen, front ribs, throat, face and eyes – take the load. The strain may be imperceptible, but little by little postural imbalance can lead to full-blown problems.

The Legs

The legs are the pillars which hold the body up. Unlike solid pillars, however, they are articulated for movement. Therefore the ankles, shanks, knees and thighs must individually have tremendous upward force to counteract the force of gravity. Time, poor deportment, injuries and lack of exercise all contribute to the waning of this upward energy. When the support weakens, the structure above it is threatened with collapse. Without strong legs the trunk and the organs housed in it become compressed and invite disease.

The Knees

The knee is the principal joint of the leg, enabling it to bend and straighten. When the leg is straight, the knee-cap acts like a cap or seal to hold the upper and lower legs firmly in line. In bending, the joint must flex evenly and deeply so that the two halves of the leg fold back on each other. When the shin and thigh are not in the same plane the knee has to rotate. When the knee is unable to straighten completely, to bend completely or to rotate to its proper degree, degeneration sets in and mobility is impaired.

The Ankles

The ankles act as grippers which support the legs at the bottom. If the ankles are lax or collapse, the legs lack a strong base from which to lift or stretch upwards.

HOW THE *ĀSANAS* WORK

This programme consists mainly of standing poses. In Āyurvedic terms it increases *kapha* and *pitta* and balances *vāta*. The balancing of *vāta* continues as the programme ends with resting poses: the inversion of the legs and relaxation.

Standing Poses (*kapha* +, *pitta* +, *vāta* =)

Standing poses train the feet and legs to regain alignment, strength, upward lift and sensitivity. As no part of the body functions in isolation from the rest, in so doing they are helped by strong extensions of the trunk and arms. They also restore firmness to the knees.

Sitting Poses (*kapha* +, *pitta* +, *vāta* =)

Sitting poses train the knees to regain their full flexion.

Inverted Poses (*kapha* –, *pitta* +, *vāta* =)

Inverted poses rest the legs.

Relaxation (*kapha* +, *pitta* –, *vāta* =)

Apart from giving rest, relaxation gives time for the retraining of muscles and joints to be assimilated.

PROPS

Wall, ledge, mat, brick, bolster, blanket

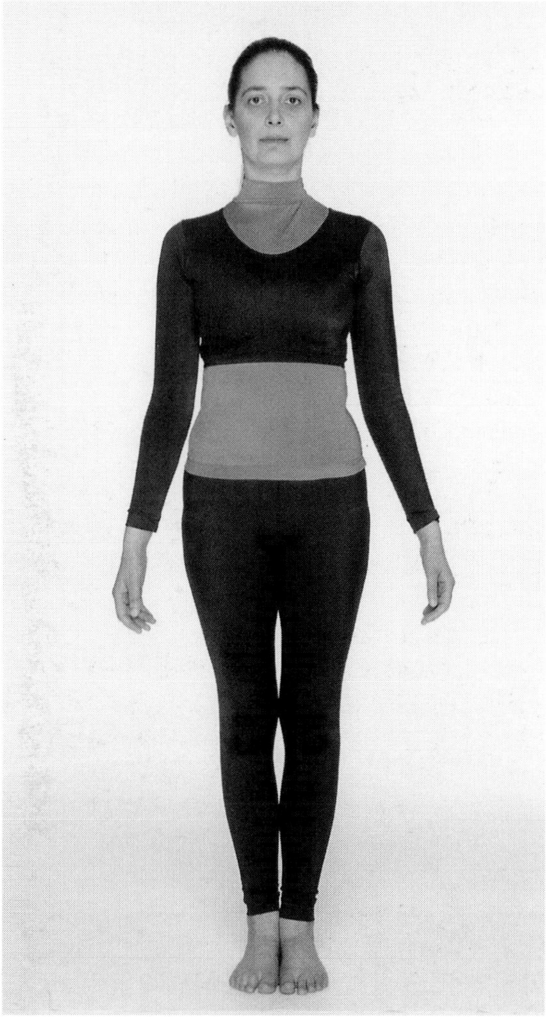

ताडासन

Tāḍāsana Palm Tree Pose

tāḍa = Palmyra palm tree; āsana = posture

Method

Stand against the wall with the feet together, the big toes, ankles and heels touching.

Stretch the soles of the feet and the toes. Tighten the knee-caps and pull the thigh muscles (quadriceps) strongly up. Then stretch the legs up from the ankles. Tighten the buttocks and stretch the trunk up against the wall. Press the shoulders to the wall. Let the arms and hands hang naturally. Stretch the sides of the neck and lift the base of the skull. Rest the back of the head against the wall.

While activating the various muscles do not tense the face or abdomen. Draw the whole body towards the wall, so that the plumb-line of its weight falls along the back of the head, the back of the trunk, the backs of the legs and the heels. Maintain the relaxation of the face, eyes and throat. Breathe normally.

Stay for 30 seconds to 1 minute.

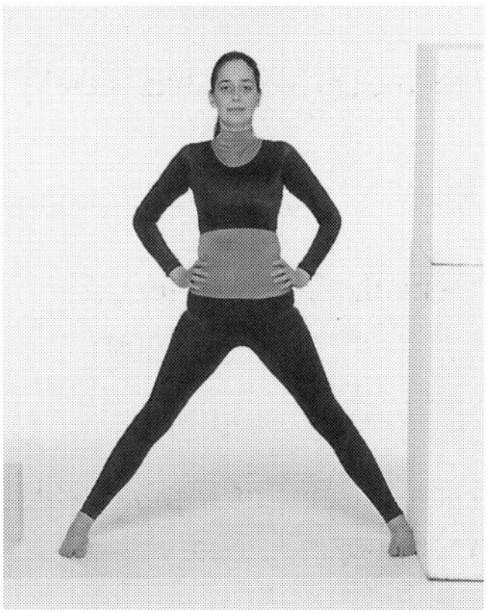

1

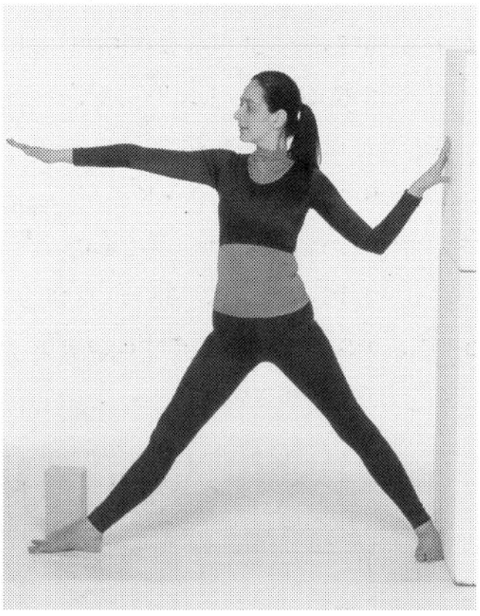

2

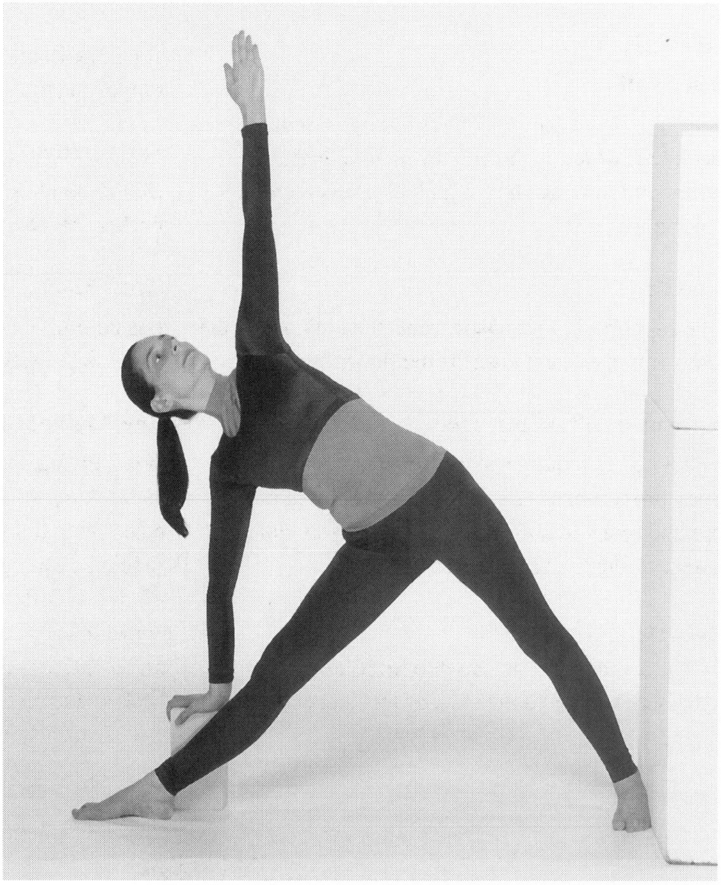

3

त्रिकोणासन

Trikoṇāsana Triangle Pose

trikoṇa = triangle

Method

Stand in *Tāḍāsana* with the left side facing the wall. Spread the legs 3½ to 4 feet apart and place the outer edge of the left foot against the wall. Align the feet so that the toes are level. Stretch the legs and trunk up. Place the hands on the hips (1).

Turn the right foot 90° out and align the heel with the left instep. In turning the foot revolve the leg also: the shin, knee and femur (thigh bone). With the help of the buttock turn the femur in the socket; grip the muscles at the outer top thigh to keep the bone in its turned position. Press the outer left foot into the corner and rotate the left leg outwards towards the wall. Keep both knees firm. Raise the arms, extending the right to shoulder level and placing the fingertips of the left hand on the wall for support. Turn the head to the right (2).

Exhale and go sideways down to the right, resting the hand on the brick placed beside the right outer foot. Raise the left arm up, with the palm facing forwards and fingers together. Keep both arms straight. Revolve the trunk upwards. Turn the head and look up [at the right thumb]. Keep the face relaxed and breathe normally (3).

Stay for 20–30 seconds. Inhale and come up. Turn the feet to the front, exhale and bring them together. Repeat on the left side.

NOTES

The Wall

The support of the wall gives strength to the back leg, which is the anchor in all standing poses and in relation to which all movements are made.

The Brick

The support of the brick prevents the collapse of the trunk into itself and towards the floor.

Measurement of Distance

The postures require a subjective understanding of body proportions. The distance in feet cited in the method refers to human feet; a tall person will spread wider than a short person.

For Knee Pain

Do the standing poses with the front foot raised against the wall and the back of the heel extended along the floor. This lifts the ankle and shin, thereby supporting the knee.

For Sciatica

Do the standing poses with the front foot turned further than 90°.

Repetition

It is helpful to repeat each standing pose twice. This ingrains the actions in the body.

The Arch of the Foot

When the supports of an arch are close together, the arch is high. When the supports are far from each other, the arch is low. For a high instep, the weight should be carried close to the arch. To achieve this, lift the foot off the floor, stretch it forward and reposition it, placing the weight on the back of the ball of the foot near the arch. Then lift the heel, stretch it back and replace it, standing on the front of the heel.

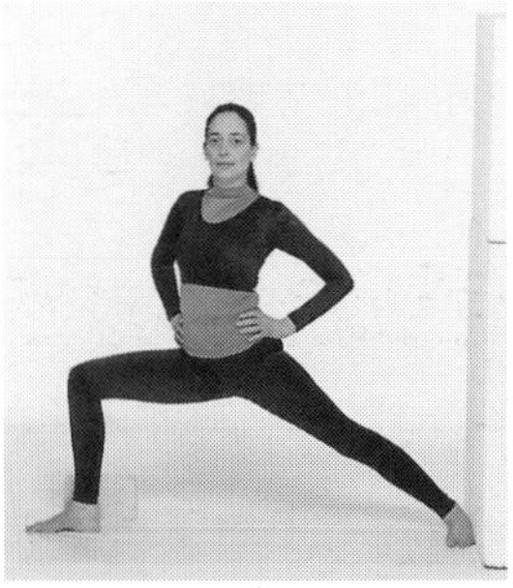

1

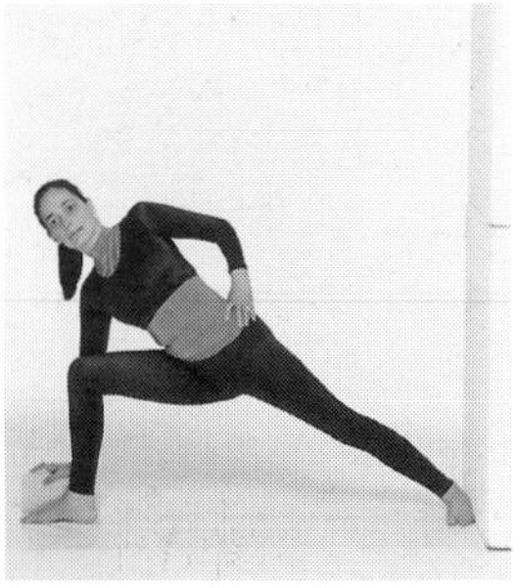

2

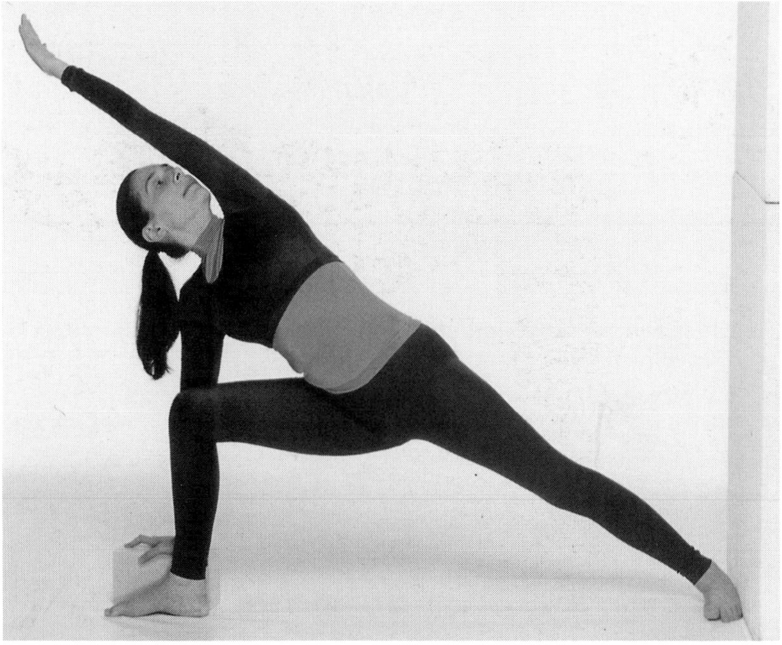

3

पार्श्वकोणासन

Pārśvakoṇāsana Lateral Angle Pose

pārśva = side; koṇa = angle; āsana = posture

Method

Stand in *Tāḍāsana* with the left side facing the wall. Spread the legs 4 to 4½ feet apart and place the outer left foot against the wall. Align the feet so that the toes are level. Stretch the legs and trunk up. Place the hands on the hips.

Turn the right foot 90° out and align the heel with the left instep. In turning the foot revolve the whole leg as in *Trikoṇāsana*. Turn the buttock strongly. Grip the muscles at the outer top thigh to keep the femur in and well turned. Keeping the back leg firm and turning towards the left, bend the right leg to form a right-angle with the shin perpendicular and thigh parallel to the floor. Control the bend by holding firm at the socket; do not put weight or strain on the knee (1).

Exhale and go sideways down, placing the right hand on the brick beside the foot (2).

Extend the left arm over the head in line with the ear, with the palm facing down and fingers together. Turn the head and look up, as if through the arm. Revolve the trunk upwards. Pressing the outer edge of the left foot down, stretch the whole left side of the body right up to the fingertips. Breathe normally and keep the face relaxed (3).

Stay for 20–30 seconds. Inhale and come up. Turn the feet to the front, exhale and bring them together. Repeat on the left side.

Note

The Right-Angle Bend

The vertical and horizontal stretches meet in the knee joint, which remains spacious and tension-free. To achieve this, place the weight on the heel, rotate the ankle in a little to hold the shin firmly and lift the shin and calf, and hold the femur head firmly in the socket and extend the thigh towards the knee.

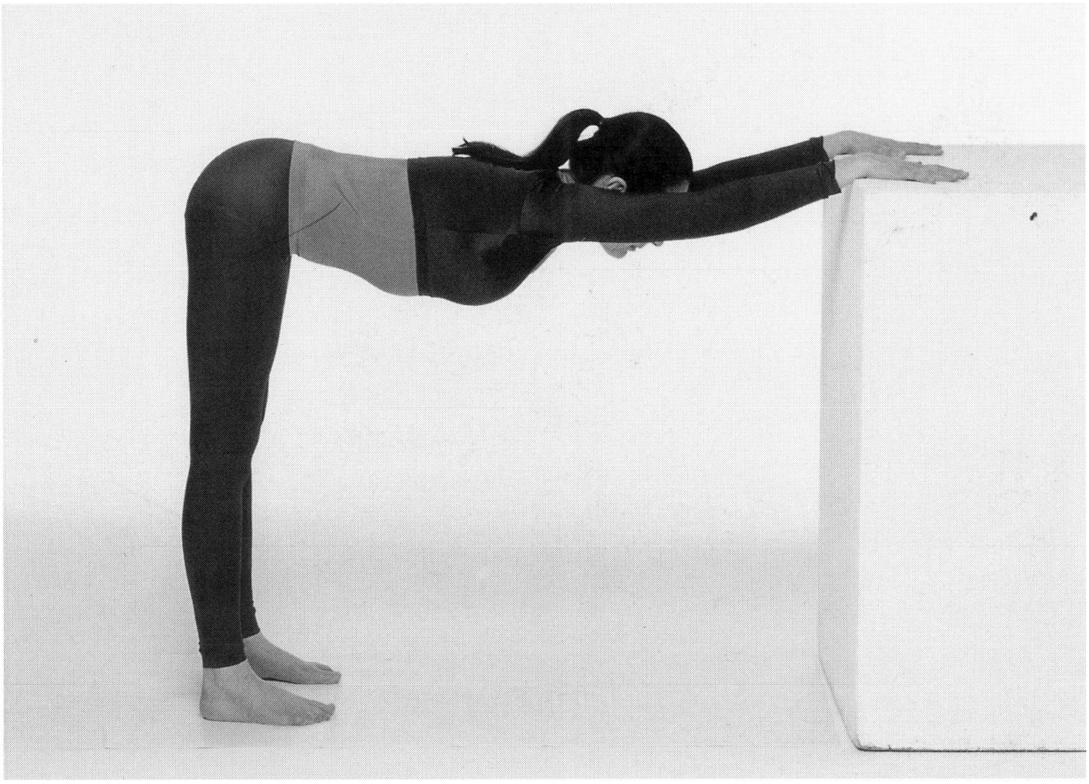

अर्ध-उत्तानासन

Ardha-Uttānāsana Half Stretching Pose

ardha = half; uttāna = stretching

Method

Stand in *Tāḍāsana* near a ledge of hip height. Take the feet one foot apart. Bend forward from the hips and place the hands on the ledge, palms facing down and fingers stretched. Keep the legs vertical, with the hips above the ankles, and stretch them strongly up. Keeping the tops of the thighs back, stretch the trunk and arms forward. Keep the head level.

Stay for 20–30 seconds. Inhale and come up.

Note

The Vertical Straight Leg

In the straight leg the two halves act as one limb. The shin bone (tibia) and the thigh bone (femur) align vertically, held in place by the knee joint. They then bear the weight of the body correctly and effortlessly. To achieve the unity and vertical axis of the leg: (a) keep the weight on the heel, (b) tighten the kneecap and press it back, at the same time stretching the back of the knee, (c) pull up the quadriceps and lift the shin, and (d) press the front thigh towards the back thigh and the shin towards the calf. Do these actions smoothly, without jerking. There should be no strain on the knee.

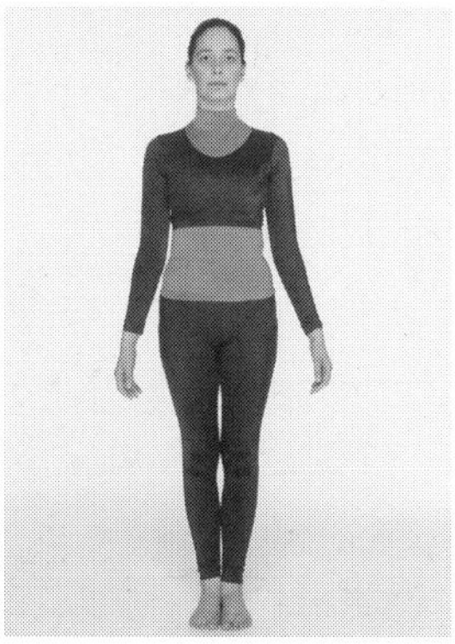

1

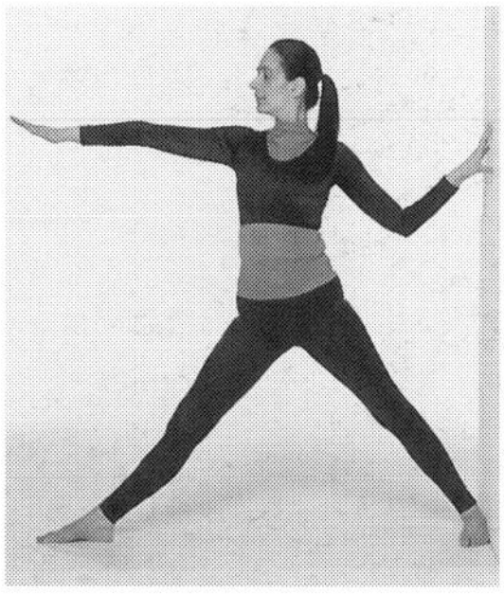

2

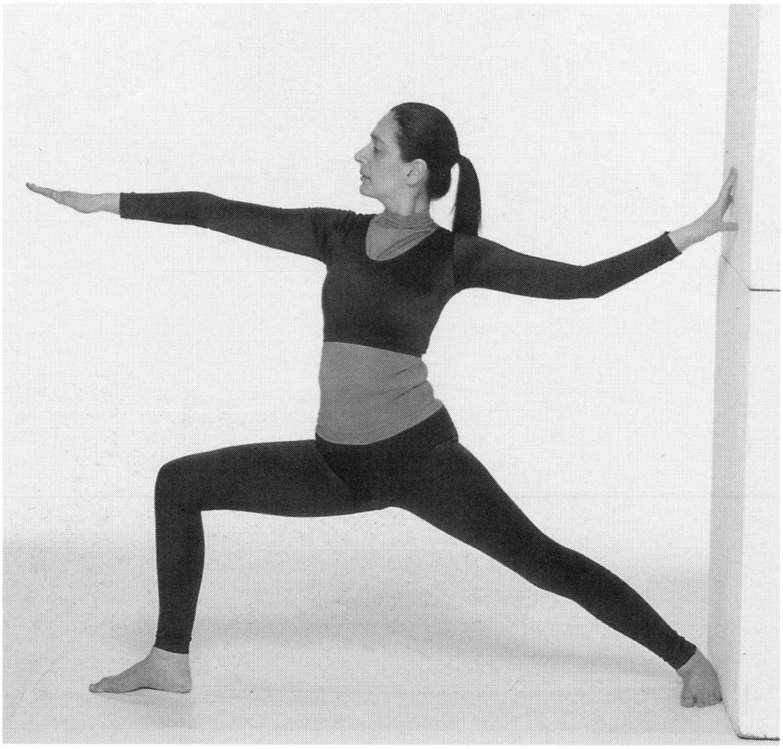

3

वीरभद्रासन २

Vīrabhadrāsana II Warrior Pose II

Vīrabhadra = name of a warrior, attendant of the god Śiva

Method

Stand in *Tāḍāsana* (1) with the left side facing the wall. Spread the legs 4 to 4½ feet apart and place the outer edge of the left foot against the wall. Align the feet. Press the outer edges of the feet down and revolve the legs away from each other. Stretch the legs and trunk up.

Turn the right foot 90° out and align the heel with the left instep. Lift the arches of the feet. Turn the whole leg together with the foot. Keep the femur head deep within the socket. Keep the knees firm and thigh muscles pulled up. Raise the arms, extending the right to shoulder level with the palm facing down and fingers together. Place the fingertips of the left hand on the wall. Turn the head to the right (2).

Exhale and, keeping the back leg firm, bend the right leg to a right-angle as in *Pārśvakoṇāsana*. Bend the leg from the hip, not the knee. With the help of the left fingertips pressing against the wall keep the trunk upright and centred between the legs. Gaze to the right with the eyes level. Breathe evenly (3).

Stay for 20–30 seconds. Inhale and come up. Turn the feet to the front, exhale and bring them together. Repeat on the left side.

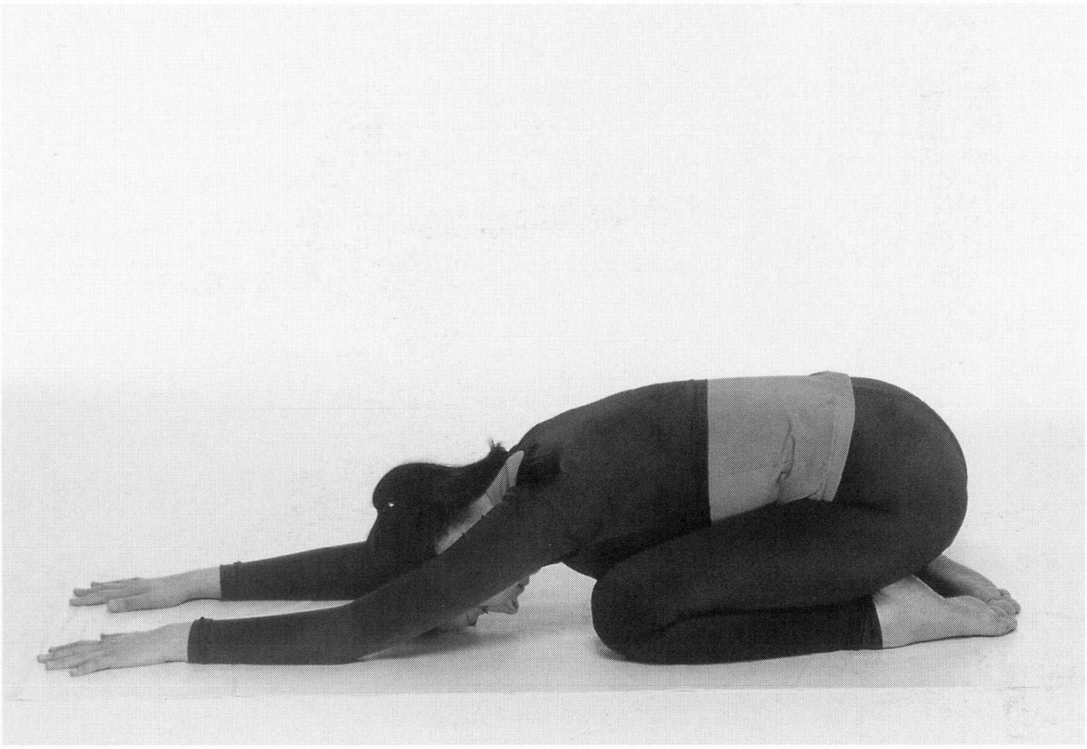

अधोमुख-वीरासन

Adhomukha-Vīrāsana Hero Pose with Head Down

adho = downwards; mukha = face, mouth; vīra = hero

Method

Kneel and bend forward with the feet together and the knees apart. Take the arms forward and rest the head on the floor. Do not widen the knees too much, just enough for the trunk to touch the legs.

If the buttocks do not rest on the heels, place a folded blanket, cushion or bolster on the heels so that the hips can act as a ballast for the stretch of the trunk and arms. If the head does not reach the floor, support it.

Stay for 20–30 seconds. Inhale and come up.

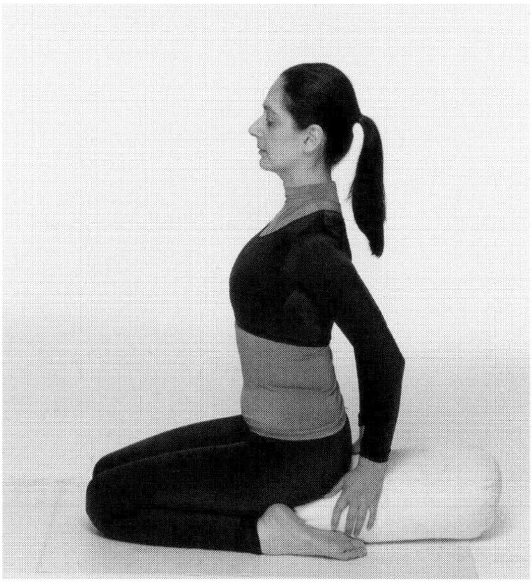

1

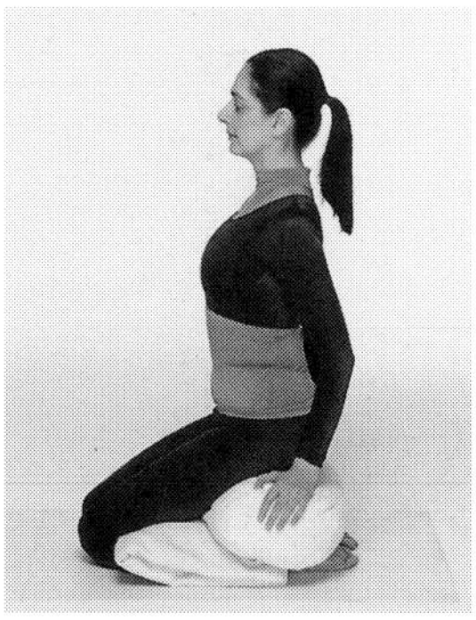

2

वीरासन

Vīrāsana Hero Pose

vīra = hero

Method

Sit on the heels. Then take the feet further apart and sit between them, placing a support (bolster or folded blankets) under the buttocks. If the thighs or calves feel tight increase the height of the support. Place the hands beside the hips and sit straight. Stretch the trunk up, lift the chest and take the shoulders back (1).

Stay for 30 seconds to 1 minute. Straighten the legs gently. With practice it will be possible to stay longer.

Note

Knee Flexion and Knee Pain

Because of the range of movement of the hip joint, the leg is able to flex outward, backward and upward in one plane, and inward in two planes, as in the lotus pose (*Padmāsana*). To fold efficiently, completely and without distortion (a) the inner and outer knee tendons should bend simultaneously to the same degree, (b) the flesh at the back of the knee should be smoothed into the joint, as into a corner, and (c) the median lines of the calf and thigh should align against each other. To re-train the knee and reduce stiffness and compression, it is helpful to place a pad at the back of the joint (a thinly folded blanket or small towel or bandage). The knee should feel relaxed and spacious (2).

Ankle Pain

Roll a blanket or towel and place it under the ankles for support. Alternatively, place the feet on a bolster, with the toes hanging free.

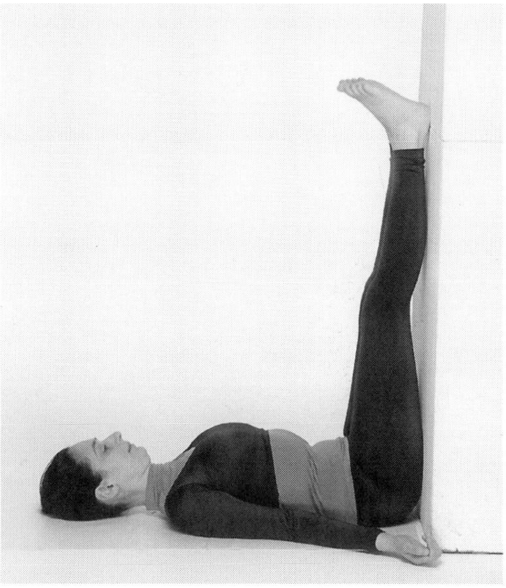

ऊर्ध्व-प्रसारित-पादासन

Ūrdhva-Prasārita-Pādāsana Upward Extended-Leg Pose

ūrdhva = upwards; *prasārita* = spread out; *pāda* = foot, leg

Method

Sit sideways near the wall with the knees bent. Bring the buttocks close to the wall. Lie back and straighten the legs up against the wall. They should be supported from buttocks to heels. Relax the arms beside the body, palms facing up. Relax the legs. Support the head with a blanket if it tilts backwards.

Stay for 1 to 5 minutes. Bend the knees, slide backwards away from the wall, turn to the side and get up.

Note
Stiffness
When the lower back is stiff and the hamstrings are tight, it may not be possible to touch the buttocks to the wall; with practice the joints and muscles become more limber.

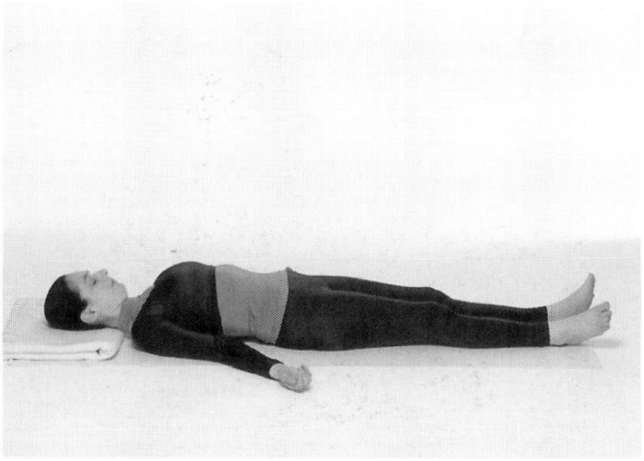

शवासन

Śavāsana Corpse Pose

śava = corpse

Method

Lie on the back in a straight line, with a folded blanket under the head and neck. Keep the head straight. Stretch the arms and legs away from the trunk, then let them relax. Let the legs and feet drop to the sides. Turn the palms to face up. Press the shoulders down and move the shoulder-blades into the body so that the chest lifts. Close the eyes and relax. Breathe softly, without strain. Feel the front of the body resting on the back of the body. Breathe softly.

Stay for 5 minutes or longer. Open the eyes, bend the knees, turn to the side and get up.

The Hips and Pelvis

The Hips

The hips are the upper part of the thighs at the joint with the pelvis. The hip joints control the direction, speed and quality of movement of the legs. As they bear the weight of the trunk, they tend to become compressed and the femurs become misaligned within the socket. The hip joint (at the outer thigh) acts together with the groin (at the inner thigh). When it is stiff the groin is hard; when it becomes supple, the groin softens. The misalignment of the hip joint – a degree of dislocation – has repercussions both for the legs and for the pelvic organs.

The Pelvis

The pelvis is the bony girdle containing the base of the spine and the hip crests. When it is upright the abdomen and pelvic organs are supported by the back. When the body tilts forward the organs lose that support. Instead of being relaxed they become compressed and are forced to bear weight. Sustained strain in the pelvis leads to all sorts of health difficulties.

HOW THE *ĀSANAS* WORK

This programme begins with a twist which increases *pitta* and *vāta* and continues with standing poses and leg stretches which increase *kapha* and *pitta* and bring *vāta* into balance. It ends with inverted poses which enhance *pitta* and bring calmness to *vāta*. *Vāta* is pacified completely in relaxation.

Standing Poses (*kapha* +, *pitta* +, *vāta* =)

In standing poses the spread of the legs, the rotation of the femur in the socket, the turn of the hips and the gripping of the muscles at the joint increase the mobility and firmness of the hip joints.

Leg Extensions (*kapha* +, *pitta* +, *vāta* =)

In addition to the above, strain is removed from the abdominal organs. This is because the pelvis is kept in one plane, vertically or horizontally, and the body weight is carried by the back. Similarly, the widening from one hip crest to the other creates space in the abdominal cavity, encouraging healthy circulation.

Twists (*kapha* –, *pitta* +, *vāta* +)

The rotation of the trunk from its base increases the flexibility of the hip joints, as in standing poses.

Inverted Poses (*kapha* –, *pitta* +, *vāta* =)

The topsy-turvy position of the trunk gives relief from the gravitational weight of the body on the hips. The upward stretch of the legs elongates the hip joints.

Relaxation (*kapha* +, *pitta* –, *vāta* =)

Lying flat on the floor with the limbs extended and relaxed rests the hips and the pelvic organs.

Props

Wall, ledge, stool or chair, mat, blanket, belt

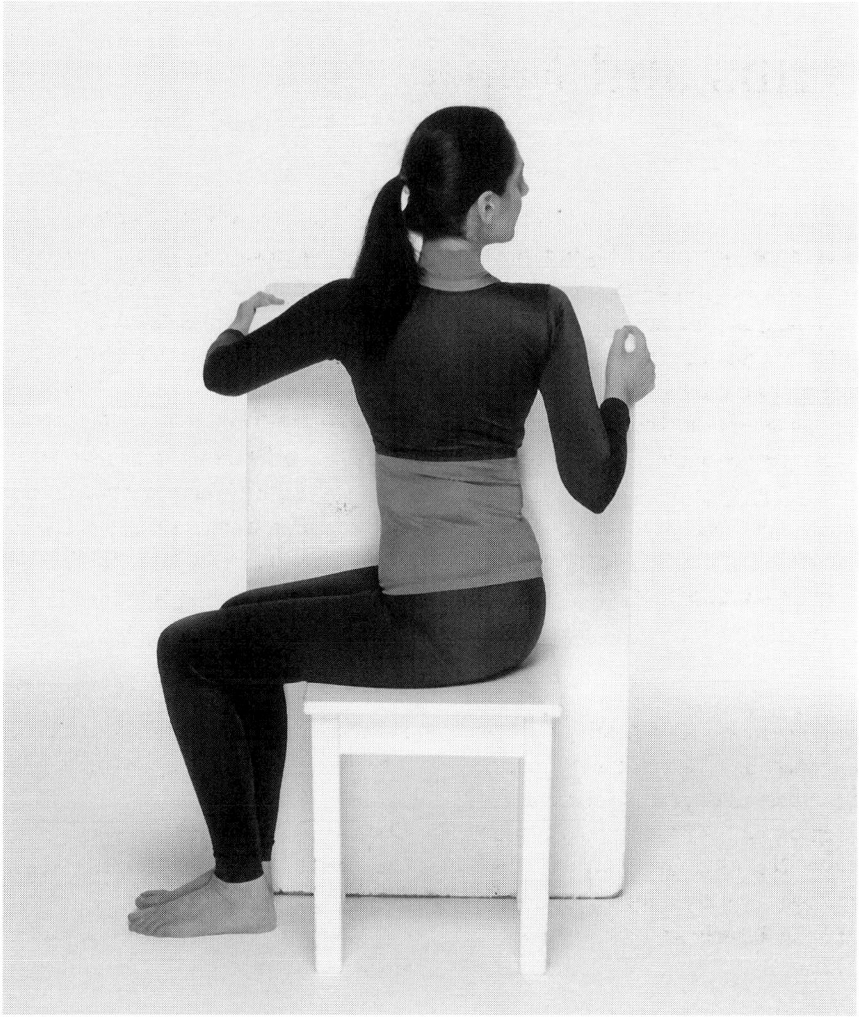

थरद्वाजासन

Bharadvājāsana Bharadvāja's Pose (on chair)

Bharadvāja = name of a sage

Method

Place a stool or chair against a wall or solid piece of furniture, preferably with a ledge. Sit sideways on the stool, with the right hip and thigh against the wall. Stretch the trunk up, lift the chest and turn towards the wall. Hold the ledge and use the hands to turn the trunk more. Start the turn from the hips, then turn the waist, rib cage and shoulders. Turn the head to the right.

Stay for 20–30 seconds. Repeat on the left.

Note

Improvising props

If the feet do not reach the floor, place a solid object underneath them.

To improvise a ledge, use a solid piece of furniture, the corners of an alcove, a door frame, banisters, etc. Otherwise use a flat wall.

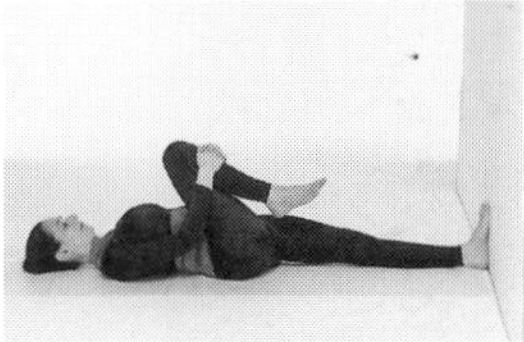

1

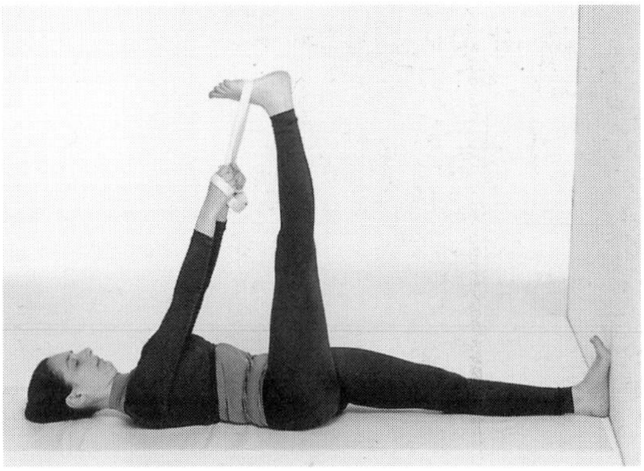

2

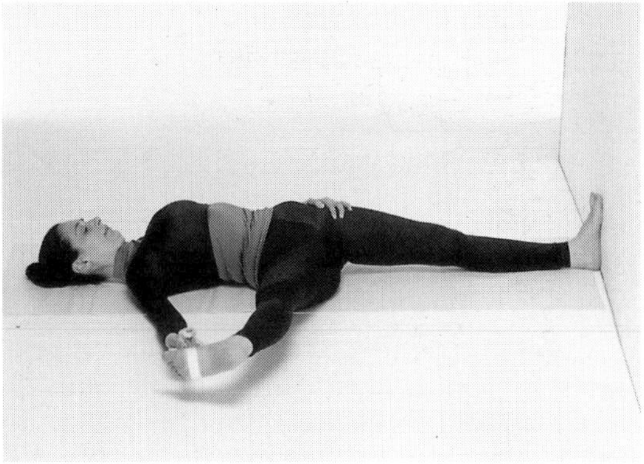

3

सुप्त-पादङ्गुष्ठासन १, २

Supta-Pādāṅguṣṭhāsana I & II Supine Thumb-to-Foot Pose I & II

supta = supine, lying; pāda = foot; aṅguṣṭha = thumb or big toe

Method

I Lie down in a straight line with the feet against the wall. Bend the knees a little and move nearer to the wall, lengthening the lower back away from the waist. Then straighten the legs by pressing them carefully down towards the floor. Do not jerk the knees.

Exhale and bend the right knee over the abdomen; hold the shin and press it down (1). Put a belt round the foot and hold the two ends separately with the two hands. Keep the shoulders down and the chest lifted.

Inhale and raise the leg to vertical, without contracting the hip towards the waist. Straighten the leg by tightening the knee cap and pressing the thigh and shin back. Stretch the foot up against the belt. Press the left foot into the wall and the leg down towards the floor (2).

Stay for 20 to 30 seconds. Exhale, bend the leg and bring it down. Repeat on the left.

II Follow the method above for *Supta-Pādāṅguṣṭhāsana* I (paras 1–3). Hold both ends of the belt with the right hand. Press the left thigh or hold the mat with the left hand. Revolve the right leg outwards in the socket. Exhale and take it down to the right. Do not rest it on the floor. Keep the kneecap tight and the thigh and shin pressed back. Stretch the foot. Control the right leg by the firm downward action of the left and its contact with the wall (3).

Stay for 20 to 30 seconds. Inhale and raise the leg. Exhale, bend it and bring it down. Repeat on the left.

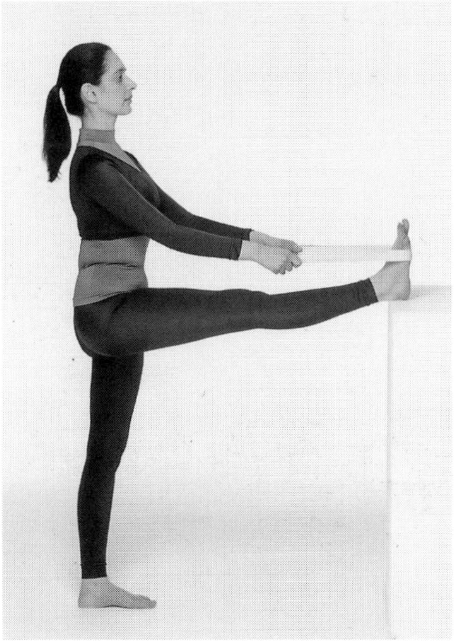

1

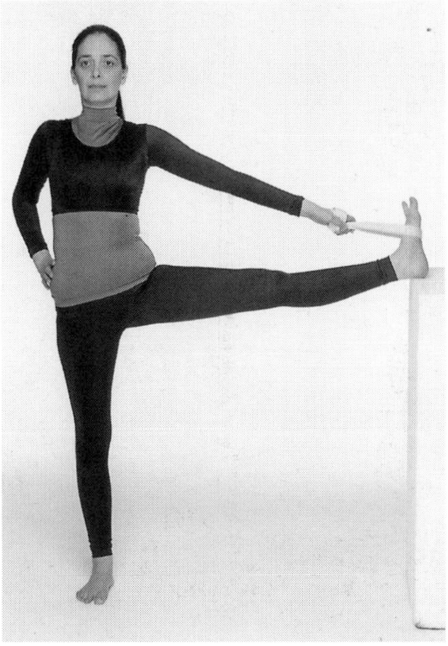

2

उत्थित-पादाङ्गुष्ठासन १, २

Utthita-Pādāṅguṣṭhāsana I & II Upright Thumb-to-Foot Pose I & II

utthita = standing up, upright

Method

I Stand in *Tāḍāsana* facing a ledge, about 3 to 4 feet away from it. Inhale, bend the right leg and place the heel on the ledge. Do not rest the Achilles tendon on it, otherwise the heel and leg cannot stretch. Place a belt round the foot and hold the ends separately with both hands. Keep the left leg perpendicular to the ground. Straighten both the legs. Press the right one down and stretch it from buttock to heel. Press the left one back and stretch it from ankle to buttock. Make sure the left foot is still facing forward. Stretch the trunk up, lift the chest and take the shoulders back (1).

Stay for 20 to 30 seconds. Exhale, bend the leg and bring it down. Repeat on the left.

II Stand in *Tāḍāsana* with the right side facing the ledge, 3 to 4 feet away from it. Inhale, bend the right leg, turn it outwards in the socket and place the heel on the ledge in line with the hip. Do not rest the Achilles tendon on the ledge. Place a belt round the foot and hold it with the right hand. Place the left hand on the hip. Straighten both the legs. Keep the left leg vertical. Press the right one down and stretch it from buttock to heel. Press the left one back and stretch it from ankle to buttock. Keep the trunk upright. Stretch it up, lift the chest and take the shoulders back (2).

Stay for 20 to 30 seconds. Exhale, bend the leg and bring it down. Repeat on the left.

Note
Stability
In both of these poses the foot that is against the wall or on the floor has to remain firm. The vertical leg in standing and the horizontal leg in lying down give the stability against which the other leg moves.

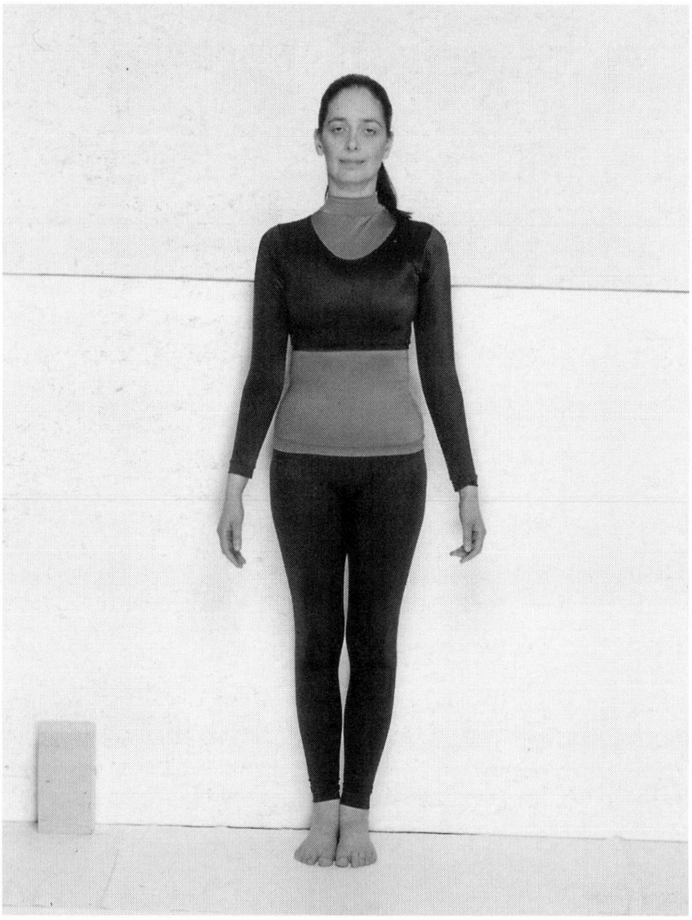

ताडासन

Tāḍāsana Palm Tree Pose

tāḍa = Palmyra palm tree

Method

Stand against the wall with the feet together, the big toes, ankles and heels touching. Stretch the soles of the feet and the toes. Tighten the knee-caps and pull the thigh muscles (quadriceps) strongly up. Then stretch the legs up from the ankles. Tighten the buttocks and stretch the trunk up against the wall. Press the shoulders towards it. Let the arms and hands hang naturally. Stretch the sides of the neck and lift the base of the skull. Rest the back of the head against the wall.

While activating the various muscles do not tense the face or abdomen. Draw the whole body towards the wall, so that the plumb-line of its weight falls along the back of the head, the back of the trunk, the backs of the legs and the heels. Maintain the relaxation of the face, eyes and throat. Breathe normally.

Stay for 30 seconds to 1 minute.

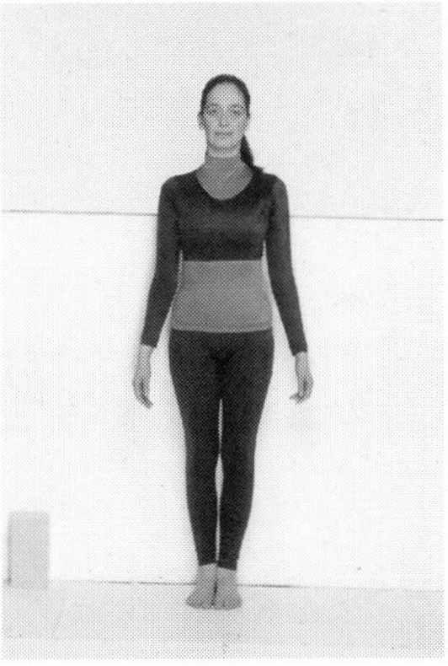

1

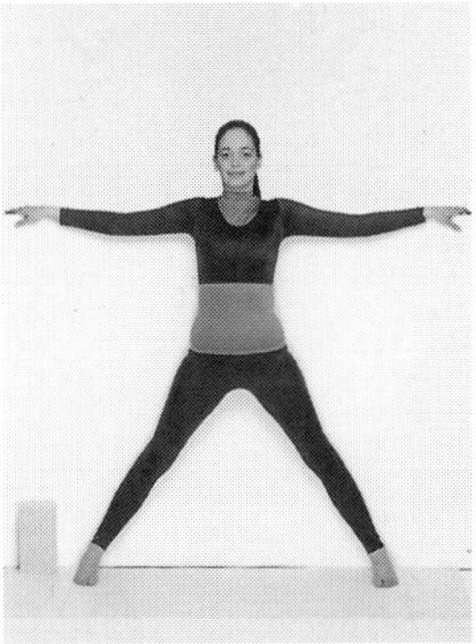

2

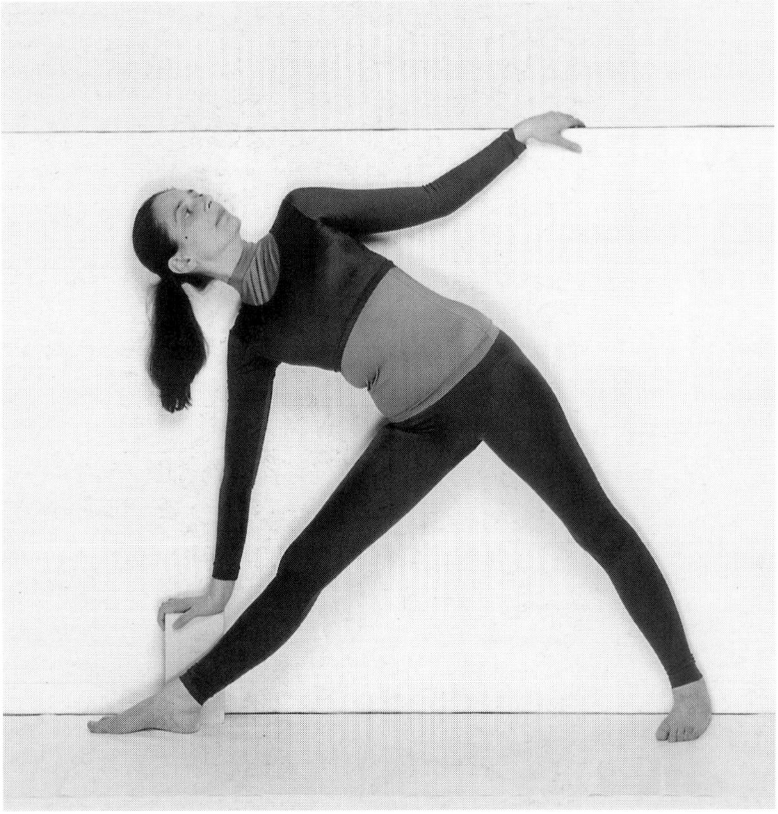

3

त्रिकोणासन

Trikoṇāsana Triangle Pose

trikoṇa = triangle

Method

Stand in *Tāḍāsana* against a wall with a ledge (1).

Take the feet 3½ to 4 feet apart. Raise the arms to shoulder level, holding the ledge if possible. Stretch the legs and trunk up (2).

Turn the left foot in a little (15°), at the same time revolving the leg outwards. Turn the right foot 90° out, at the same time revolving the whole leg. Line up the right heel with the left instep. The right hip and left heel should be against the wall, the right foot away from it. Exhale and go sideways down to the right, bending from the hip joint. Place the right hand on a brick beside the outer foot. Hold the ledge with the left hand and revolve the trunk upwards and towards the wall. Press the left thigh towards the wall. Turn the head, resting it on the wall, and look up. Breathe normally and relax the face (3).

Stay for 20 to 30 seconds. Inhale and come up. Repeat on the left.

Note

The Wall

The wall support gives a sense of direction: instead of leaning forward the various parts of the body are pulled back into the vertical plane.

The Ledge

The ledge helps to give leverage for the lift and turn of the pelvis.

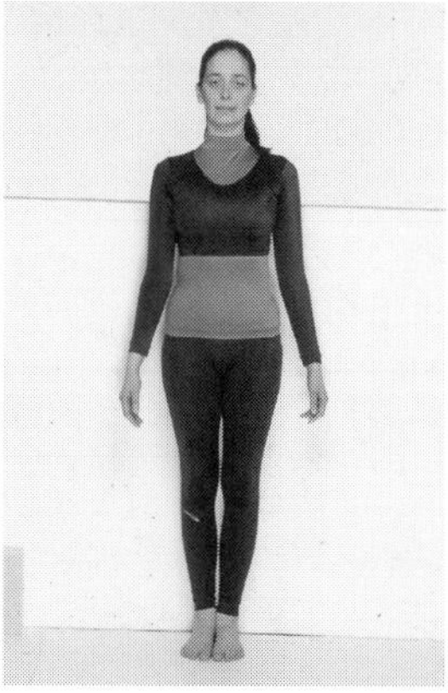
1

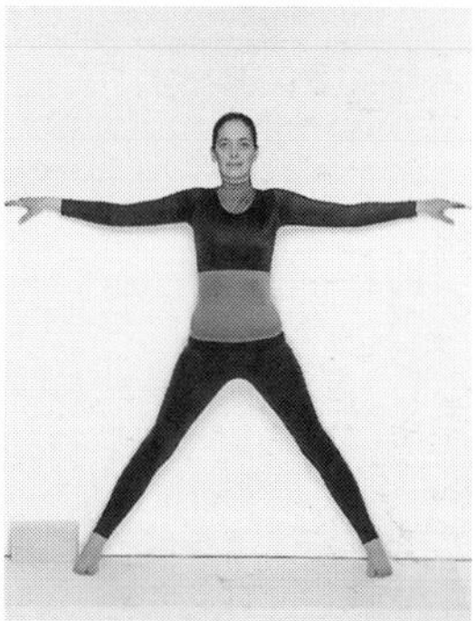
2

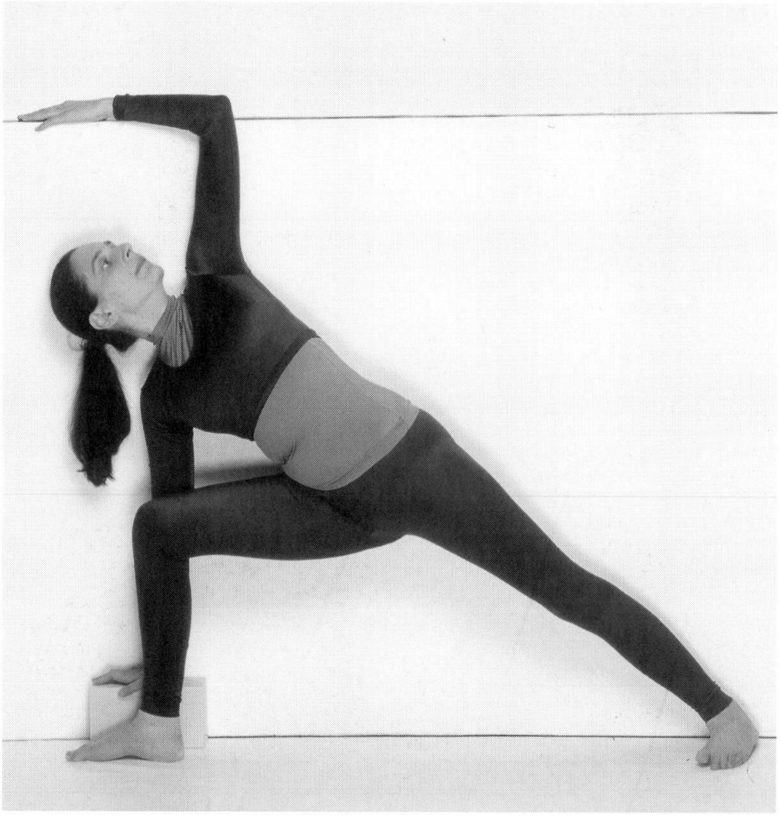
3

पार्श्वकोणासन

Pārśvakoṇāsana Lateral-angle Pose

Method

Stand in *Tāḍāsana* against a wall with a ledge (1).

Take the feet 4 to 4½ feet apart. Raise the arms to shoulder level, holding the ledge if possible. Stretch the legs and trunk up (2).

Turn the left foot in a little (15°), at the same time revolving the leg outwards. Turn the right foot 90° out, at the same time revolving the whole leg. Line up the right heel with the left instep. The right hip and left heel should be against the wall, the right foot a little away from it.

Exhale, bend the right leg to a square and go sideways down to the right, placing the right hand on a brick beside the outer foot. Hold the ledge with the left hand and revolve the hip and trunk upwards and towards the wall. Press the right knee and left thigh towards the wall. Turn the head and look up. Rest the head against the wall. Breathe quietly and remain relaxed (3).

Stay for 20 to 30 seconds. Inhale and come up. Repeat on the left.

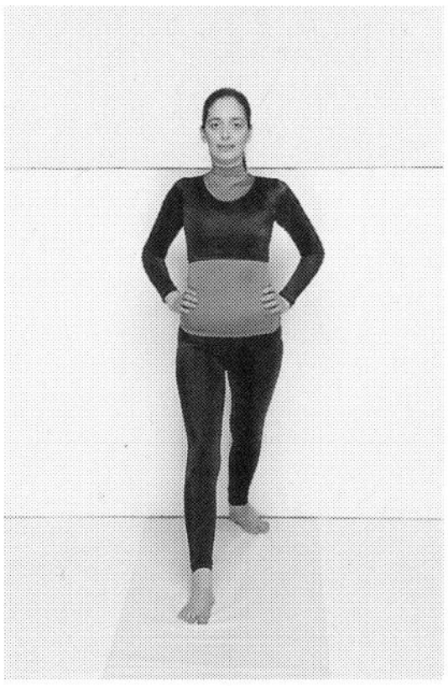

1

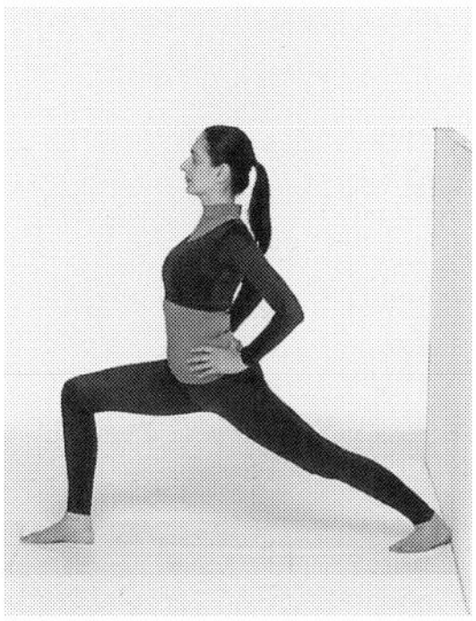

2

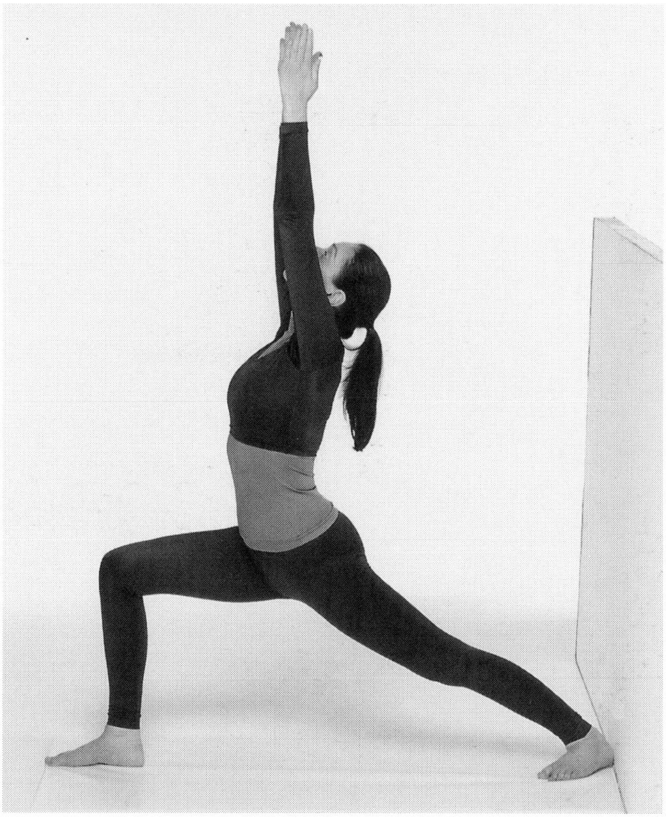

3

वीरथद्रासन १

Vīrabhadrāsana I Warrior Pose I

Method

Stand with the left side facing the wall. Take the feet 4 to 4½ feet apart and place the left foot against the wall. Then turn the left foot deep in (45 to 60°) so that only the heel is against the wall; in doing so turn the leg in also. Turn the right foot 90° out. Align the right heel and left arch. Turn the trunk 90°, to face the same way as the feet. Place the hands on the hips and turn the hips further to make them parallel (1).

Exhale and bend the right leg to a right angle. Keep the muscles at the socket gripped in and move the knee outwards. Press the left heel strongly down and lift the inner leg. Keep the trunk vertical (2).

Inhale and raise the arms, with the elbows straight. Keep the palms facing each other and the fingers stretching. Moving the thoracic spine in, take the head back and look up at the ceiling. Do not hold the breath. Do not strain the eyes and throat (3).

Stay for 20 to 30 seconds. Inhale and come up. Repeat on the left.

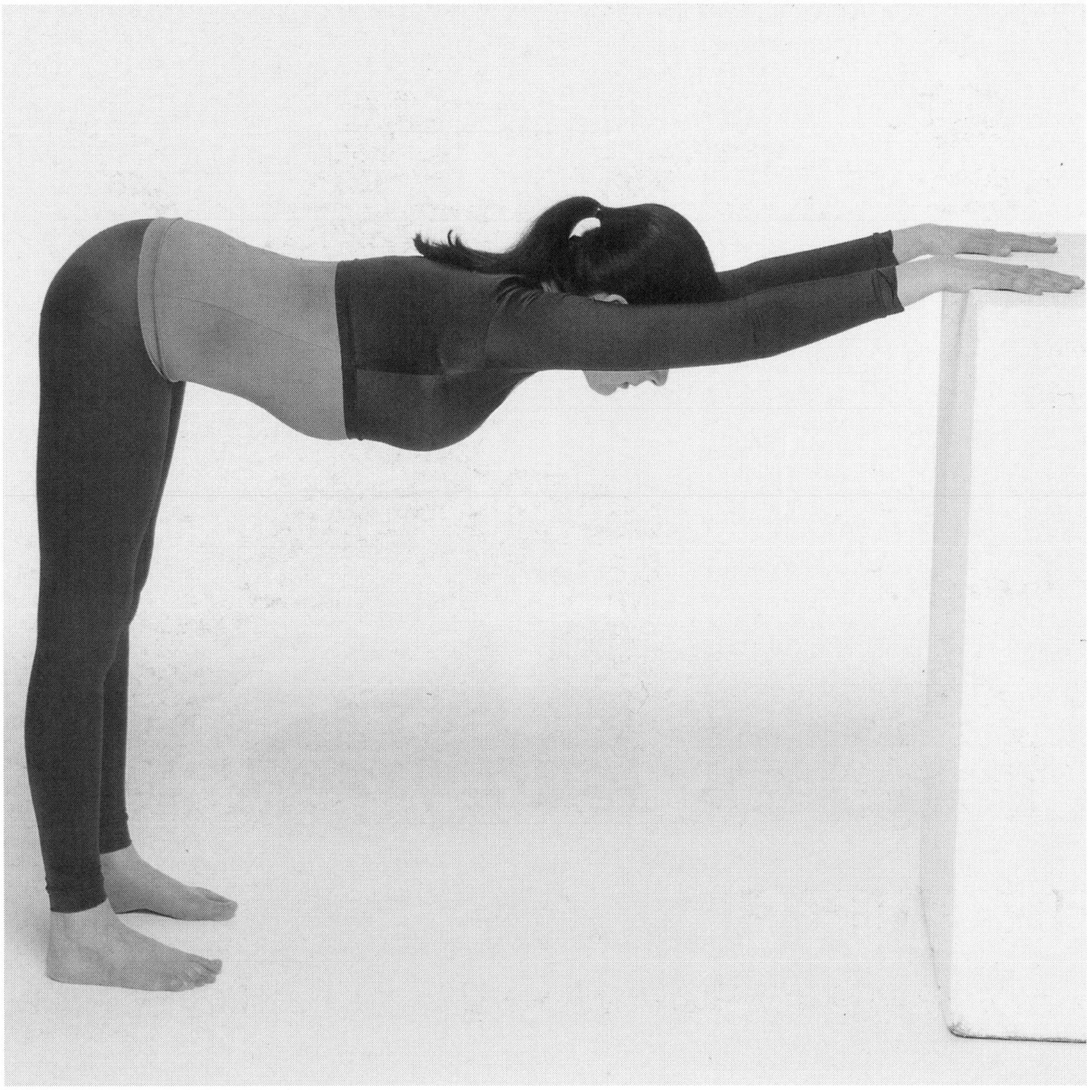

अर्ध-उत्तानासन

Ardha-Uttānāsana Half Stretching Pose

Method

Stand in *Tāḍāsana* 3 to 4 feet from a ledge of hip height. Take the feet one foot apart. Bend forward from the hips and place the hands on the ledge, palms facing down and fingers stretched. Keep the legs vertical with the hips above the ankles and stretch them strongly up. Keeping the tops of the thighs back, stretch the trunk and arms forward.

Stay for 20–30 seconds. Inhale and come up.

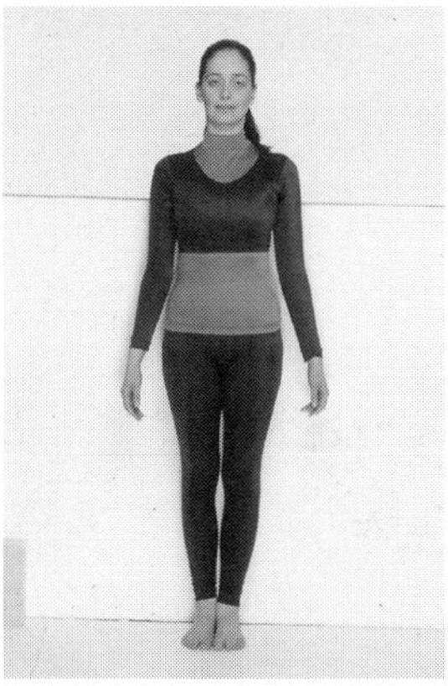
1

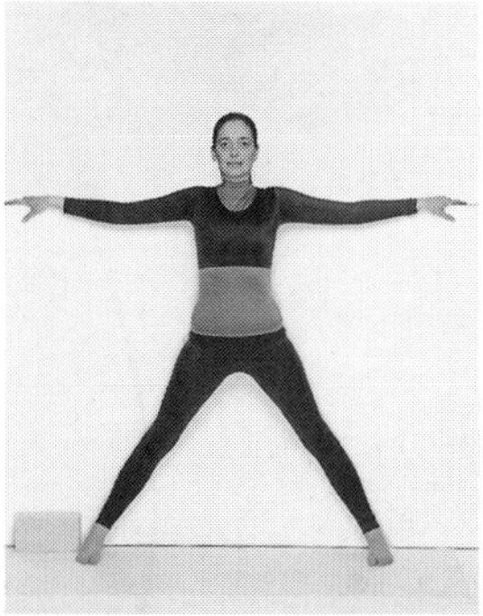
2

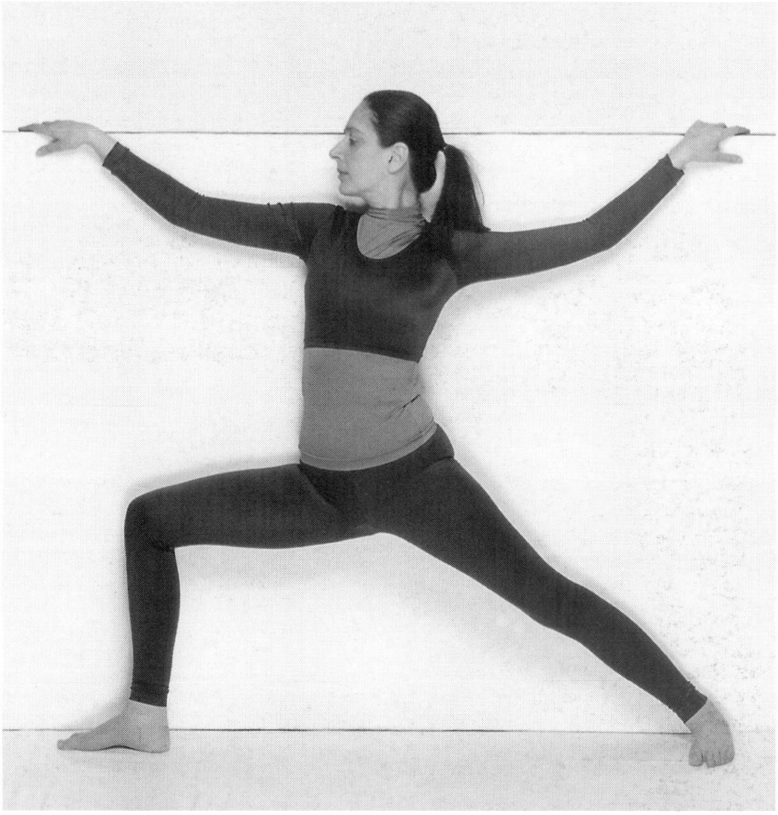
3

वीरथद्रासन २

Vīrabhadrāsana II Warrior Pose II

Method

Stand in *Tāḍāsana* against a wall with a ledge (1).

Take the feet 4 to 4½ feet apart. Stretch the legs and trunk up. Raise the arms to shoulder level and hold the ledge (2).

Turn the left foot slightly in (15°), pressing the outer foot down and revolving the leg outwards. Turn the right foot and leg 90° outwards. Line up the right heel with the left instep. Keep the right hip and left heel against the wall, the right foot a little away from it. Exhale and bend the right leg to a square. Keep the trunk vertical. Press the right knee and left thigh towards the wall. Turn the head to the right, resting it against the wall. Breathe normally. Relax the face (3).

Stay for 20 to 30 seconds. Inhale and come up. Repeat on the left.

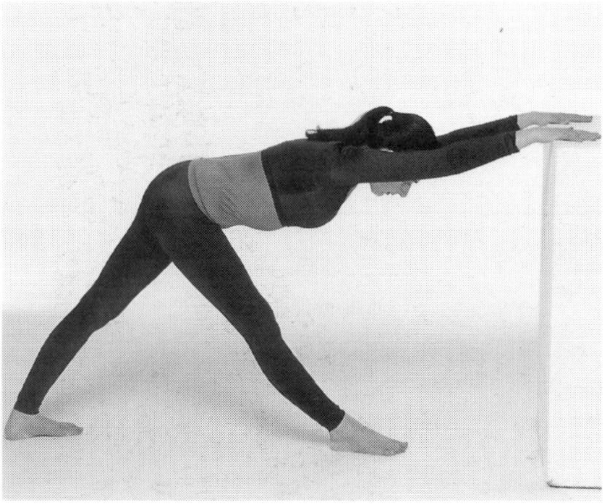

पार्श्वोत्तानासन

Pārśvottānāsana
Sideways Stretching Pose

pārśva = side; uttāna = stretching

Method

Stand with the right side facing a ledge, 2 to 3 feet away from it. Spread the legs 3½ to 4 feet apart. Place the hands on the hips. Turn the left foot deep in (45 to 60°), revolving the leg also. Turn the right foot 90° out. Turn the hips and trunk to face the ledge. Keep the knees tight and leg muscles pulled up. Exhale, bend forward from the hips, keeping them level, and place the hands on the ledge. Stretch the trunk and arms.

Stay for 20 to 30 seconds. Inhale and come up. Repeat on the left.

Later on, bend down further over the right leg. Place the hands on either side of the foot, on the floor or on bricks. Keep the legs straight and the hips level. Relax the head.

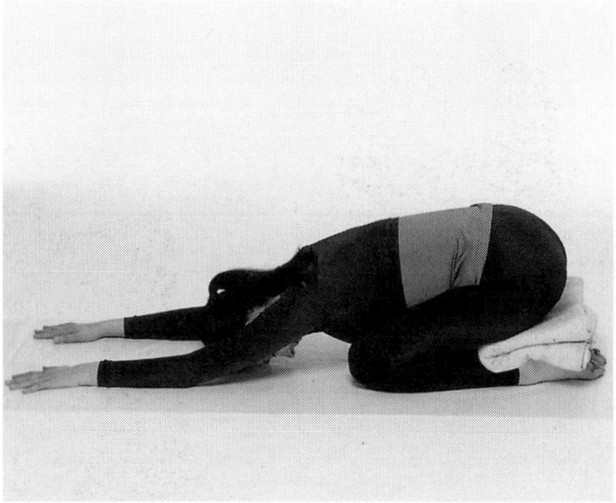

अधोमुख-वीरासन

Adhomukha-Vīrāsana
Hero Pose Face Down

Method

Kneel and bend forward with the heels together and the knees apart with just enough room for the trunk. Take the arms forward and rest the head on the floor. To relieve compression of the hips, place a folded blanket or bolster on the heels. If the head does not reach the floor, support it.

Stay for 20–30 seconds. Inhale and come up.

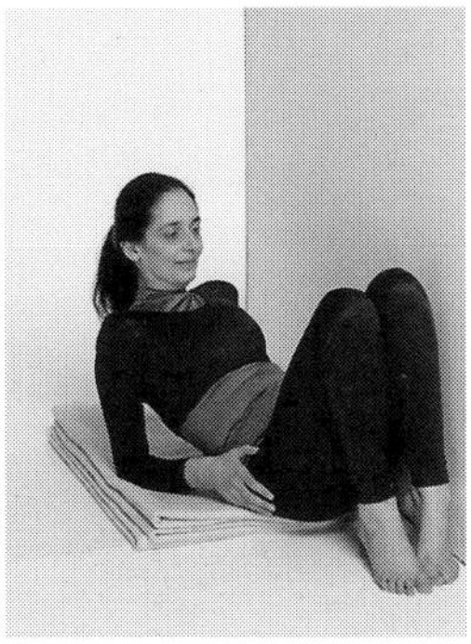
1

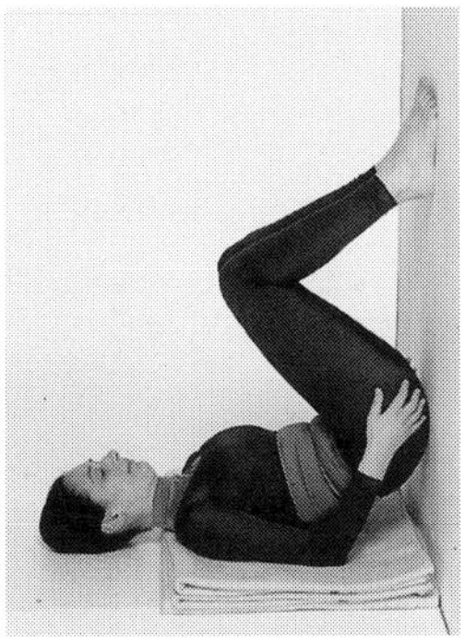
2

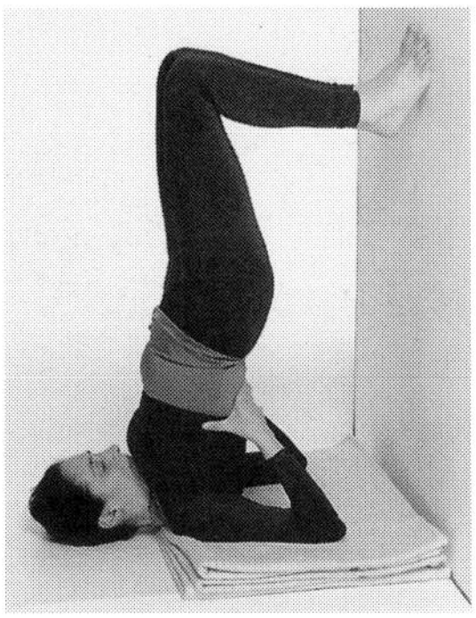
3

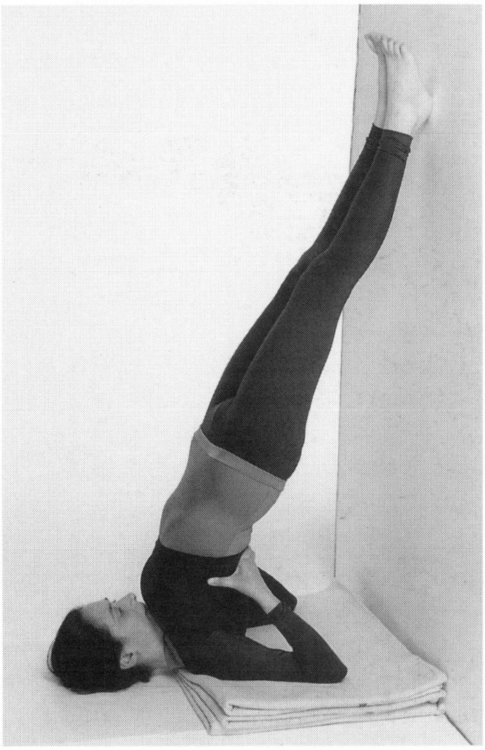
4

सर्वाङ्गासन

Sarvāṅgāsana Shoulder Balance

sarva = all; aṅga = body, limb

Method

Place two or three neatly folded blankets near the wall with the folded edges away from the wall. Lie sideways against the wall, propped up on the elbows and with the knees bent, in preparation for taking the legs up the wall (1).

Swivel the body round so that the shoulders remain on the blankets but the head is on the floor. Lay the trunk flat and take the feet onto the wall. Keep the knees bent. Align the head, trunk and legs. Move the shoulders away from the neck and the shoulder-blades into the body (2).

Exhale, press the feet against the wall and lift the trunk up, immediately supporting the back with the hands. Bring the chest forward (3).

Straighten the legs, keeping the feet against the wall. Bring the elbows in. Continue to move the chest forward (4).

Note

Cautions

Do not do this (or any inverted) pose during menstruation.

There should be no pressure in the head (temples, forehead, eyes, ears) or throat. Pressure may be due to unfamiliarity with the pose or an incorrect position. If the problem persists or is due to a serious condition such as high blood pressure or eye problems, consult a teacher.

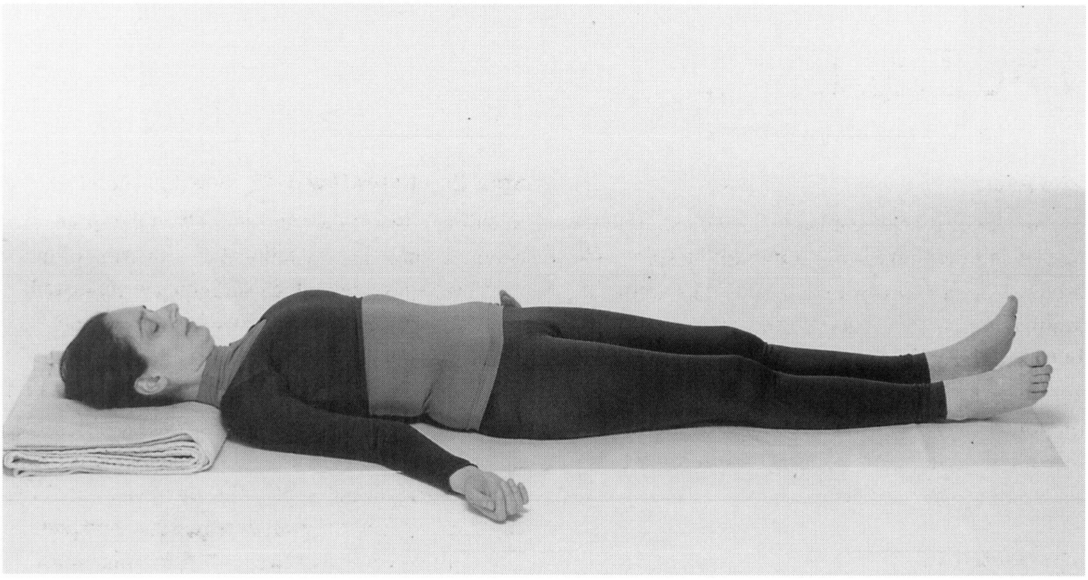

शवासन

Śavāsana Corpse Pose

Method

Lie on the back in a straight line, with a folded blanket under the head and neck. Stretch the arms and legs away from the trunk, then let them relax. Let the legs drop to the sides right from the tops of the thighs. Let the feet drop further to the sides. Press the shoulders down and the shoulder-blades into the body. Keep the chest lifted. Take the arms a little further from the body. Turn the palms to face up and let the hands curl naturally. Close the eyes and completely relax the trunk, limbs and head. Breathe softly, without strain. Feel the space within the body.

Stay for 5 minutes or longer. Keep the mind on the relaxation; do not let it stray. Open the eyes gently, bend the knees and turn to the side. Get up from the side.

The Back

The Back

The back consists of the back ribs and shoulder-blades and the pelvis in addition to the spine. The broad structures protect the spine and support its multifarious movements. As the spine is closely linked to the nervous system the back of the body controls the front of the body. A healthy spine is the fount of youth. Impairment or degeneration of the spinal vertebrae is not only debilitating but risks damage to the nerves.

The Back Ribs

The back ribs hold the spine in place and support the more mobile front ribs which expand during respiration. The support comes from holding the back ribs in a concave position. When they take a convex shape the lungs become compressed.

HOW THE *ĀSANAS* WORK

This programme consists mainly of twists which, increase *pitta* and *vāta*, and standing poses, which increase *pitta* and *kapha*. It is a vigorous programme and therefore ends with a supported inverted pose and relaxation so as to bring *vāta* quietly into balance.

Standing Poses (*kapha* +, *pitta* +, *vāta* =)

Standing poses stretch and strengthen the spine, counteracting the gravitational compression of the vertebrae. In so doing they straighten accentuated curves resulting from age or wear and tear, and restore the natural curves. They relieve backache.

Twists (*kapha* –, *pitta* +, *vāta* +)

In twists the lateral rotation of the spine increases its mobility and blood supply. The altered aspect of the vertebrae to each other relieves pressure and pain. In order to be effective twisting of the spine must always follow extension.

Inverted Poses (*kapha* –, *pitta* +, *vāta* =)

Inverted poses decompress the spine and allow it to rest.

Relaxation (*kapha* +, *pitta* –, *vāta* =)

Relaxation allows the body and mind to return to normal after exertion.

Props

Wall, ledge, table, chair, stool, mat, brick, bolster, blanket.

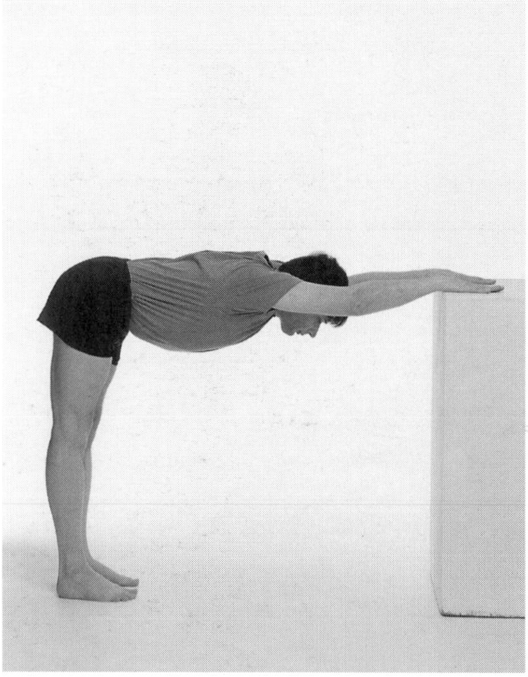

उर्ध-उत्तानासन

Ardha-Uttānāsana
Half Stretching Pose

Method

Stand in *Tāḍāsana* near a ledge of hip height. Take the feet one foot apart or further if the lower back is stiff or painful. Bend forward and place the hands on the ledge, palms facing down and fingers stretched. Keep the legs vertical, with the hips over the ankles. Tighten the knees and pull the thigh muscles strongly up. Press the tops of the thighs back and stretch the trunk and arms forward. The stronger the stretch of the legs, the better the stretch of the trunk. Keep the back of the head in line with the spine.

Stay for 20–30 seconds. Inhale and come up.

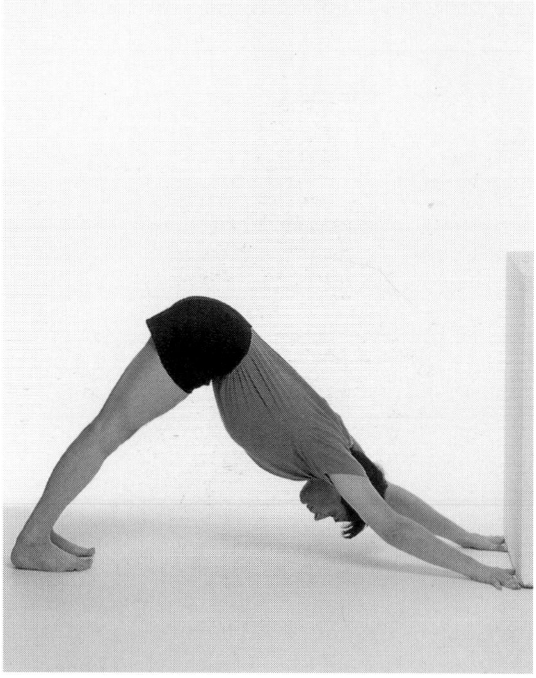

अधोमुरव-श्वासन

Adhomukha-Śvāsana
Dog Pose, Head Down

adho = downwards; mukha = face, mouth; śva(n) = dog

Method

Kneel near the wall, 2 or 3 feet away from it. Place the hands on the floor against it, turning them outwards so that the index fingers and thumbs touch the wall. Place them the same distance apart as the shoulders.

Curl the toes in. Exhale, raise the hips and straighten the legs and arms. Take the feet hip-width apart. Tighten the knees and elbows. Pressing the thumbs and index fingers against the wall, move the arms and trunk towards the legs. At the same time press the legs strongly back. Stretch the arms up and lift the shoulders and hips higher. Relax the head and neck.

Stay for 20–30 seconds. Exhale, bend the knees and go down.

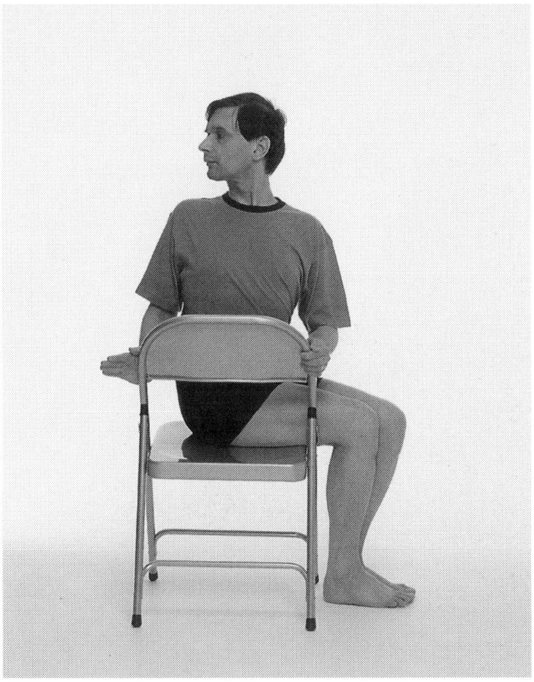

थरद्वाजासन

Bharadvājāsana

Bharadvāja's Pose (on chair)

Method

Sit sideways on a chair, with the right side facing its back. Join the feet. Stretch the trunk up, turn to the right and hold the chair back. Keep the spine vertical. Exhale and turn the hips, waist, rib cage and shoulders. Finally turn the head and neck.

Stay for 20–30 seconds. Inhale and come to the centre. Repeat on the left.

Note

For Backache

Place a brick or book between the thighs and keep the feet apart. This creates space in the lower back and relieves pinching.

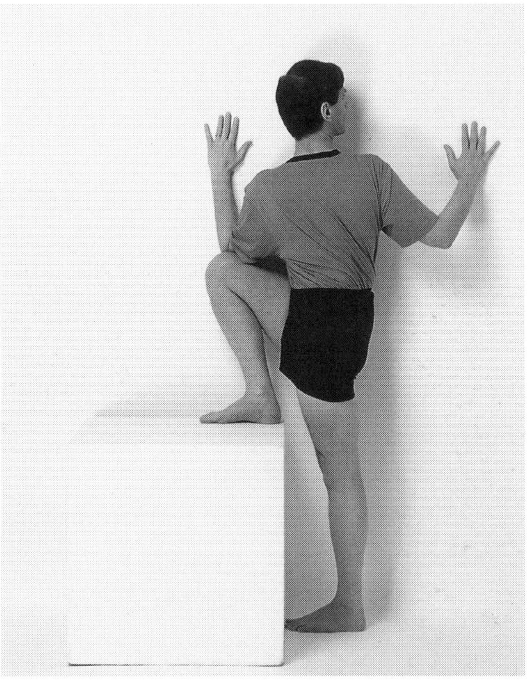

उत्थित-मरीच्यासन

Utthita-Marīcyāsana

Marīci's Pose (standing)

utthita= standing, upright; Marīci = name of a sage

Method

Place a low table or high stool against the wall. Stand in *Tāḍāsana* in front of it with the right side near the wall. Place the right foot on the table. Keep the hip and thigh against the wall. Turn towards the wall. Hook the left elbow behind the right knee and place the hands on the wall. Keep the left leg vertical and the hip drawn in. Exhale and turn the trunk, using the help of the arms. Turn the head and neck.

Stay for 20–30 seconds. Inhale and come to the centre. Repeat on the left.

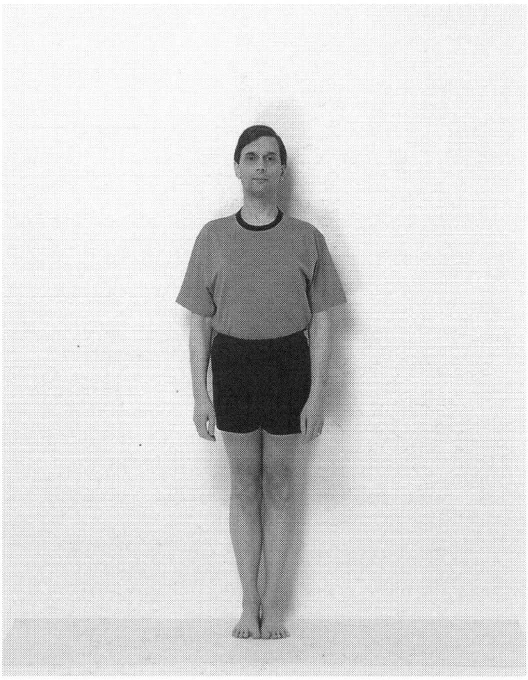

ताडासन

Tāḍāsana Palm Tree Pose

Method

Stand against the wall with the feet together. Keep the heels, ankles and big toes touching. Stretch the soles and the toes. Lift the inner ankles and the arches. Tighten the knee caps and stretch the legs up from the ankles. Pull up the quadriceps strongly. Tighten the buttocks, stretch the trunk up and lift the chest. Lift the sides of the rib cage. Roll the shoulders back towards the wall, move the shoulder blades in and lengthen the arms downwards. Stretch the neck and lift the base of the skull. Balance evenly on the two feet. Breathe quietly.

Stay for 20 to 30 seconds.

> **Note**
> *The Wall*
> The wall supports the back, preventing any strain due to independent movements.

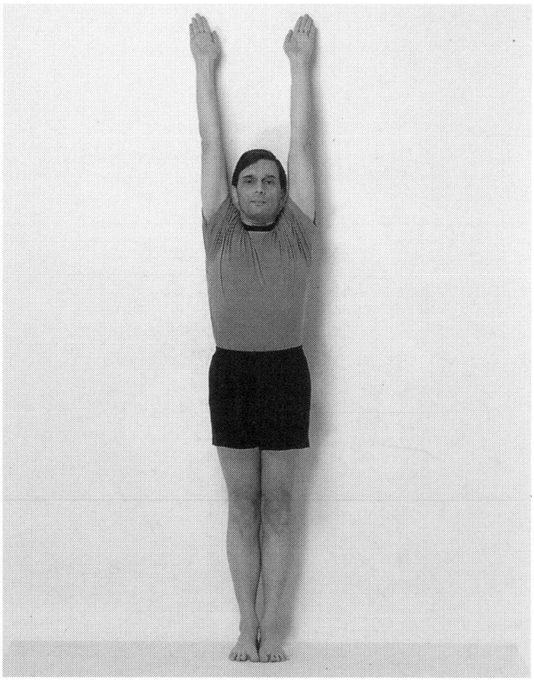

ऊर्ध्वहस्त-ताडासन

Ūrdhvahasta-Tāḍāsana Palm Tree Pose with Arms Up

ūrdhva = upwards; hasta = hand

Method

Stand in *Tāḍāsana* against the wall. Inhale and raise the arms over the head, keeping the elbows tight and fingers together. Rest the backs of the hands against the wall. Stretch from the upper arms to the fingertips. With the help of the arms pull the sides of the trunk up.

Stay for 20 to 30 seconds. Exhale and bring the arms down.

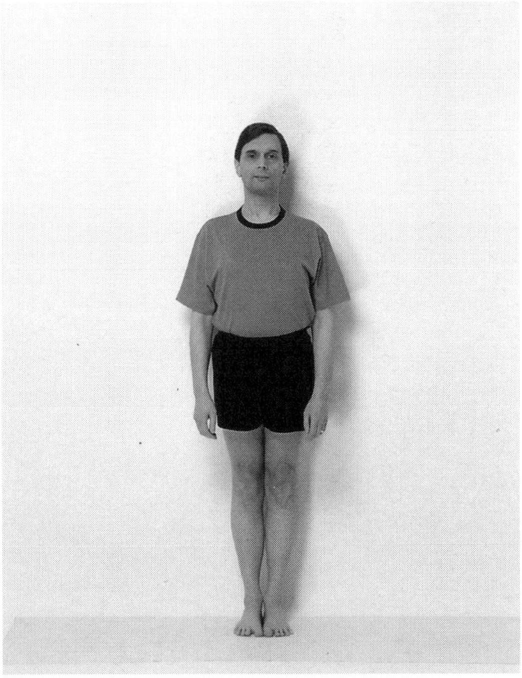

1

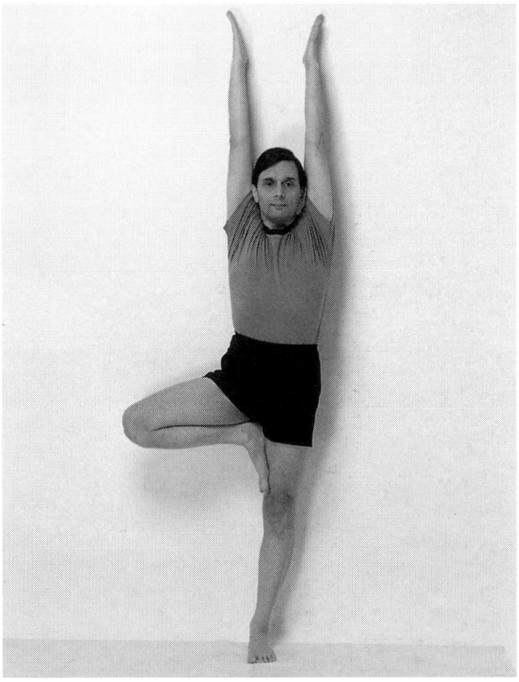

2

वृक्षासन

Vṛkṣāsana Tree Pose

vṛkṣa = tree

Method

Stand in *Tāḍāsana* against the wall (1). Bend the right leg to the side and place the foot at the top of the inner left thigh. Place the heel in the groin. Inhale and stretch the arms up with the palms facing each other. Keep the left leg firm and vertical. Stretch the sides of the trunk. Press the right buttock forward and the right knee back. Move the shoulder-blades in and press the arms towards the wall. Breathe evenly (2).

Stay for 20 to 30 seconds. Exhale and bring the arms and leg down. Repeat on the left.

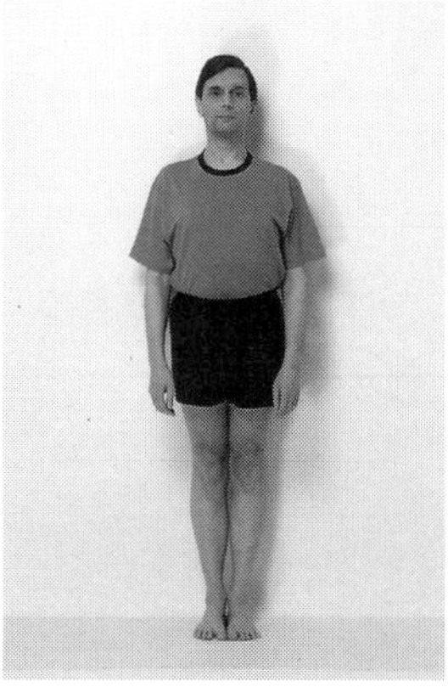
1

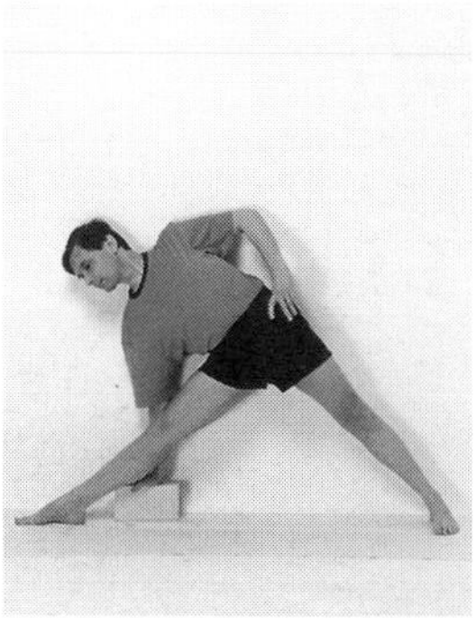
2

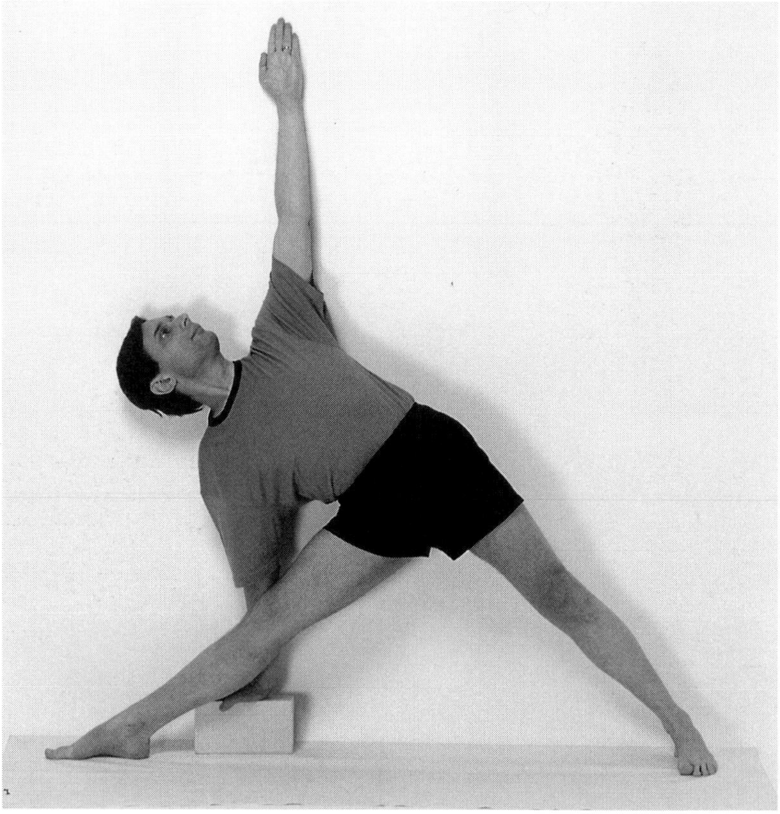
3

त्रिकोणासन

Trikoṇāsana Triangle Pose

Method

Stand in *Tāḍāsana* against the wall (1).

Take the feet 3½ to 4 feet apart. Raise the arms to shoulder level. Stretch the legs and trunk up.

Turn the left foot in a little (15°), at the same time revolving the leg outwards. Turn the right foot and leg 90° out. Align the right heel and left instep. The right hip and left heel should touch the wall. Exhale and go sideways down to the right, placing the right hand on a brick beside the outer foot. Placing the left hand on the hip crest, pull the hip back towards the wall (2).

Stretch the left arm up against the wall, palm facing forward. Lift the trunk and revolve it upwards towards the wall. Press the left thigh towards the wall. Rest the head on the wall and look up. Keep the face and breathing relaxed (3).

Stay for 20 to 30 seconds. Inhale and come up. Repeat on the left.

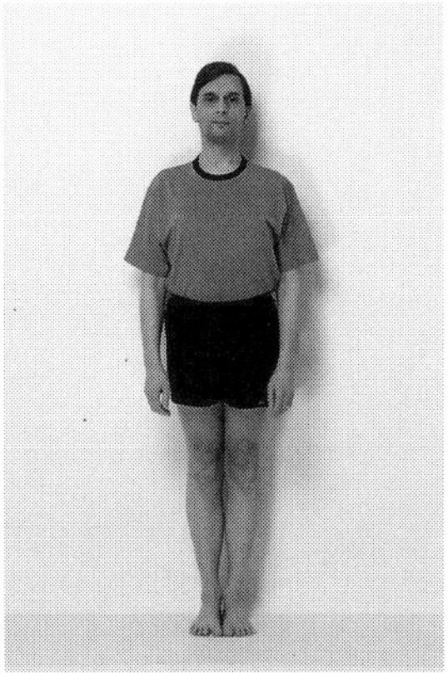
1

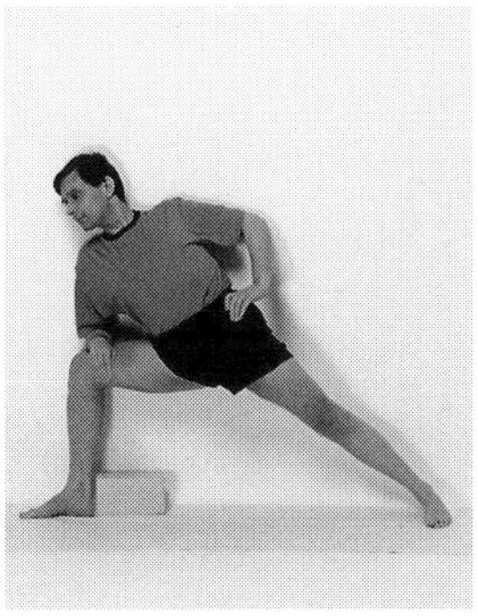
2

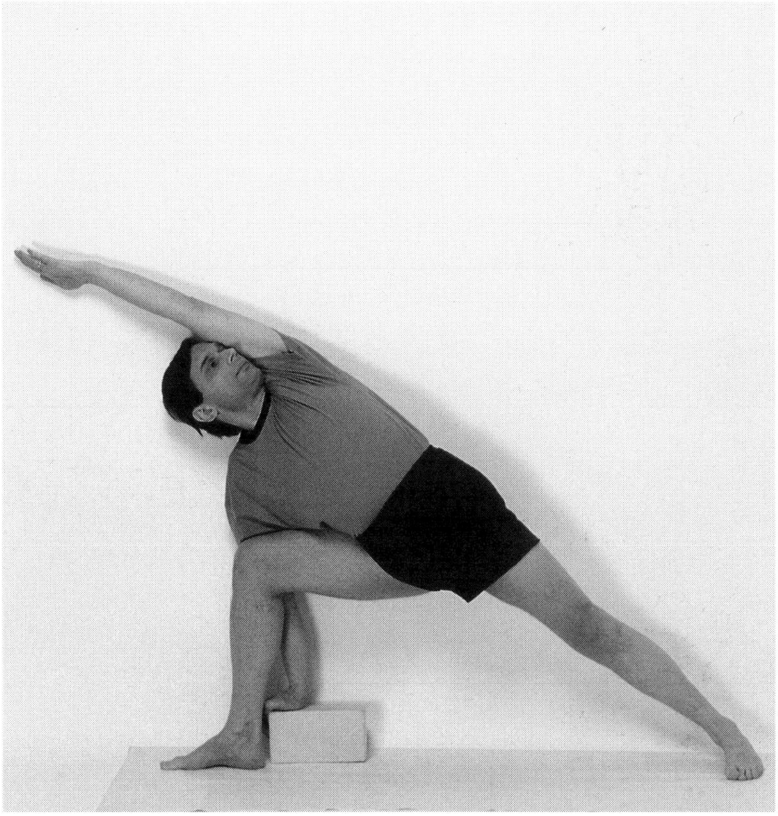
3

पर्श्वकोणासन

Pārśvakoṇāsana Lateral Angle Pose

Method

Stand in *Tāḍāsana* against a wall (1).

Take the feet 4 to 4½ feet apart. Raise the arms to shoulder level. Stretch the legs and trunk up.

Turn the left foot in a little (15°), at the same time revolving the leg outwards. Turn the right foot 90° out, together with the leg. Line up the right heel with the left arch. The wall supports the right hip and left heel. Exhale, bend the right leg to a square and go sideways down to the right, placing the right hand on a brick beside the outer foot. Place the left hand on the hip and pull the hip back towards the wall (2).

Stretch the left arm up and over the head, palm facing down. Revolve the trunk upwards press it back towards the wall. Press the right knee and left thigh towards the wall. Turn the head and look up. Rest the head against the wall. Breathe normally and relax the face (3).

Stay for 20 to 30 seconds. Inhale and come up. Repeat on the left.

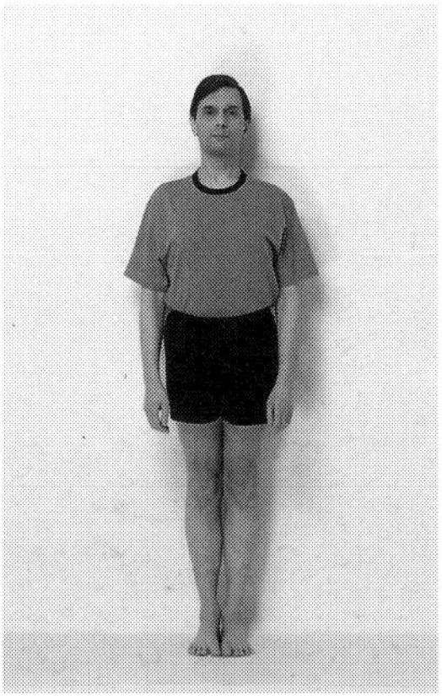

1

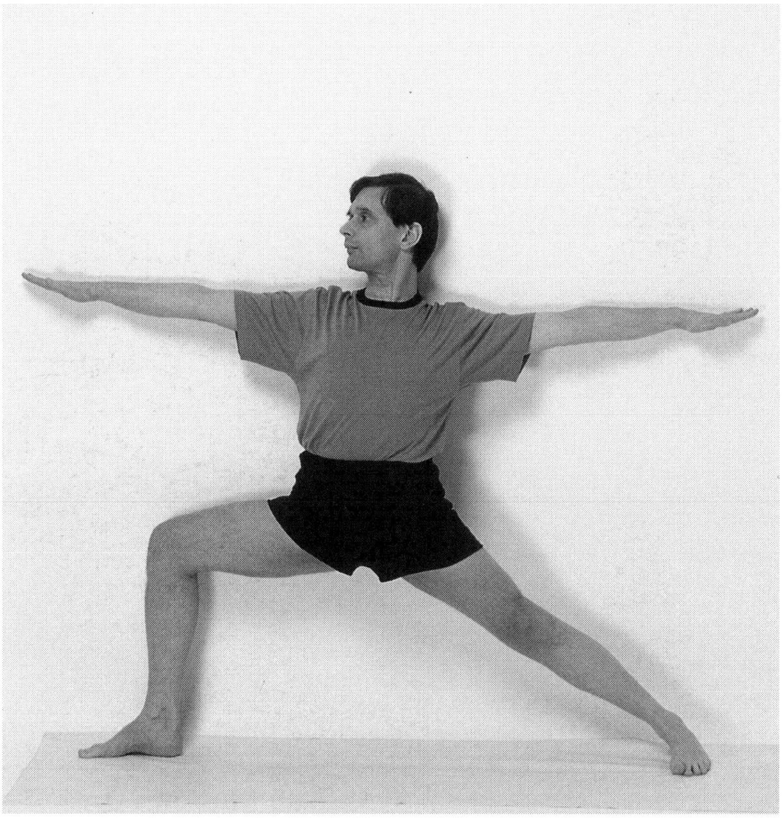

2

वीरभद्रासन २

Vīrabhadrāsana II Warrior Pose II

Method

Stand in *Tāḍāsana* against a wall (1).

Take the feet 4 to 4½ feet apart. Stretch the legs and trunk up. Raise the arms to shoulder level, with the little fingers touching the wall. Turn the left foot slightly in (15°). Press the outer edge of the foot down and lift the inner ankle. Revolve the leg outwards. Turn the right foot and leg 90° out. Align the right heel with the left instep. Keep right hip and left heel against the wall, the right foot away from it. Exhale and bend the right leg to a square. Keep the trunk vertical. Press the right knee and left hip and thigh towards the wall. Turn the head to the right, resting it against the wall. Breathe normally (2).

Stay for 20 to 30 seconds. Inhale and come up. Repeat on the left.

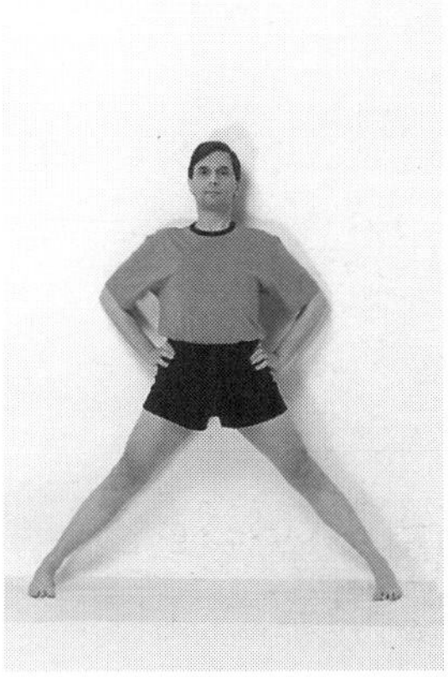
1

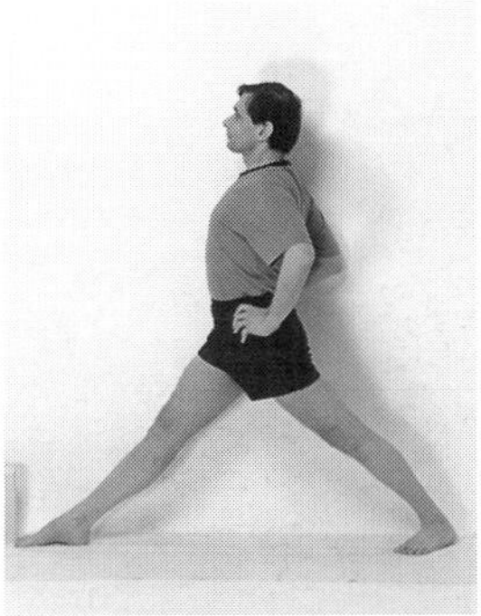
2

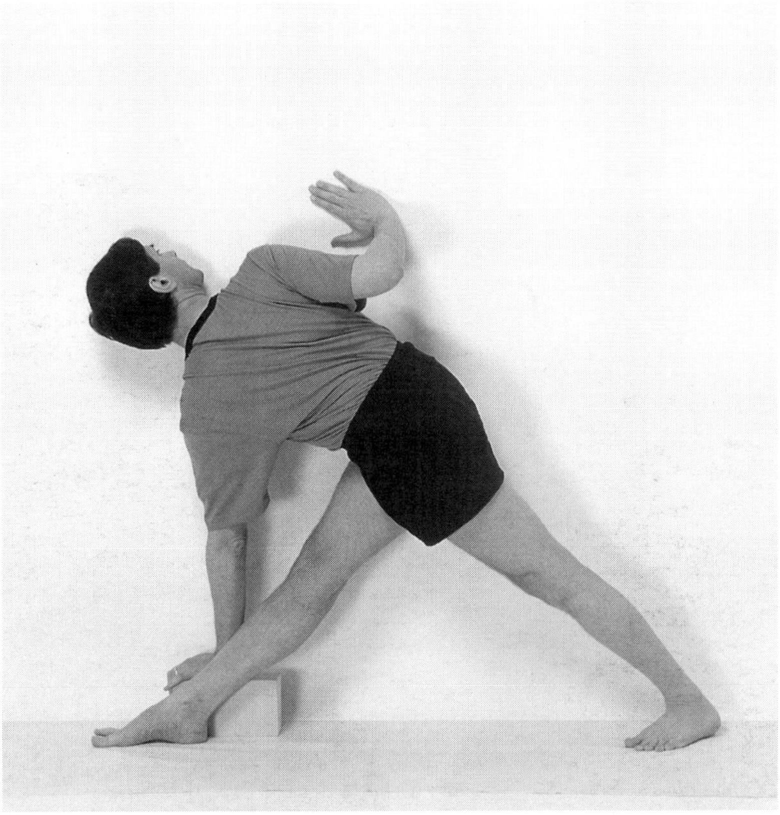
3

परिवृत्त-त्रिकोणासन

Parivṛtta-Trikoṇāsana Revolved Triangle Pose

parivṛtta = revolved; trikoṇa = triangle

Method

Stand in *Tāḍāsana* against a wall.

Take the feet 3½ to 4 feet apart. Place the hands on the hips. Stretch the legs and trunk up (1).

Take the left foot deep in (45 to 60°) and the right foot 90° out. Turn the left leg in the same direction as the foot. Turn the hips and trunk to the right (2).

Exhale and take the trunk sideways down, continuing the rotation. Place the left hand on the brick. Bend the right arm and place the hand on the wall. Keep the trunk in the vertical plane but allow room for the right hip to rest against the wall. Keep the left hip drawn in, as if pressed to the wall. With the help of the hands turn the trunk further. Turn the head and look up (3).

Stay for 20 to 30 seconds. Inhale and come up. Repeat on the left.

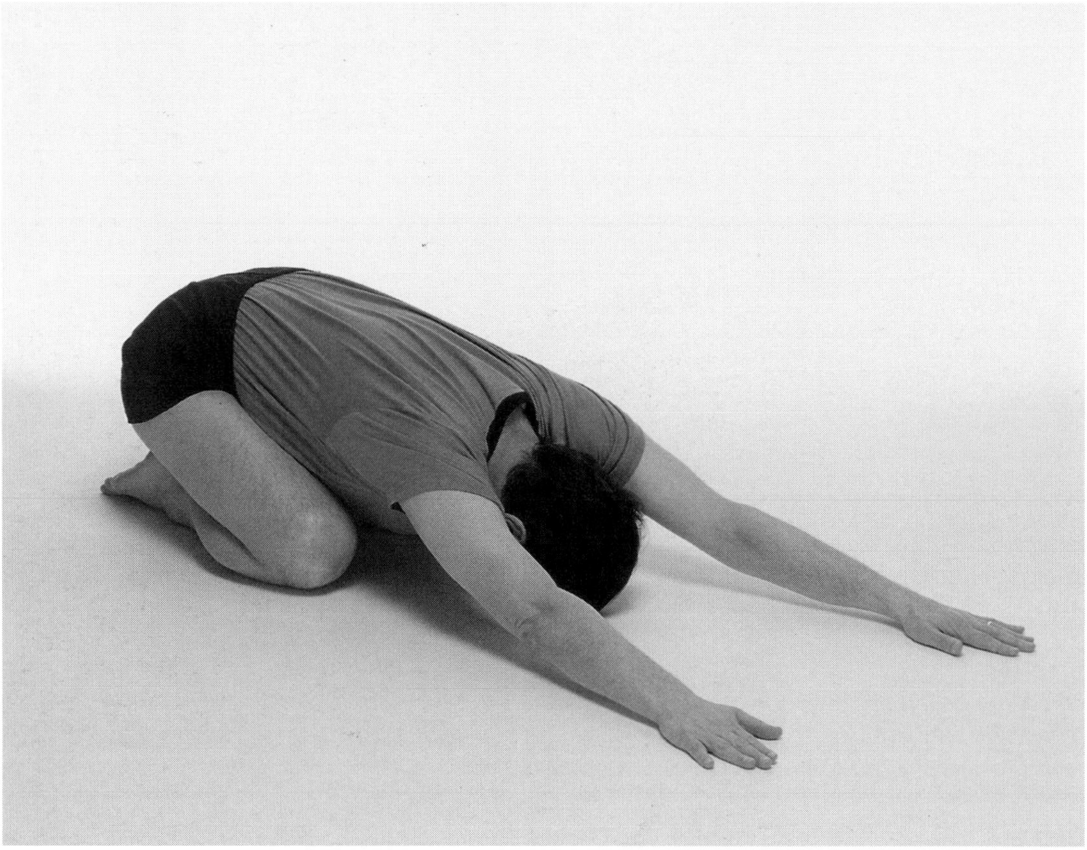

अधोमुख-वीरासन

Adhomukha-Vīrāsana Hero Pose Face Down

Method

Kneel with the toes together and the knees apart. Place a rolled blanket across the top thighs, tucking it into the groins. Press the blanket down and extend the trunk up. Exhale and bend down, maintaining the length of the trunk. Rest the head on the floor. Stretch the arms forward.

Stay for 20 to 30 seconds. Inhale and come up.

Note

For back pain

The support of the rolled blanket frees the lower back, giving relief from pain.

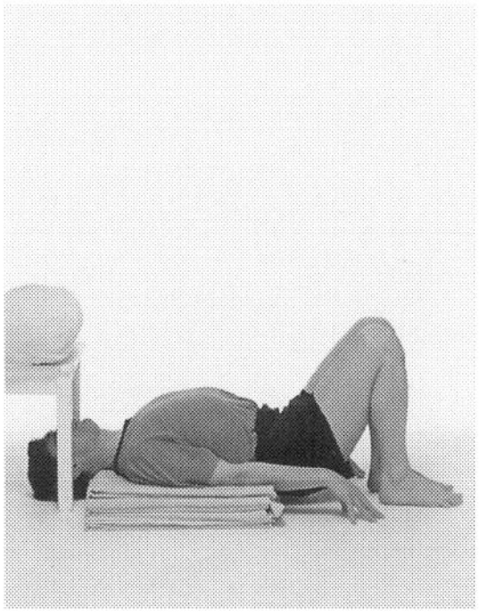
1

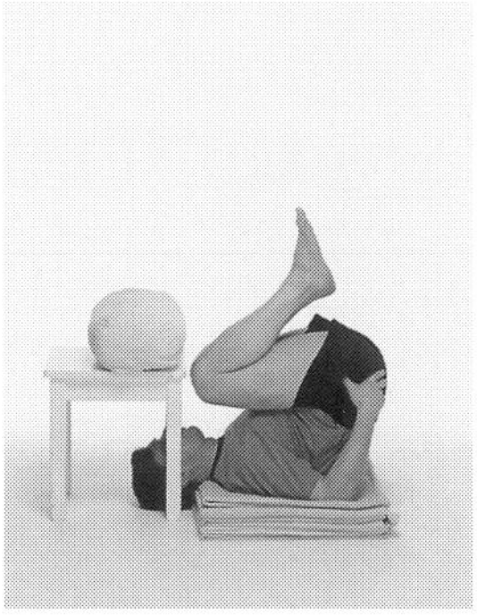
2

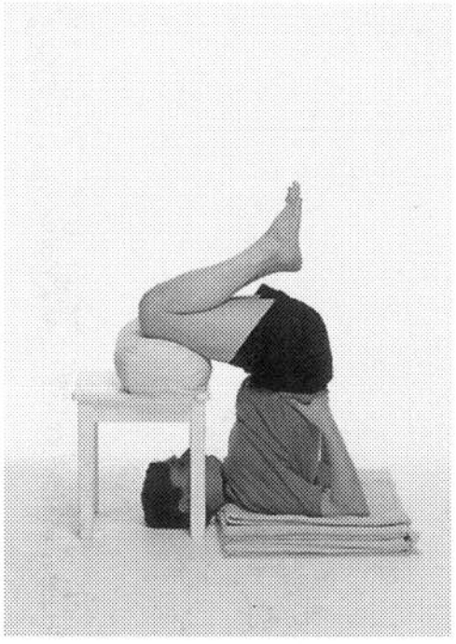
3

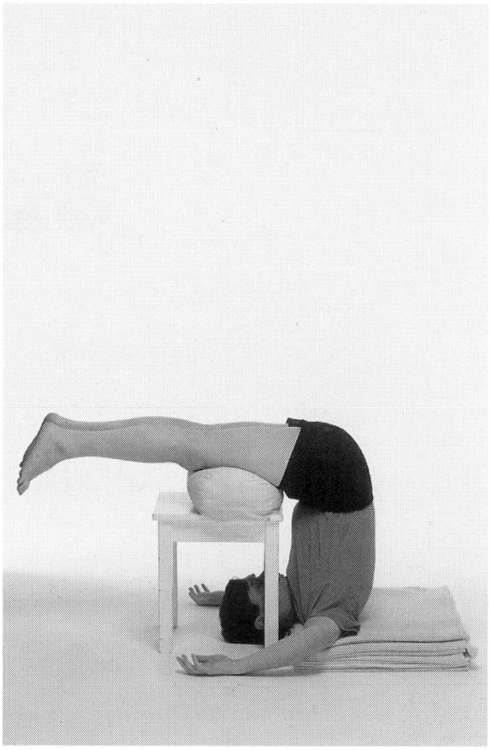
4

अर्ध-हलासन

Ardha-Halāsana Half Plough Pose

ardha = half; hala = plough

Method

Place 3 or 4 folded blankets on the floor, with the neat edges together. Place a stool the height of the trunk in front of them. If it is too low place a bolster or folded blankets on top. Lie down with the shoulders on the blankets and the head off the neat edge of the folded blankets. Draw the stool carefully over the head. Bend the knees. Press the shoulders down and the shoulder blades in. Lift the chest and lengthen the arms, keeping the palms down (1).

Exhale and swing the legs up over the abdomen. At the same time support the back with the hands (2).

Raise the back further and lift the thighs onto the bolster or stool (3).

Inch the thighs further onto the support and then straighten the legs. Be securely on the tops of the shoulders so as not to slide off the blankets. Take the arms over the head and relax (4).

Stay for 2 to 5 minutes. Ease the legs slowly backwards and push the stool away. Exhale and come down slowly. Be careful not to fall with a thump.

Note

Improvisation of Props

For this pose to be effective, there should be length in the trunk. Experiment with the height of the support to find what is comfortable.

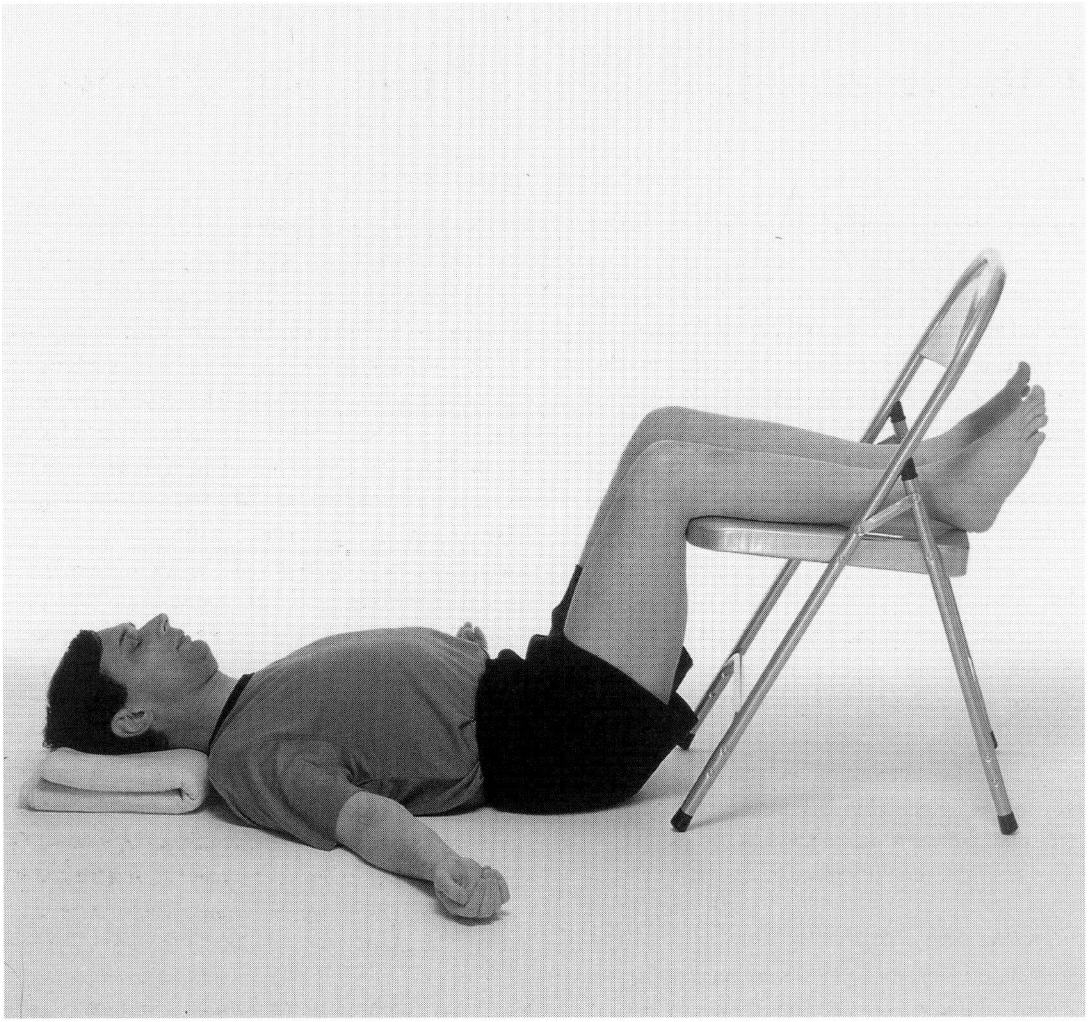

शवासन

Śavāsana Corpse Pose (with chair)

śava = corpse

Method

Lie on the floor with the calves resting on the seat of a chair. Bring the chair in so that the edge of the seat reaches the knees. Place a folded blanket under the head and neck. For extra ease of the back place a folded blanket under the sacrum (lower back). Close the eyes. Relax.

Stay for 5 minutes or longer. Open the eyes, bring the legs down, then turn to the side and get up.

The Neck, Shoulders, Arms and Hands

The Neck

The neck holds up the head and acts as a pivot for it. The weight of the head and a stooping posture pull the skull forward of its fulcrum, creating pressure inside the head and strain on the sense organs. The cervical vertebrae, being delicate, should be moved with the help of the strong thoracic vertebrae which form their base. Then the natural length and curvature of the neck are maintained. If this is not done, compression and tension ensue. A collapsed neck places stress on the throat.

The Shoulders

The shoulder is the joint of the arm and the body. The shoulder blades support the upper trunk and together with the collar bones keep the upper trunk erect. If the shoulder blades are not pressed towards the rib cage, the shoulders hunch and the sternum (breast bone) sinks. This reduces the girth of the rib cage and therefore the expansion of the lungs. Stiffness of the shoulder incapacitates the arms.

The Arms

The arms are used for lifting, carrying and enabling the work of the hands. Being constantly in motion they lack stability, and through the repeated muscle contraction involved in lifting objects they become short. If the arms are moved from the shoulder without the support of the shoulder blades they become strained.

The elbows divide the arm into two for greater range of movement. As with the knees, they both keep the extended arm firm or flex it upon itself. They also allow the arms to turn, giving a blend of power and dexterity. When movements are done repeatedly with contracted arms or with the upper- and fore-arm out of alignment, the elbow becomes strained.

The wrists link the hands to the arms and give them strength like a bandage support. Weak and strained wrists impede the functioning of the hands.

The Hands

The hands are a wonder of nature, matching the resourceful mind. The versatility and sensitivity of the fingers becomes dulled through habitual contraction and awkward or restricted movements.

HOW THE *ĀSANAS* WORK

This programme starts with arm work, which increases *vāta* and therefore mobility. It moves on to twists, which have the same *doṣic* effect of enhancing *pitta* and *vāta*. One or two standing poses are included to increase stamina (*kapha*) and bring about a better balance of *vāta*. The strong action of these poses is balanced by a supported inverted pose followed by relaxation, which quietens *vāta*.

Armwork (*kapha* –, *pitta* +, *vāta* +)

The arm actions stretch, straighten, flex and turn the arms and hands in various directions, promoting the flow of blood and energy. This creates space in the neck, shoulders and upper back, releasing tension.

Twists (*kapha* –, *pitta* +, *vāta* +)

The lateral turning of the spine/trunk after extension relieves pressure due to compression and strain. The rotation starts at the base and continues upward with a spiraling effect. As each part is eased and refreshed it helps the one above it to turn more. Thus maximum freedom of movement is gained for the neck.

Standing Poses (*kapha* +, *pitta* +, *vāta* =)

Standing poses lengthen the spine. In *Ardha Candrāsana* the spine is horizontal and resistance to gravitational force is achieved by the vertical arms and leg. Therefore the neck can elongate and turn freely.

Inverted Poses (*kapha* –, *pitta* +, *vāta* =)

In this variation of *Sarvāṅgāsana* with a chair the body weight is taken by the lower back on the chair. The shoulders are supported on a height and the head hangs down, giving length and freedom to the neck in an inverted position and restoring its natural curve.

Relaxation (*kapha* +, *pitta* –, *vāta* =)

The curve of the neck is supported by a rolled blanket so that tense muscles can relax.

Props

Wall, ledge, stool, chair, blanket

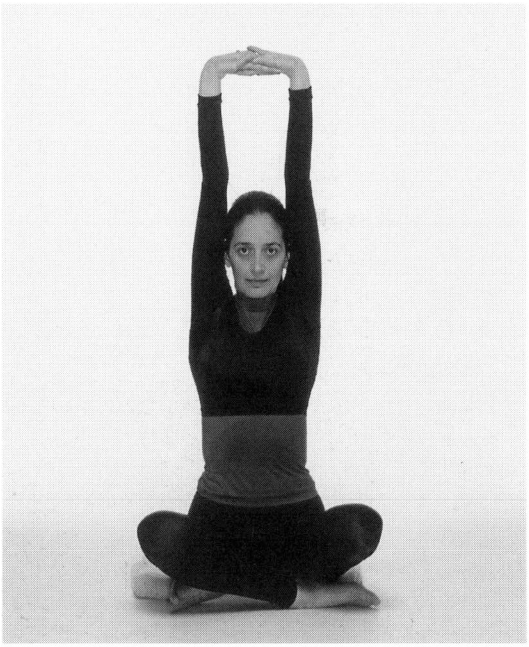

पर्वतासन

Parvatāsana Mountain Pose

parvata = mountain

Method

Sit on one or two folded blankets with the legs simply crossed (*Sukhāsana* – Easy Pose). Interlock the fingers and turn the palms out. Inhale and stretch the arms up. Tighten the elbows. Pull up the sides of the trunk with the help of the arms. Do not tense the throat.

Change the interlock of the fingers by placing the right fingers in front of the left ones or vice versa. Repeat.

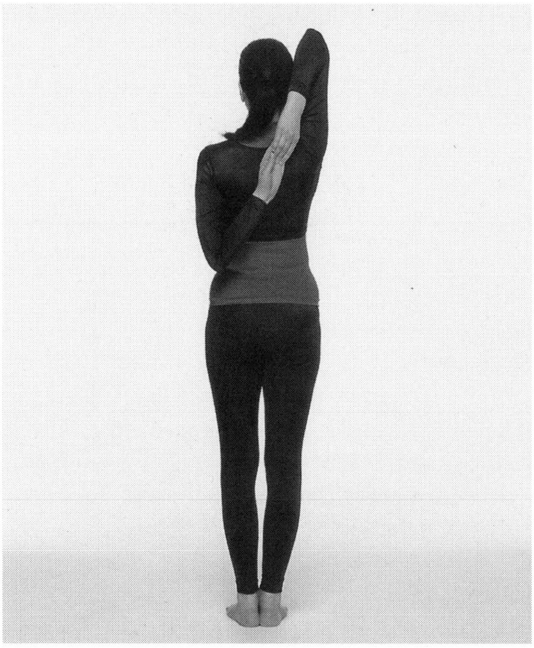

अर्ध-गोमुखासन

Ardha-Gomukhāsana Half Cow-Head Pose (arms only)

ardha = half; gomukha = face of cow

Method

Stand in *Tāḍāsana*. Take the right arm behind the back, hold the elbow and, with the help of the left hand, move the forearm up along the spine. Stretch the left arm forward and up, turn it in the socket so that the palm faces back, then bend the elbow and catch the right hand. Grasp a belt if it is not possible to catch the hands. Keep both upper arms vertical. Do not tilt the trunk. Catch further and further.

Stay for 20 to 30 seconds. Exhale, bring the arms down. Repeat the other way.

Note

Armwork

Armwork may be done either standing or sitting in any position.

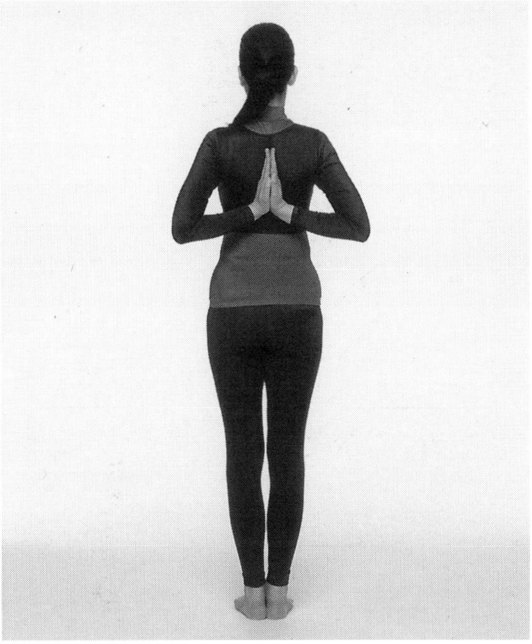

पृष्ठ-नमस्कार

Pṛṣṭha-Namaskāra Salutation at the Back

pṛṣṭha = back; namaskāra = salutation

Method

Stand in *Tāḍāsana*. Take the hands behind the back and join the palms, with the fingers pointing down. Keep the arms relaxed. Turn the hands in and take them up the spine as high as possible between the shoulder blades. Roll the shoulders back, press the shoulder blades in and lift the chest. Take the elbows back.

Stay for 20 to 30 seconds. Release the hands; if the wrists pain turn them slowly out and in.

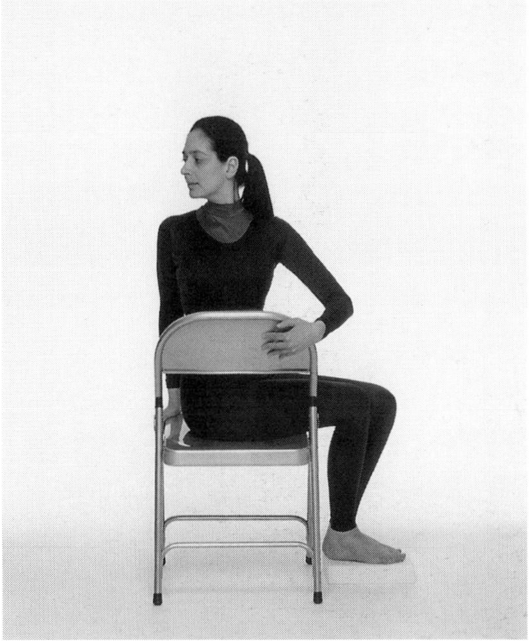

भरद्वाजासन

Bharadvājāsana *Bharadvāja's* Pose (on Chair)

Method

Sit sideways on a chair with the right hip and thigh against the back [of the chair]. Lift the trunk. Turn to the right and hold the back rest of the chair. Exhale and turn further, on the axis of the spine. Take the right arm behind the trunk to grip the seat of the chair. Turn the head and neck. Breathe normally.

Stay for 20 to 30 seconds. Inhale and come to the centre. Repeat on the left.

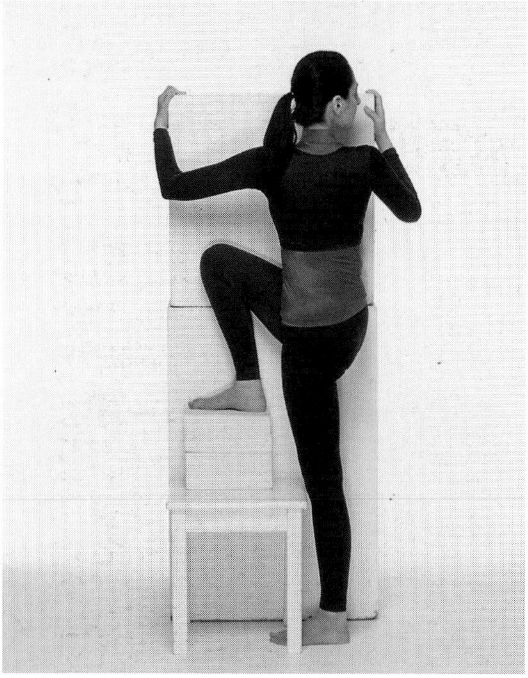

उत्थित-मरीच्यासन

Utthita-Marīcyāsana
Marīci's Pose (standing)

Method

Place a low table or high stool against a wall, preferably with a ledge. Build up the height level with the mid-thigh using blocks. Stand in *Tāḍāsana* in front of it with the right side near the wall. Place the right foot on the support. Keep the hip and thigh against the wall. Turn towards the wall. Grip the ledge or wall. Keep the left leg vertical and pulled up strongly. Draw the hip in. Exhale and turn the trunk, using the help of the arms. Turn the head and neck. Breathe evenly and stay relaxed.

Stay for 20–30 seconds. Inhale and come to the centre. Repeat on the left.

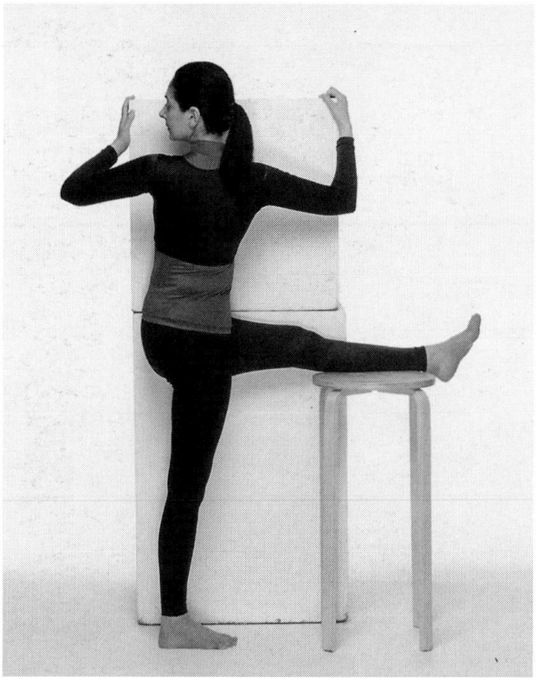

उत्थित-पादाङ्गुष्ठासन ३

Utthita-Pādāṇguṣṭhāsana III
Upright Thumb-to-foot Pose III

Method

Place a stool or table of hip height against a wall, preferably with a ledge. Stand in *Tāḍāsana* with the right side near the wall, 1½ to 2 feet in front of the stool. Raise the right leg and rest the calf on it. Turn towards the wall and hold onto the ledge. Stretch the left leg up and keep the hip pressed in. Lift the trunk, then exhale and turn further, using the hands to lever the trunk round. Move the back ribs and shoulder blades in. Turn the head and neck.

Stay for 20–30 seconds. Inhale and come to the centre. Repeat on the left.

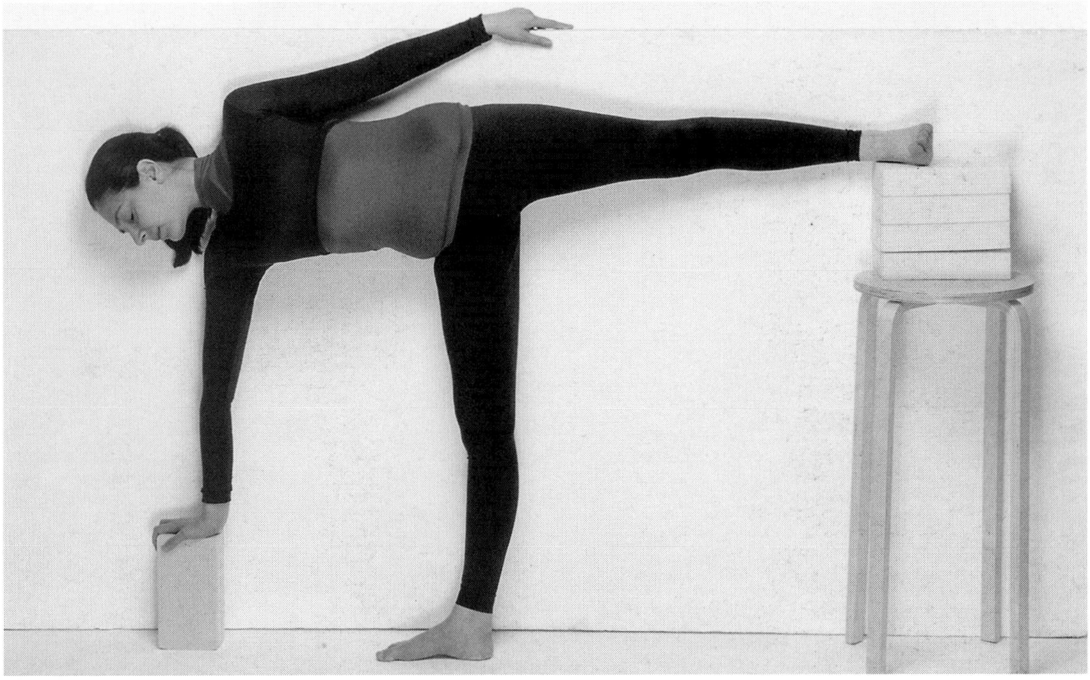

अर्ध-चन्द्रासन

Ardha-Candrāsana Half-Moon Pose

ardha = half; candra = moon

Method

Place a high stool or table against a wall, preferably with a ledge. Build it up to hip height using blocks. Stand in *Tāḍāsana* against the wall with the stool on the left. Spread the legs 3½ to 4 feet apart. Turn the feet to the right, exhale and go into *Trikoṇāsana* (see page 67). Place the right hand on a brick and the left hand on the ledge. Revolve the trunk upwards.

Exhale, bend the right leg and bring the bodyweight forward onto the right foot and hand. Simultaneously bring the left leg in and raise it up onto the stool.

Straighten and stretch the right leg, keeping it vertical. Stretch the left leg and foot. Gripping the ledge strongly with the left hand, lift the left hip and press it back towards the wall. Rest the trunk and head against the wall; revolve the trunk upwards. Move the shoulder blades in. Look down to keep the throat passive. If there is no strain, turn the head to look up.

Stay for 20–30 seconds. To come down, exhale, bend the right leg and lower the left leg. Go into *Trikoṇāsana*. Inhale and come up. Repeat on the left.

Note

The pose may be done with only the wall as a support.

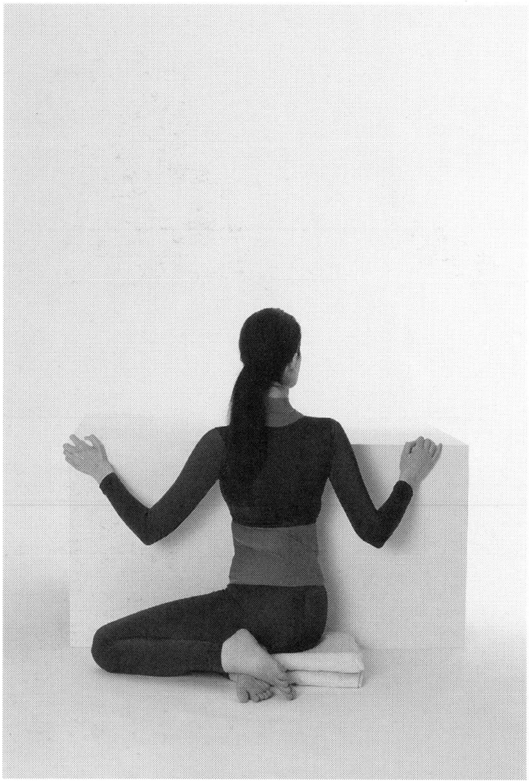

भरद्वाजासन

Bharadvājāsana Bharadvāja's Pose

Method

Place two folded blankets near a wall with a ledge. Sit on the edge of the blankets with outstretched legs, with the right hip against the wall. Bend the legs to the left, placing the left foot on the right instep. Keep the knees close together. Rest the knees on the floor and press the left thigh down. Turn to the right, keeping the trunk vertical. Hold the ledge but take the shoulders back and lift the chest. Exhale and turn the hips, waist, rib cage and shoulders. Turn the head and neck. Breathe evenly and stay relaxed.

Stay for 20–30 seconds. Inhale and release. Come to the centre. Repeat on the left.

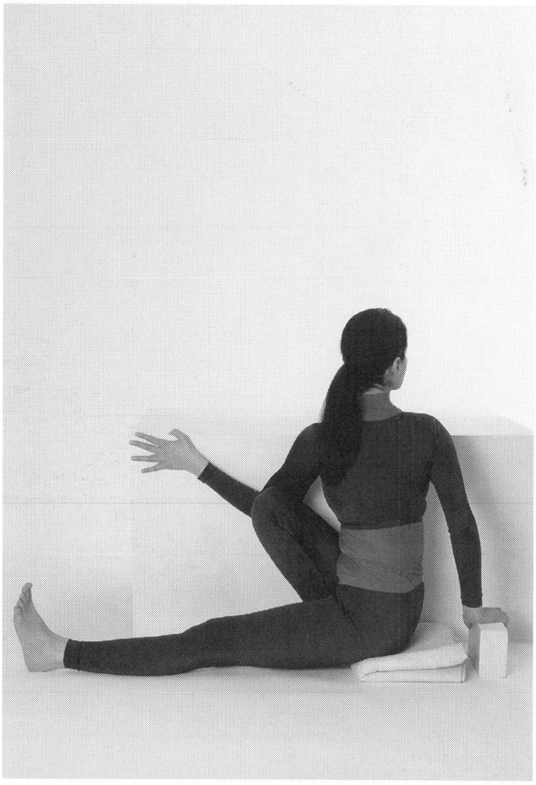

मरीच्यासन ३

Marīcyāsana III Marīci's Pose III

Method

Place two folded blankets near a wall with a ledge. Sit on the edge of the blankets with outstretched legs, with the right hip against or close to the wall. Bend the right leg up and bring the foot back towards the thigh. It should touch the left inner thigh. Exhale and turn towards the wall, bending the left elbow and hooking it behind the right knee. Hold the ledge. Place the right hand on a brick behind the hips (or hold the ledge). Lift the trunk and stretch the left leg and foot. Use the pressure of the right knee against the left arm, and the leverage of the right arm, to turn more. Turn the head and neck. Breathe normally.

Stay for 20–30 seconds. Inhale and release. Come to the centre. Repeat on the left.

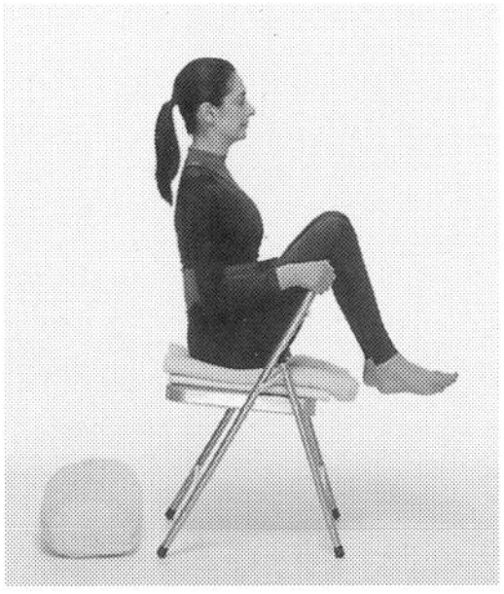
1

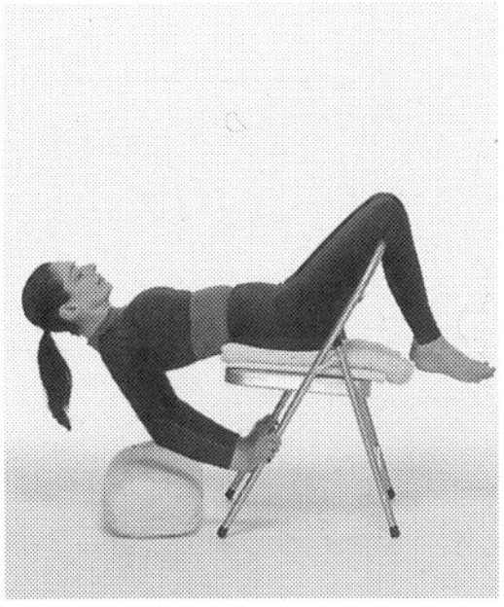
2

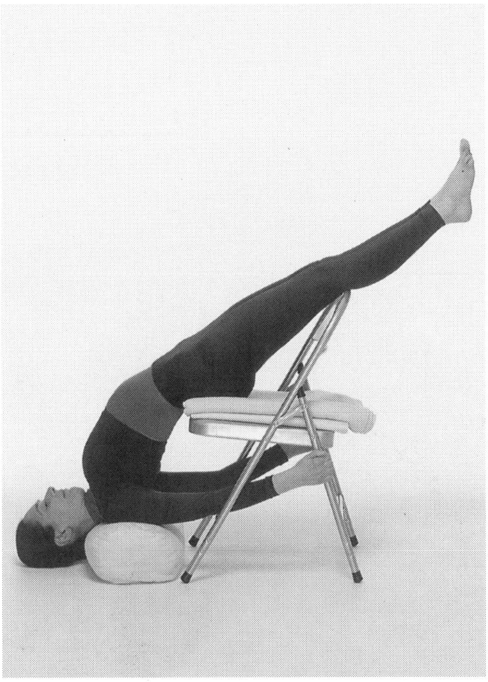
3

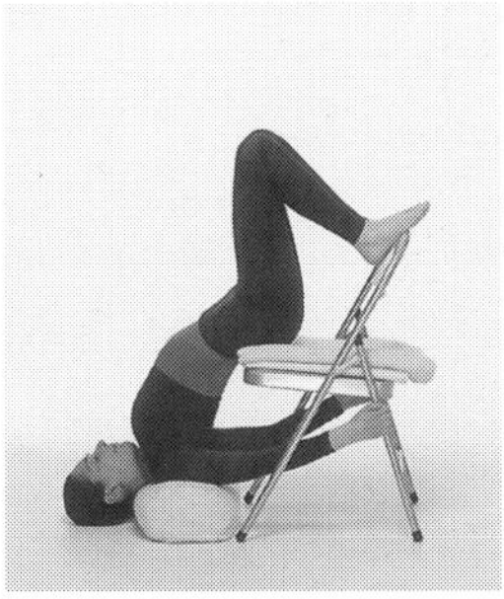
4

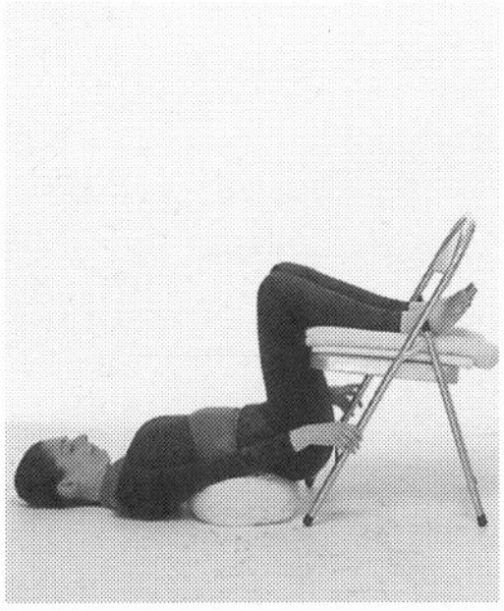
5

सर्वाङ्गासन

Sarvāṅgāsana Shoulder Balance (on chair)

sarva = all, entire; aṅga = body, limb

Method

Place a mat and blanket on a sturdy chair. Place a bolster or folded blankets lengthwise on the floor in front of it. Sit backwards astride the chair and take the legs over the back rest of the chair. Move the buttocks nearer to the back rest (1).

Lean back so that the waist can curve over the front edge of the seat. **While going down hold firmly onto the front legs or seat of the chair (2).**

Curving the waist over the front of the seat, lower the trunk towards the floor and rest the shoulders on the bolster. Rest the head on the floor. Keep the lower back securely on the seat of the chair. Take the arms inside the legs of the chair and hold the back legs of the chair. Straighten the legs against the back rest of the chair. Move the shoulders away from the neck and lift the chest, pressing the shoulder blades in (3).

Stay for 3 to 5 minutes. To come down, bend the legs and rest the feet on the back of the chair (4).

Ease the sacrum (lower back) off the chair onto the bolster, at the same time releasing the hands and holding the front legs. (Or, slide the chair a little away and come down [5].)

Note

Adjustments to the Pose

If the head feels heavy, place a folded blanket beneath it to raise it.

If the chair back cuts into the legs, place a blanket over it.

If it is strenuous for the back, place the chair about 1 to 1½ feet way from the wall so that the feet can rest on the wall with the legs in a more upright position.

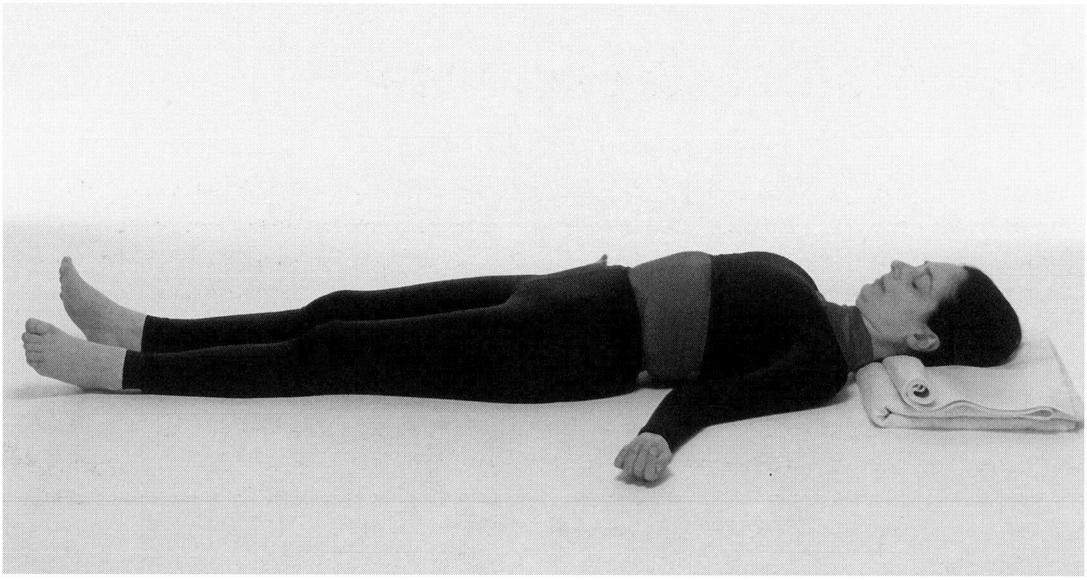

शवासन

Śavāsana Corpse Pose

Method

Lie down in a straight line, with a folded blanket under the head and neck. If there is discomfort in the neck, roll a second blanket a little and place the rolled portion under the neck so as to support the curve. Lengthen the legs away from the trunk, then let them relax outwards from the tops of the thighs. Let the feet drop further to the sides. Lengthen the arms. Press the shoulders down and the shoulder-blades into the body. Keep the chest lifted. Turn the upper arms so that the biceps face up, then relax the arms and hands. Close the eyes and relax the face. Let the eyeballs sink down into their sockets. Let the tongue rest on the floor of the mouth. Relax the throat. Do not let the mind wander but be attentive to the relaxation. Breathe softly, without strain.

Stay for 5 minutes or longer. Open the eyes gently, bend the knees and turn to the side. Get up from the side.

Physiological Efficiency

The systems of the body are designed to work in concord. Their individual functions are dependent on each other and the impairment of one system affects the others. Therefore the proper maintenance of all systems is of paramount importance for health.

The body is built to function efficiently, but like any machine it needs to be provided with the right fuel, in the right quantity and of the right quality. Over-eating, under-eating and eating wrong foods habitually all impair the smooth functioning of the body systems, starting with digestion. Partial digestion, assimilation and elimination create the build up of toxins which remain in the body and circulate in the various tissues. Āyurveda considers that the colon is the main breeding ground of all diseases. Apart from self-induced causes, environmental and genetic or congenital factors also impair physiological function.

Yoga practice can help greatly to counter the deterioration of body tissues, alleviate discomfort and restore efficiency to the physiological systems.

The Digestive Tract

A well-functioning digestive system is essential for health. Faulty diet has a deleterious effect in many ways. It can overtax it through overeating, through eating heavy foods or eating before the complete digestion of a previous meal. It can create too much gas through the consumption of the wrong types of foods for the constitution. Various Yoga *āsanas* speed up the digestive process, increase the power of the digestive fire and encourage peristaltic action and the passing of trapped flatus.

The Respiratory Tract

Coughs, colds, congestion, bronchitis, dyspnoea, asthma and a predisposition to lung infections may be due to an unsuitable diet, which ultimately weakens the immune system, as well as to external causes. Yoga postures expand the chest and increase the capacity of the lungs, thereby strengthening the whole respiratory system. Where the condition is severe the postures are done with support so that the expenditure of energy is minimized.

The Cardio-vascular System

The functioning of the cardio-vascular system can be impaired by wrong food habits: improperly digested elements remain in the body and coat the arteries instead of being excreted. Other non-traumatic causes are a sedentary lifestyle and overstrain.

When the heart is at risk no other risks should be taken. The supported postures that expand the chest and improve oxygenation are also beneficial for the heart. The feeling of oppression in this region is removed and is substituted by lightness and ease.

The Circulatory System

Impairment to the circulatory system results in the scarcity of energy in the body. This affects all the systems, producing a range of effects from lethargy and irritability to organic disorders due to the reduced supply of blood to the tissues. Poor circulation may have dietary causes or may be the symptom of other diseases which weaken the immune system. Yoga postures done in swift succession generate heat which radiates through the body. When these sequences are done regularly over time they "jump start" the body.

The Reproductive System

Impairment of the reproductive organs and female monthly cycle may be due to improper food and poor elimination, to strain or to external or genetic factors. Yoga practice tones the pelvic organs. For women especially, it is effective in ameliorating many menstrual disorders (irregularity of menses, amenorrhea, dysmenorrhea) and in relieving the discomfort of endometriosis, cysts, etc. Similarly, it is beneficial during pregnancy and the post-natal period, although a newcomer to yoga requires the supervision of an experienced teacher. In later life it helps to alleviate the hot flushes and mood swings of menopause and to counter osteoporosis.

The Immune System

Chemical additives to food, pollution, continued stress and infections all weaken the immune system. Yoga restores strength and stamina in a non-aggressive way. Supported inverted poses increase the intake of oxygen and nourish the brain and nerves.

The Abdominal Organs: Stomach, Liver and Intestines

A healthy digestive tract is the key to the body's well-being. Food taken in is converted into body tissue; good nutrition and a digestion that works well result in healthy tissues. Although digestion starts in the stomach, it continues in the small bowel, which is the longest part of the intestine. Ideally the stomach breaks down food without heartburn or reflux; the liver metabolizes nutrients without producing nausea and intestinal peristalsis is not impeded by too much gas or by lax muscle tone. A faulty diet and diseased or damaged organs impair the efficiency of the digestive system. So does poor posture, in which the organs are compressed. Yoga practice strengthens the digestive organs and alleviates discomfort and pain. It also increases metabolic efficiency.

HOW THE *ĀSANAS* WORK

This programme begins with supine poses which increase physiological energy (*pitta*) and channelise *vāta*. Supported back-bending poses further increase *pitta* and energisze *vāta*. They are followed by supported forward bends which also stimulate *pitta* but reduce any agitation of *vāta*. The long sequence of inverted poses continue the stimulation of *pitta* while at the same time balancing *vāta*. The final relaxation calms *pitta*.

Supine poses (*kapha* +, *pitta* +, *vāta* =)
Supine poses stretch the front of the body and therefore the whole digestive tract. This increased space enhances their efficiency and discourages pockets of congestion. Digestion is faster and bloating is reduced. These poses are safe to perform after meals.

Backbends (*kapha* –, *pitta* +, *vāta* +)
Backbends give a strong extension to the stomach and liver. This stretch increases the flow of blood; thereby stimulating the secretion of digestive juices and hormones.

Forward Bends (*kapha* +, *pitta* +, *vāta* –)
In forward bends the digestive organs are supported in a horizontal position and are able to rest. The abdomen becomes soft. This encourages the passing of flatus.

Inverted Poses (*kapha* –, *pitta* +, *vāta* =)
Inverted poses relieve the pressure of gravity on the digestive organs. They become relaxed. In *Viparīta-Karaṅī* the inversion of the legs over the horizontal pelvis encourages the pooling of blood in the abdomen. This activates the gastric juices.

Relaxation (*kapha* +, *pitta* –, *vāta* =)
Relaxation rests and stabilizes the body and mind.

Props
Chair, stool, bench, bolster, mat, blankets

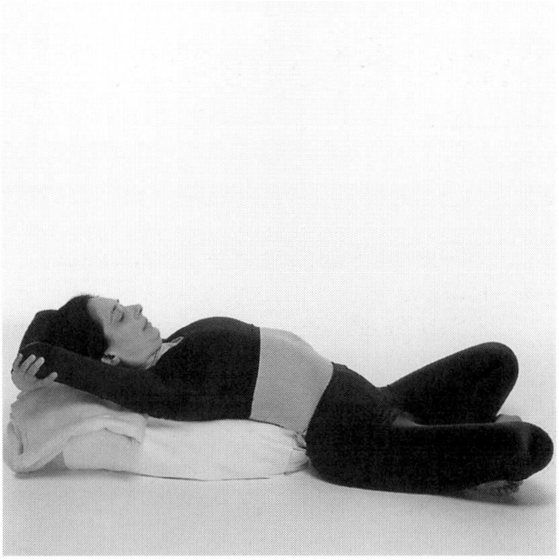

मत्स्यासन

Matsyāsana Fish Pose

matsya = fish

Method

Sit in simple cross-legs (*Sukhāsana*) in front of a bolster placed lengthwise on the floor. Hold the bolster against the body and lie back on it. Place a folded blanket under the head and neck. Fold the arms over the head.

Stay for 3 to 5 minutes. Come up, change the cross-legs and repeat.

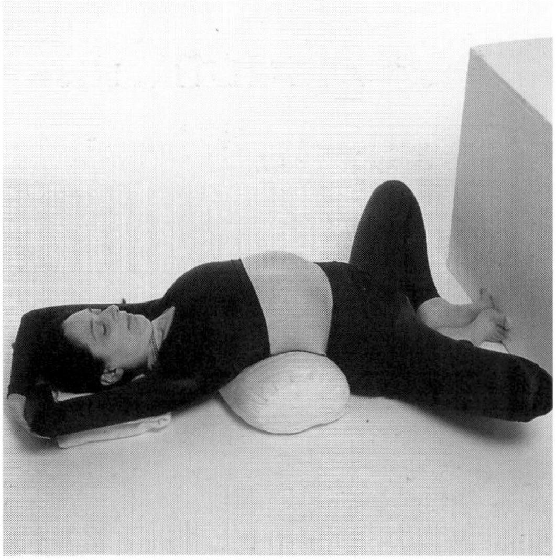

सुप्त-बद्धकोणासन

Supta-Baddhakoṇāsana Supine Cobbler's Pose (Bound-Angle Pose)

supta = supine; baddha = bound; koṇa = angle

Method

Sit in front of a wall with a bolster placed crosswise behind the back. Bend the knees to the sides and bring the soles of the feet together. (This is *Baddhakoṇāsana* – Cobbler's Pose.) Go closer to the wall. Keeping the soles joined, bend the toes outwards and press them against the wall. Bring the buttocks forward to close the space between the thighs and calves. Hold the bolster against the body and lie back over it, resting the shoulders on the ground. Place a folded blanket under the head and neck. Take the arms over the head and catch the elbows.

Stay for 3 to 5 minutes. Bring the knees together and slide away from the wall. Turn to the side and get up.

Note

For Back Pain

If the back is stiff or painful, place the bolster lengthwise.

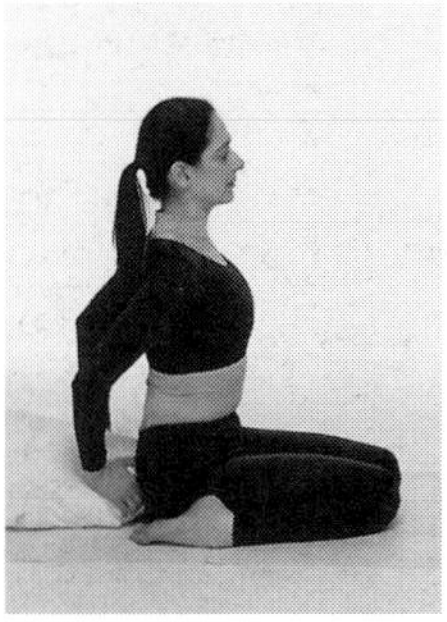

1

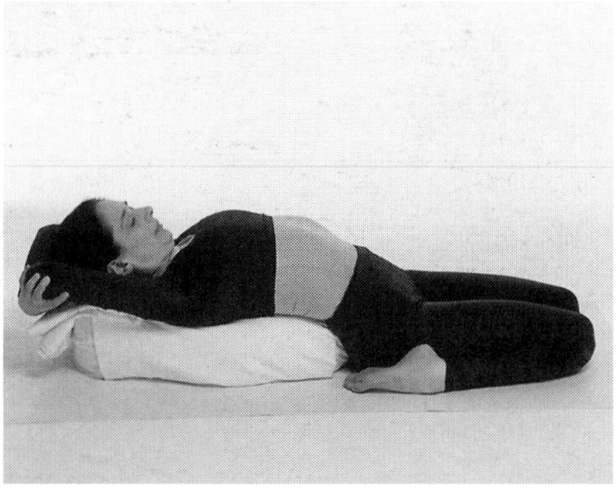

2

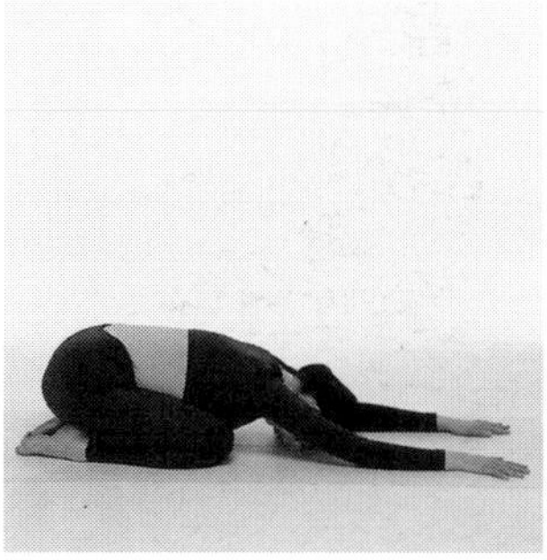

3

सुप्त-वीरासन

Supta-Vīrāsana Supine Hero Pose

supta = supine; vīra = hero

Method

Sit in *Vīrāsana* in front of a bolster placed lengthwise on the floor. Hold the bolster against the body (1).

Lie back. Place a folded blanket under the head and neck. Fold the arms over the head (2).

Stay for 3 to 5 minutes. Come up and do *Adhomukha-Vīrāsana*. Sit on the heels, spread the knees apart and bend forward (3).

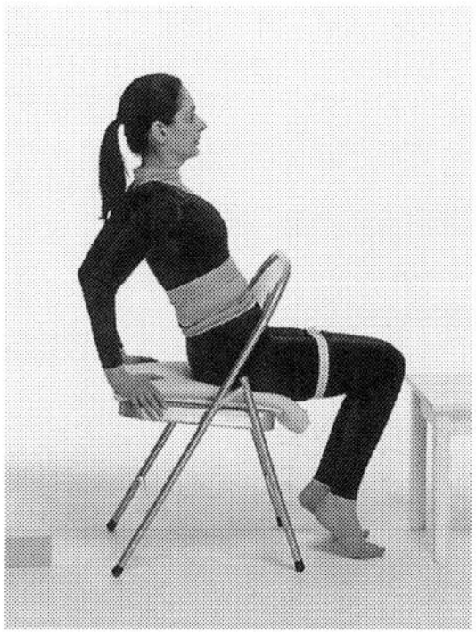

1

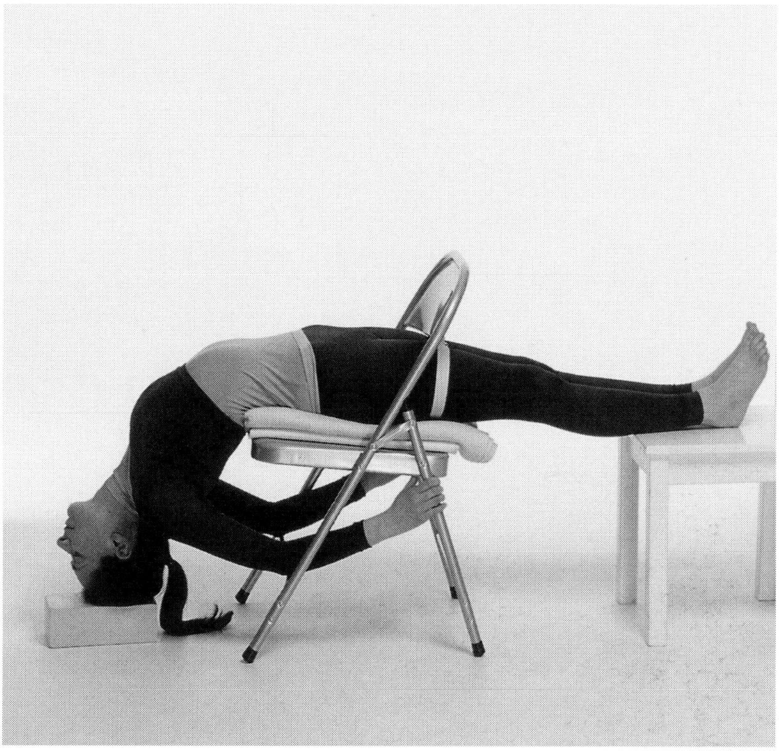

2

विपरीत-दण्डासन

Viparīta-Daṇḍāsana Inverted Staff Pose

viparīta = inverted, reverse; daṇḍa = staff, rod

Method

Place a low stool against the wall. Place a chair 1½ to 2 feet in front of it, with its back to the stool. Place a mat and blanket on the chair. Place a brick or bolster in front of the chair. Facing the back of the chair, take the legs through the gap between the seat and the back rest and sit backwards on the chair. Tie the mid-thighs together with a belt. Hold the seat and move as close to the back edge as possible (1).

Exhale and lean back, lower the trunk and curve the waist over the seat. Rest the crown of the head on the support. Raise the feet onto the stool. Take the arms inside the legs of the chair and hold the back legs. Tighten the knees and stretch the legs. Allow the chest to curve and open. Relax the face (2).

Stay for 1 to 3 minutes. To come up, bring the feet down. Release the hands and hold the top of the chair. Inhale and swing the trunk up, keeping the back concave. Bring the head up last. Lean forward on the back rest of the chair. Come out of the chair carefully.

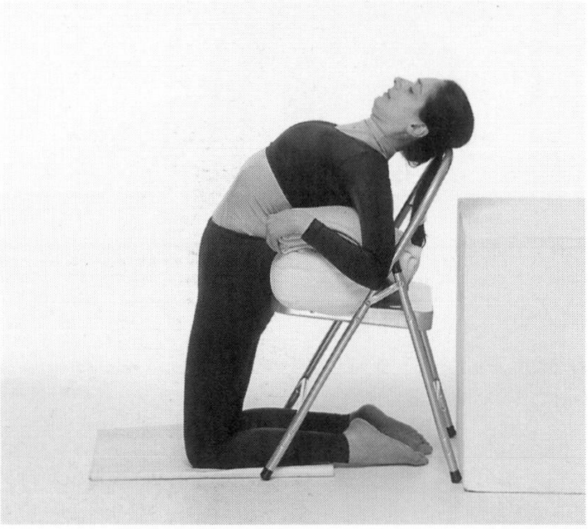

उष्ट्रासन

Uṣṭrāsana Camel Pose

uṣṭra = camel

Method

Place a chair against a wall or sturdy piece of furniture. Place a (non-slip)mat and bolster crosswise on it. Kneel with the back to the chair, taking the shins beneath the seat. Take the knees and feet a little apart. Go closer to the chair and hold the bolster against the body. Exhale and lean back over it, resting the head on the chair back.

Stay for 1 to 2 minutes. Inhale and come up. Kneel and bend forward in *Adhomukha-Vīrāsana* (see page 59).

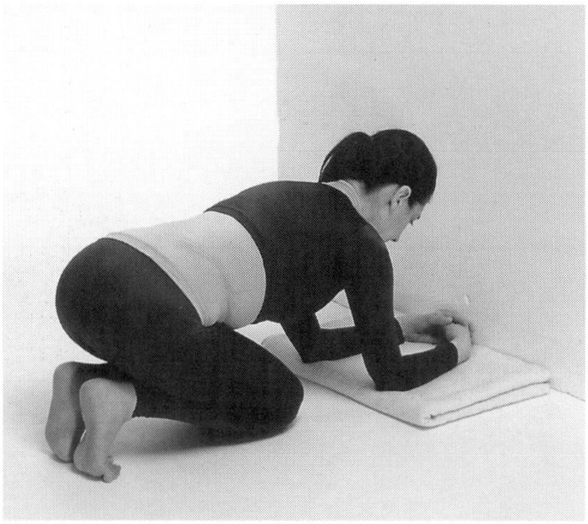

1

शीर्षासन

Śīrṣāsana Head Balance

śīrṣa = head

Method

Place a folded blanket against the wall with the neat edge inwards. Kneel in front of the blanket and align the legs and trunk. Interlock the fingers and place the forearms and hands on the blanket with the fingers touching the wall. Keep the elbows in line with the shoulders (1).

Lift the shoulders away from the neck, extend the neck and place the crown of the head on the blanket. Lift the shoulders (2).

Lift the knees and straighten the legs. Walk the feet in till the trunk is nearly vertical. Keep the shoulders lifted and move the chest forward (3).

Exhale and jump up with bent legs, if possible with both legs together (4).

Rest the feet on the wall. Lift the shoulders (5).

Straighten the legs against the wall. Lift the shoulders, tighten the buttocks and stretch the trunk and legs up. Breathe normally. Relax the face and eyes (6).

Stay for 30 seconds to 1 minute initially, then increase the time. Bend the legs, keeping the feet on the wall. Then come down. Stay kneeling with the head on the floor for a few seconds until the blood flow returns to normal.

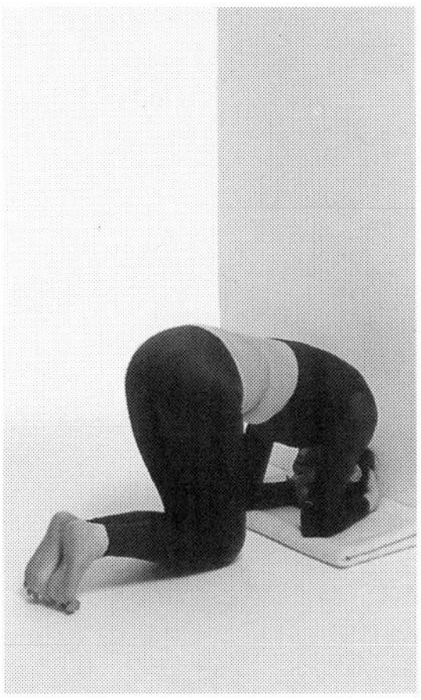

2

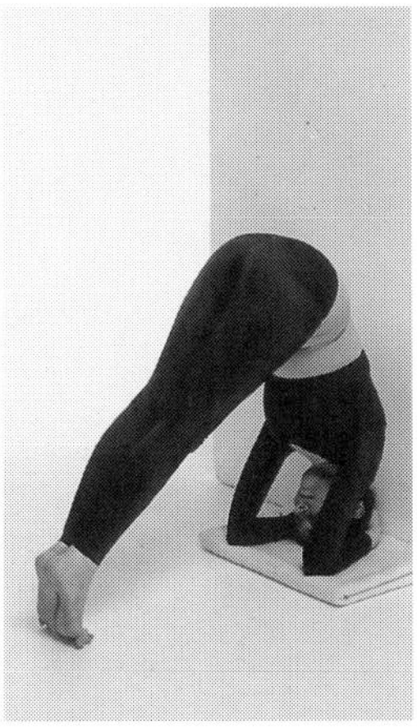

3

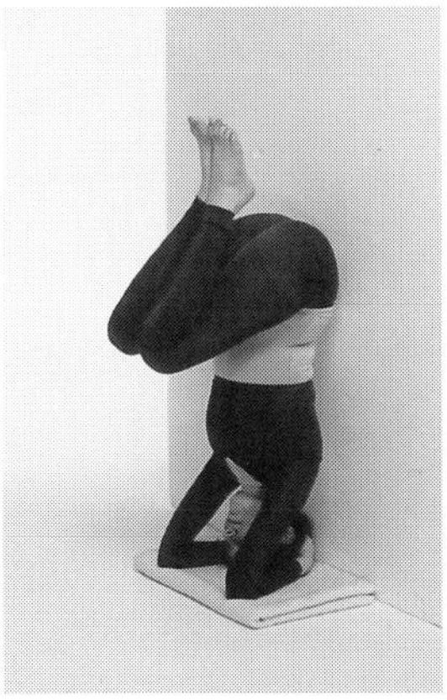

4

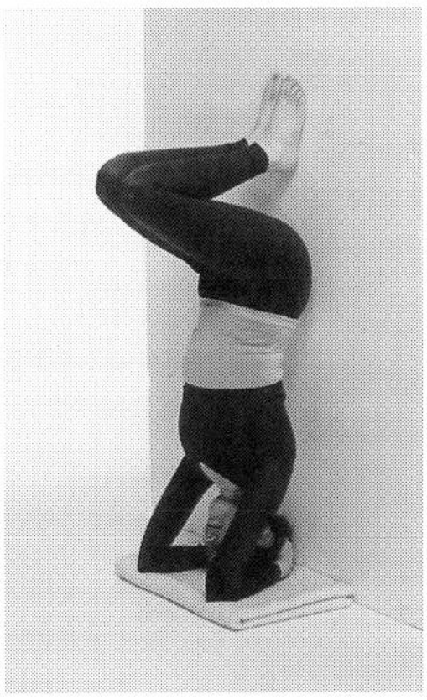

5

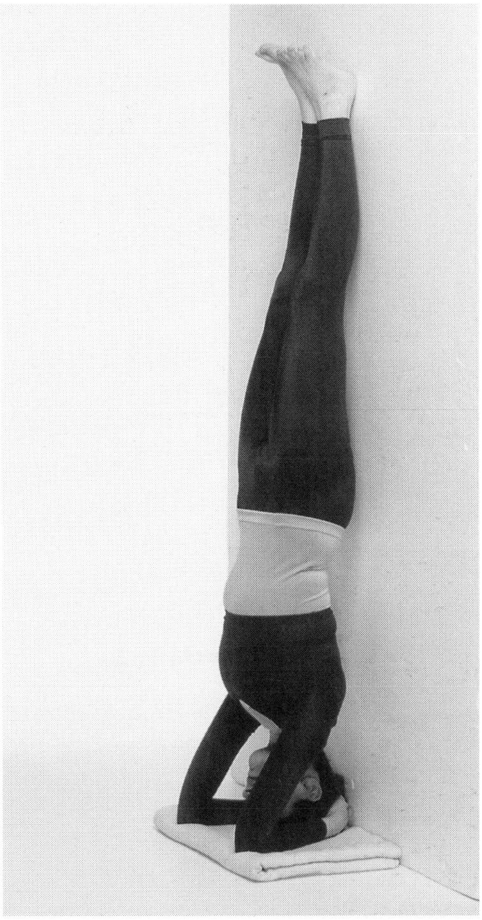

6

Note

Cautions

Śīrṣāsana should be attempted only when the neck has been strengthened by standing poses, twists, *Sarvāṇgāsana* and *Halāsana*. Beginners may prefer to postpone learning it for several months.

Śīrṣāsana should be done once only in any practice session, as going up and down repeatedly causes irritability.

If there is pressure on the neck, place the head down a little forward of the crown.

If the eyes become strained or bloodshot, do forward bends with the head supported (see pages 102–4). Only resume *Śīrṣāsana* practice when the eyes remain relaxed.

As the pressure and shape of the eyeball alters, it is safest to remove contact lenses.

Contra-indications, for which a teacher should be consulted: detached retina, hypertension, neck injuries.

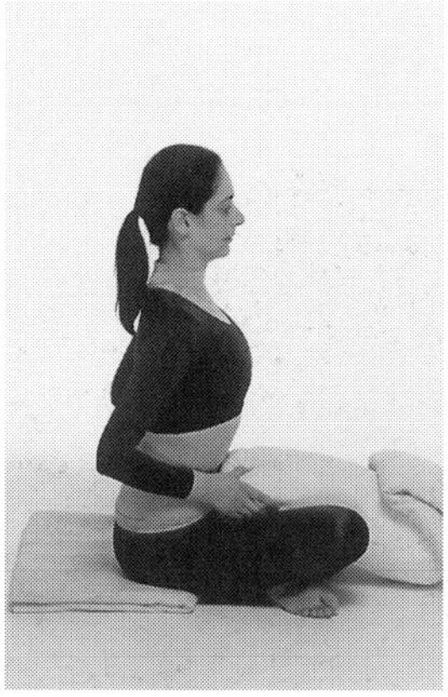
1

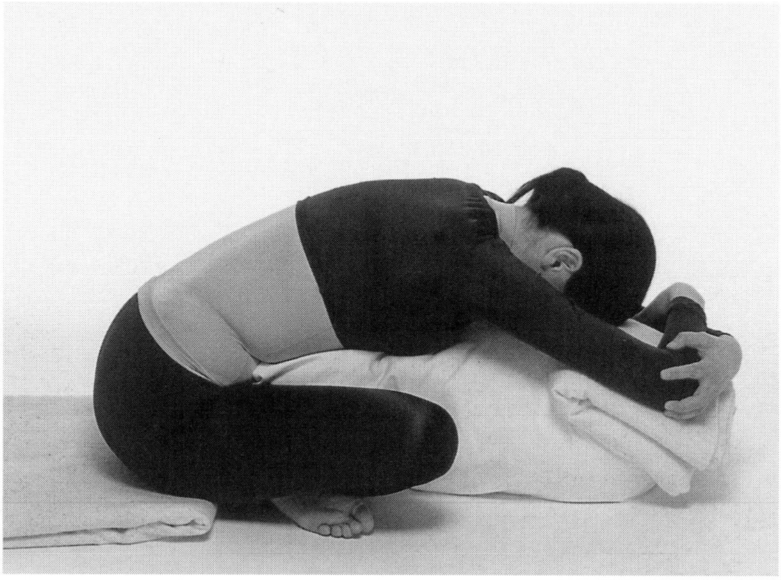
2

अधोमुख-सुखासन

Adhomukha-Sukhāsana Easy Pose, Face Down

adho = downwards; mukha = face, mouth; sukha = ease, comfort

Method

Sit on one or two folded blankets in simple cross-legs. Place a bolster lengthwise on the legs and hold it against the abdomen. Press it down and lift the trunk away from it (1).

Exhale and bend forward over the bolster so that it supports the front of the body. Rest the forehead on a blanket. Stretch the arms forward (2).

Stay for 2 to 3 minutes. Inhale, come up and change the cross-legs. Repeat on the other side.

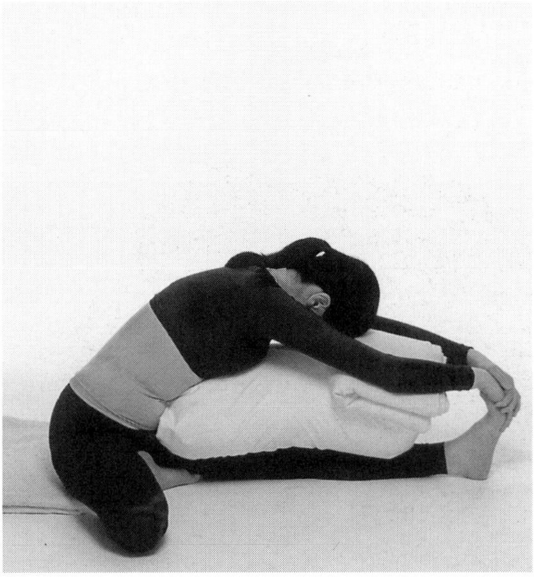

जानुशीर्षासन

Jānuśīrṣāsana Head-to-Knee Pose

jānu = knee; śīrṣa = head

Method

Sit on one or two folded blankets with the legs stretched out in front. Bend the right leg to the side and bring the heel to its own groin, with the sole facing up. Place a bolster lengthwise on the left leg, touching the abdomen. Press the bolster down and lift the trunk away from it. Keep the left leg stretched and the right leg relaxed.

Exhale and bend forward over the bolster. Rest the forehead on a blanket. Stretch the arms forward. Catch the feet if possible, or use a belt.

Stay for 1 to 2 minutes. Inhale and come up. Repeat on the other side.

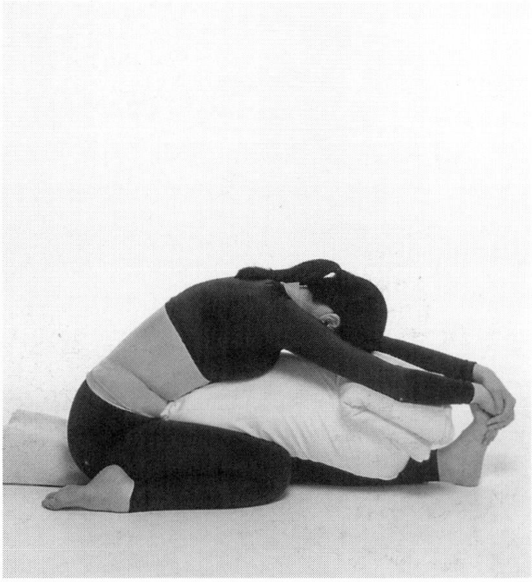

एकपाद-वीर-पश्चिमोत्तानासन

Ekapāda-Vīra-Paścimottānāsana Posterior Stretching Pose with One Leg in Hero Pose

eka = one; pāda = foot, leg; vīra = hero; paścima = posterior, west; uttāna = stretching

Method

Sit on two folded blankets with the legs stretched out in front. Move the blankets to be under the left buttock. Bend the right leg back, with the foot beside the thigh. Bring the knees together. Place a bolster lengthwise on the left leg, touching the abdomen. Press the bolster down and lift the trunk away from it.

Exhale and bend forward over the bolster. Rest the forehead on a blanket. Stretch the arms forward. Catch the feet if possible, or use a belt.

Stay for 1 to 2 minutes. Inhale and come up. Repeat on the other side.

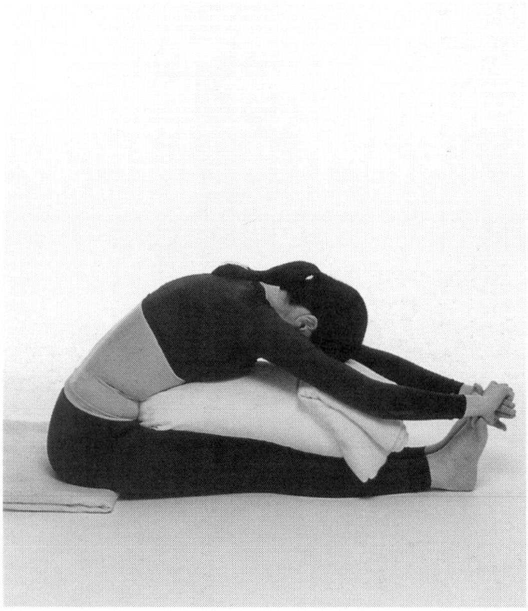

पश्चिमोत्तानासन

Paścimottānāsana Posterior Stretching Pose

paścima = posterior; uttāna = stretching

Method

Sit on one or two folded blankets with the legs stretched out in front and the feet together. Place a bolder lengthwise on the legs and against the abdomen. Press it down and lift the trunk away from it.

Exhale and bend forward over the bolster. Rest the forehead on a blanket. Stretch the arms forward. Catch the feet, or use a belt to do so.

Stay for 2 to 3 minutes. Inhale and come up.

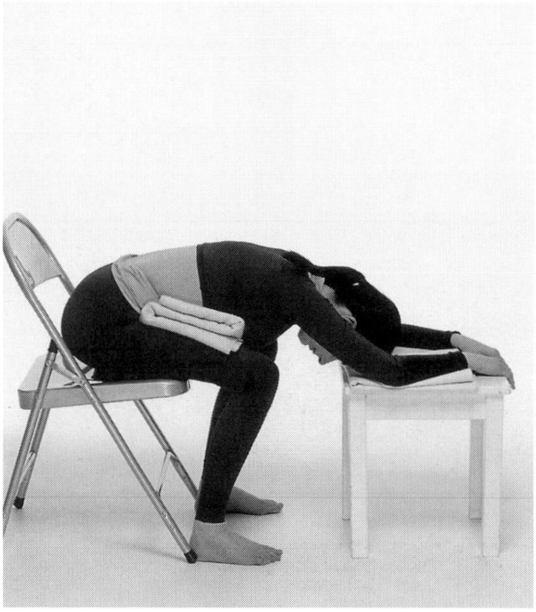

पवनमुक्तासन १

Pavanamuktāsana I Wind-Releasing Pose I

pavana = wind; mukta = released

Method

Sit on a chair with another chair or stool in front, padded with a blanket. Place a folded blanket on the thighs, tucking it back into the groins. Stretch the trunk up.

Exhale and bend forwards, resting the forehead and arms on the stool.

Stay for 2 to 3 minutes. Inhale and come up.

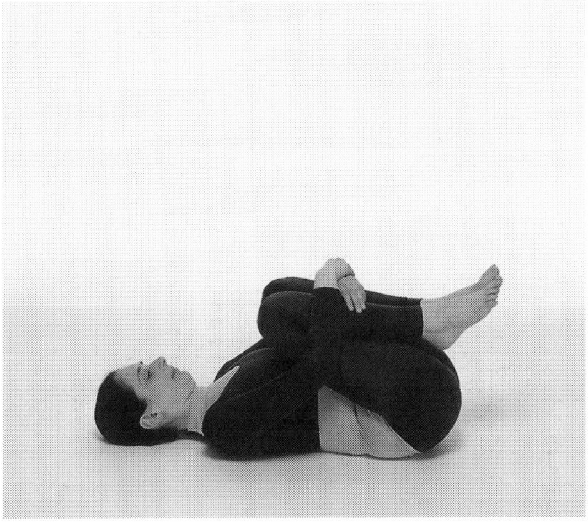

पवनमुक्तासन २

Pavanamuktāsana II
Wind-Releasing Pose II

Method

Lie on the back with the knees bent over the abdomen. Clasp the arms round the shins.

Exhale, raise the head towards the knees and rock backwards and forwards a few times.

Inhale and release the legs.

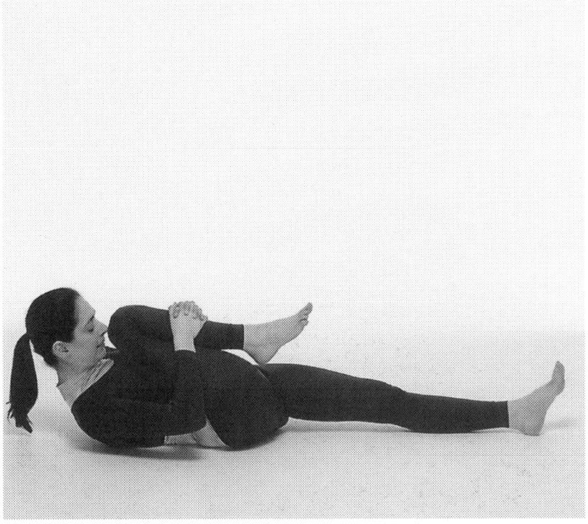

एकपाद-पवनमुक्तासन

Ekapāda-Pavanamuktāsana
One-Legged Wind-Releasing Pose

Method

Lie on the back in a straight line. Bend the right leg over the abdomen. Clasp the arms round the shin. Exhale and raise the head towards the knee. Keep the left leg stretched.

Stay for 20 to 30 seconds. Inhale and release the leg. Repeat on the left.

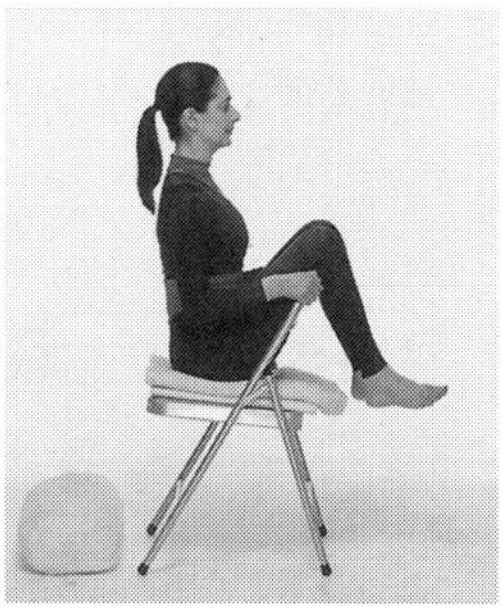
1

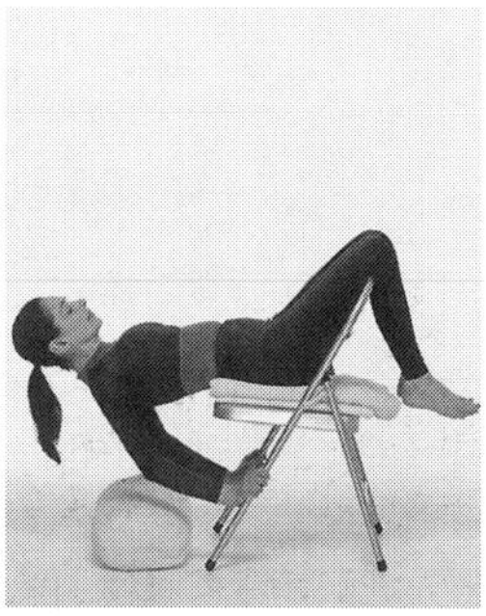
2

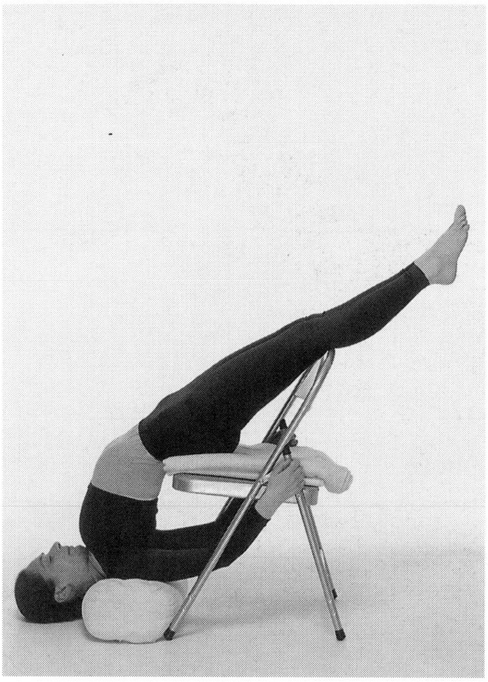
3

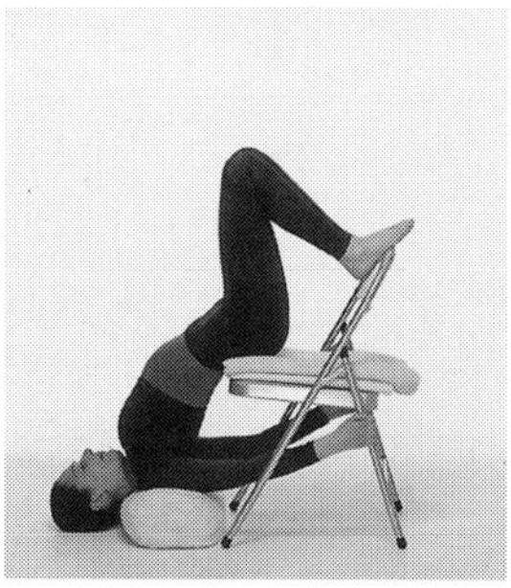
4

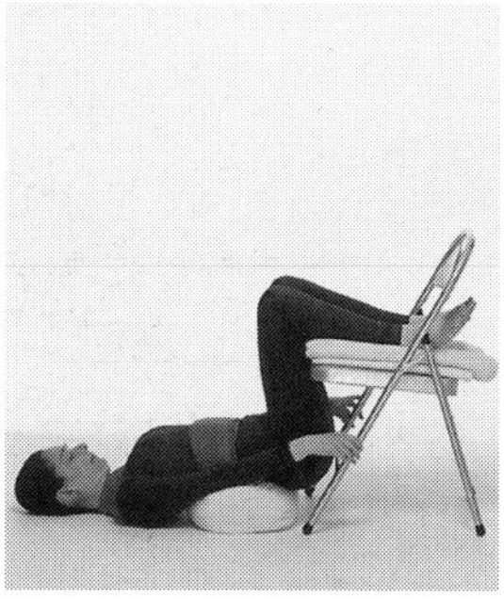
5

सर्वाङ्गासन

Sarvāṅgāsana Shoulder Balance (on chair)

Method

Place a mat and blanket on a sturdy chair. Place a bolster or folded blankets lengthwise on the floor in front of it. Sit backwards on the chair and take the legs over the back rest of the chair. Move the buttocks nearer to the back (1).

Lean back so that the waist can curve over the front edge of the seat. **While going down hold firmly onto the front legs or seat of the chair (2).**

Curving the waist over the front of the seat, lower the trunk towards the floor and rest the shoulders on the bolster. Rest the head on the floor. Keep the lower back securely on the seat of the chair. Take the arms inside the legs of the chair and hold the back legs of the chair. Straighten the legs against the back rest of the chair. Take the shoulders back and lift the chest, pressing the shoulder blades in (3).

Stay for 3 to 5 minutes. To come down, bend the legs and rest the feet on the back of the chair (4).

Ease the sacrum (lower back) off the chair onto the bolster, at the same time releasing the hands and holding the front legs. (Or, slide the chair a little away and come down [5].)

Note

Adjustments to the Pose

If the head feels heavy, place a folded blanket beneath it to raise it.

If the chair back cuts into the legs, place a blanket over it.

If it is strenuous for the back, place the chair about 1 to 1½ feet way from the wall so that the feet can rest on the wall with the legs in a more upright position.

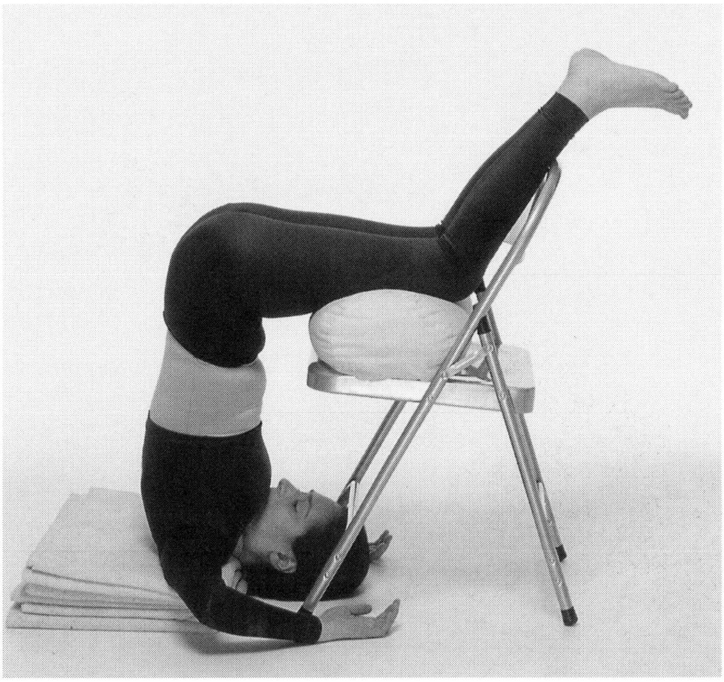

1

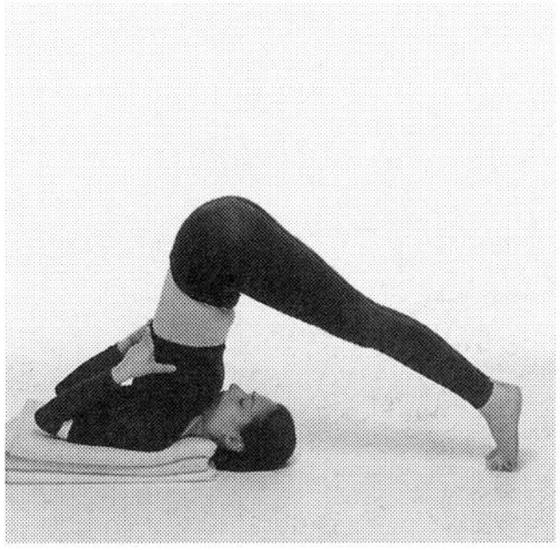

2

अर्ध-कर्णपीडनासन

Ardha-Karṇapīḍanāsana Half Pressing-the-Ear Pose

ardha = half; karṇa = ear; pīḍana = pressing, pressure, restriction

Method

Place three or four folded blankets on the floor with the neat edges together. Place a chair in front of them with a bolster or blankets on the seat. Lie down with the shoulders on and the head off the blankets. Exhale, bend the knees over the abdomen and swing them up and onto the chair (see *Ardha-Halāsana* on page 85). Pull the chair over the head. Rest the thighs on the bolster and the shins on the back of the chair. Take the arms over the head and relax them (1).

Stay for 2 to 5 minutes. Come down carefully, pushing the chair away.

Alternative for well-practised students – *Halāsana* Plough Pose

Method

Place three or four folded blankets on the floor with the neat edges together. Lie down in a straight line with the shoulders on and the head off the blankets. With the arms behind the back, place a belt around the upper arms just above the elbows to keep the elbows in. Exhale, bend the knees over the abdomen and swing them over the head to the floor. Straighten the knees. Place the hands on the back and lift the trunk and hips (2).

Stay for 2 to 5 minutes. Bend the legs and slide down carefully.

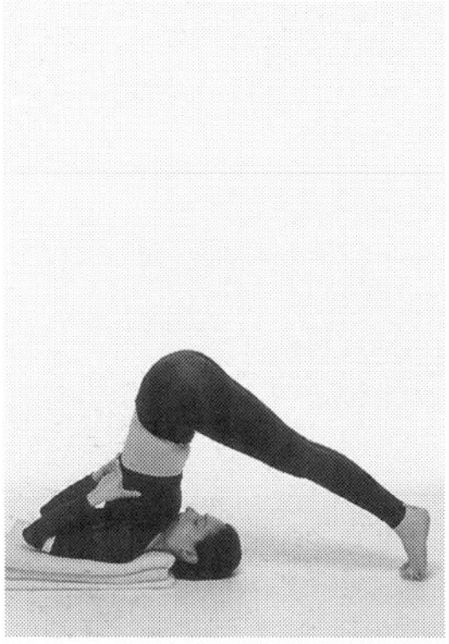

1

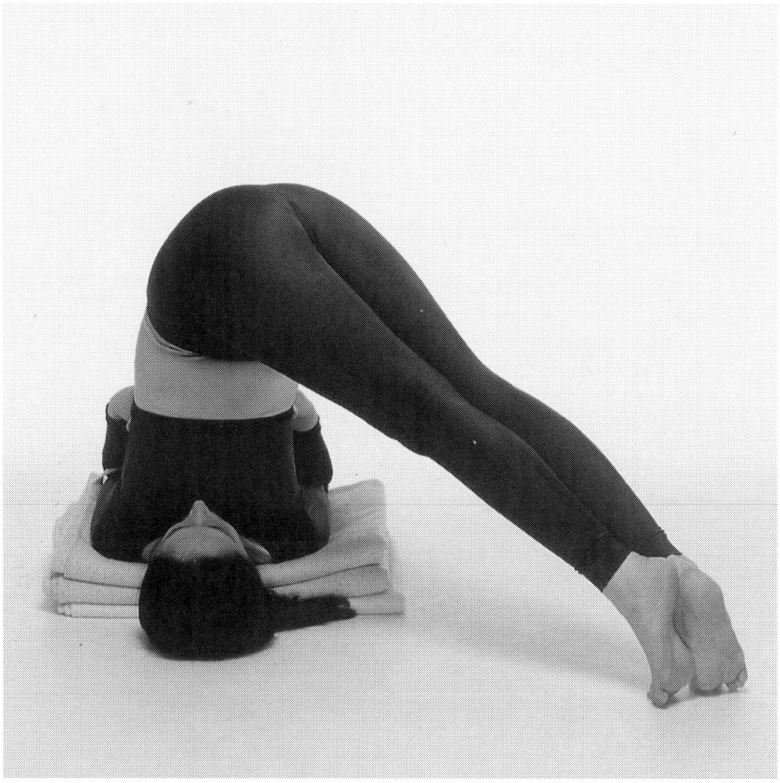

2

पार्श्व-हलासन

Pārśva-Halāsana Lateral Plough Pose

pārśva = side; hala = plough

Method

Be in *Halāsana* (1). Exhale and walk the feet to the right. Keep the trunk upright and the hips lifted. Bring the right side of the trunk forward (2).

Stay for 20 to 30 seconds. Come to the centre. Repeat on the left.

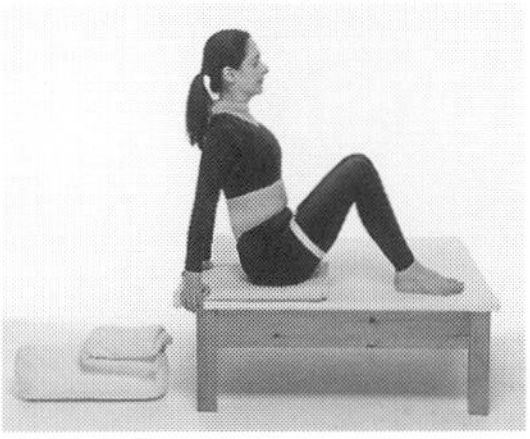

1

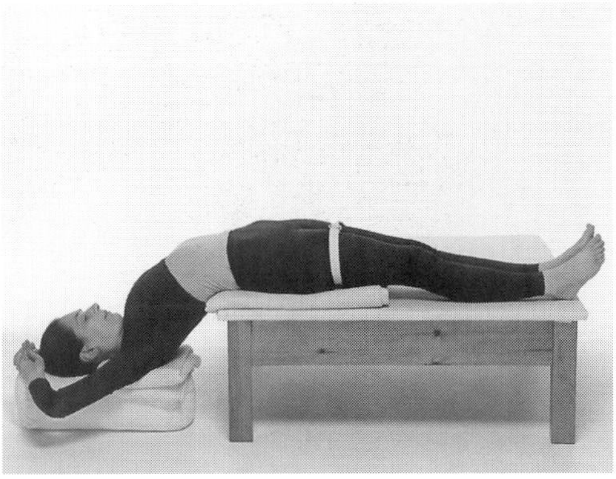

3

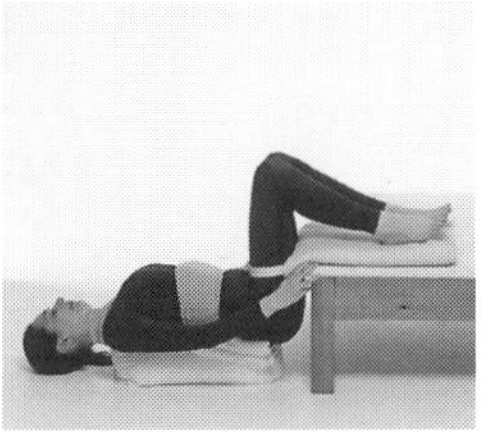

4

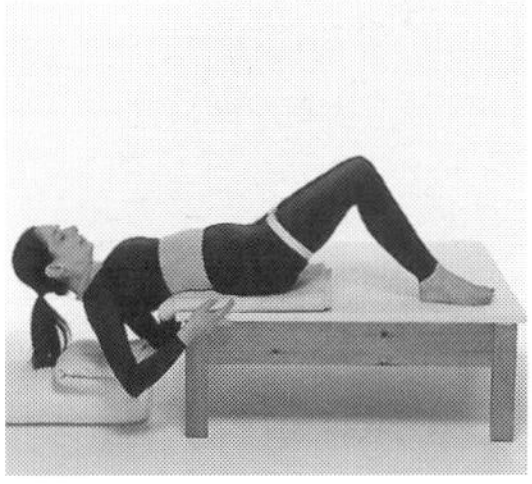

2

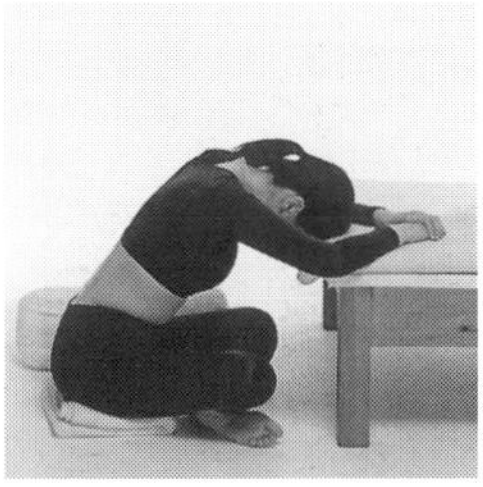

5

सेतुबन्ध-सर्वाङ्गासनासन

Setubandha-Sarvāṅgāsana Shoulder Balance Bridge (on bench)

setu = bridge; bandha = bound; sarva = all, entire; aṅga = body, limb

Place a bolster lengthwise in front of a bench, low table or bed. Place a folded blanket on the bench end of the bolster, with the neat edge away from the bench. Place a folded blanket on the bench, reaching to the edge. Sit on the bench a little away from the edge. For more comfort in the pose, tie the legs together at the mid-thigh with a belt (1).

Holding onto the bench firmly, lean back so that the waist curves over the edge (2).

Lower the trunk down so that the shoulders rest on the folded blanket and the head on the bolster. Stretch out the legs. Lift and open the chest. Take the arms over the head. Relax (3).

Stay for 5 minutes or longer. To come down, bend the knees and hold the bench. Slide backwards carefully till the lower back rests on the bolster (4).

Turn to the side, sit in simple cross-legs or on the heels and bend forwards, resting the forehead on the bench. Stay till the back is eased (5).

Note

For back pain

If the back hurts, raise the feet onto a support, decrease the drop between the bench and bolster by adding more blankets.

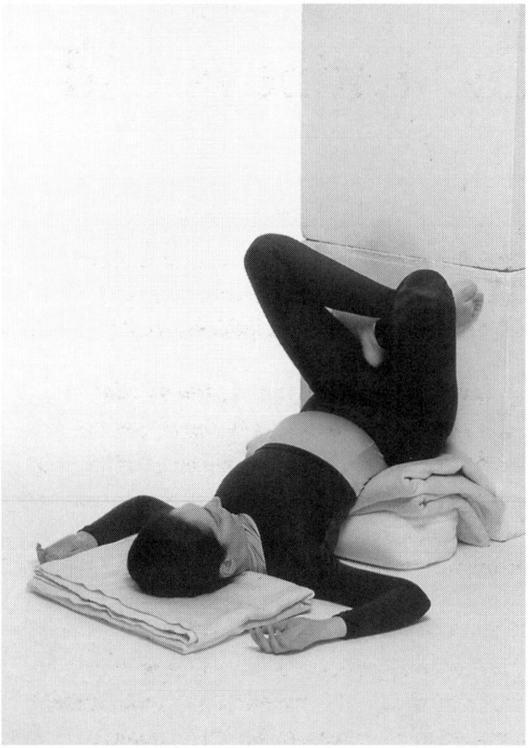

विपरीत-करणी मुद्रा

Viparīta-Karaṇī Mudrā Reverse Action Position

viparīta = inverted, reverse; karaṇī = practice, action; mudrā = position

Method

Place a bolster lengthwise a little away from the wall with a blanket on top. Sit sideways on it. Lean backwards, simultaneously turning the body to be perpendicular to the wall. (See the method given for *Ūrdhva-Prasārita-Pādāsana* on page 61.) Lie down with the lower back on the bolster and the shoulders on the floor. Keep the buttocks against the wall. Place a blanket under the head. Bend the legs into simple cross-legs and take the arms over the head. Relax.

Stay for 5 minutes or longer. Change the cross-legs. To come down, slide backwards, and turn to the side.

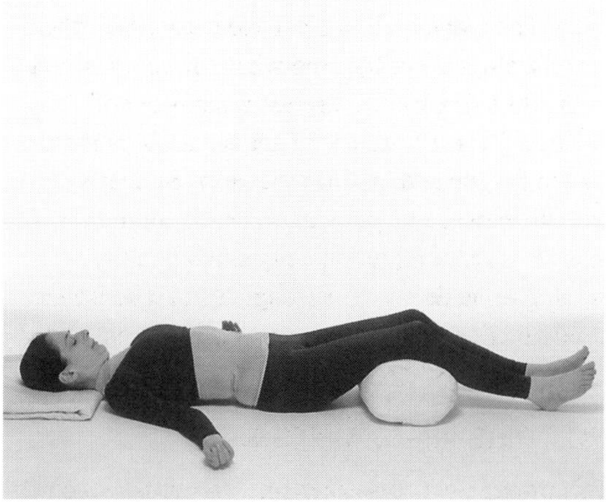

शवासन

Śavāsana Corpse Pose

Method

Lie down in a straight line with a bolster under the knees. This allows the abdomen to stay soft and relaxed. Place a folded blanket under the head and neck. Lengthen and then relax the arms and legs. Close the eyes.

The Abdominal Organs: Kidneys and Bladder

The Urinary System

An efficient system of elimination keeps the body fresh. The kidneys filter fluid and waste. The filters become sluggish or blocked when the composition of the fluid that passes through them is out of balance. Over time the constant demands on them lead to fatigue and loss of efficiency. Similarly, with the passage of years the elasticity of the bladder is reduced; its capacity and reliability of holding urine decrease. Through Yoga practice the good functioning of these organs is maintained.

HOW THE *ĀSANAS* WORK

This programme consists mainly of twists, which increase mobility (*vāta*) and physiological energy (*pitta*). They are followed by groin-opening poses which further increase *pitta* while at the same time decompressing *vāta* to balance it and reducing *kapha* by creating lightness. Inverted poses continue to increase *pitta* and to balance *vāta*; the final relaxation quietens *pitta* and brings calmness to *vāta*.

Twists (*kapha* –, *pitta* +, *vāta* +)

Twists are the key poses which activate the kidneys. In the lateral turn of the trunk the kidneys are squeezed; the release of the squeeze after returning to the centre flushes them with blood. Repeated irrigation in this way keeps the kidneys healthy.

Groin-opening Poses (*kapha* –, *pitta* +, *vāta* =)

Baddhakoṇāsana and *Upaviṣṭakoṇāsana* keep the bladder in good shape. The spreading apart of the legs and relaxing of the groin area creates space in the lower abdomen and lifts and tones the muscles supporting the bladder.

Inverted Poses (*kapha* –, *pitta* +, *vāta* =)

These are especially effective when done with the groin-opening poses. The inversions relax the whole abdomen and relieve pressure felt in the organs when the body is upright.

Relaxation (*kapha* +, *pitta* –, *vāta* =)

In relaxation the organs rest as much as the physical structure, especially when they have previously been deliberately activated.

Props

Wall, chair, bench, bolster, blankets, brick

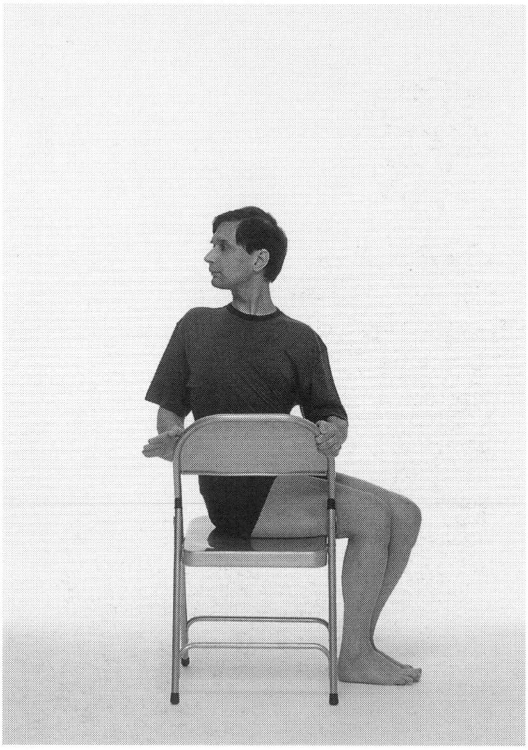

थरद्वाजासन

Bharadvājāsana
Bharadvāja's Pose (on chair)

Method

Sit sideways on a chair with the right side facing the back. Keep the feet together, the trunk up. Hold the back rest of the chair. Exhale and turn to the right. Turn the head and neck. Take the shoulders back, lift the chest and press the back ribs and the kidneys in. Breathe evenly and relax the face.

Stay for 20 to 30 seconds. Inhale and come to the centre. Repeat on the left.

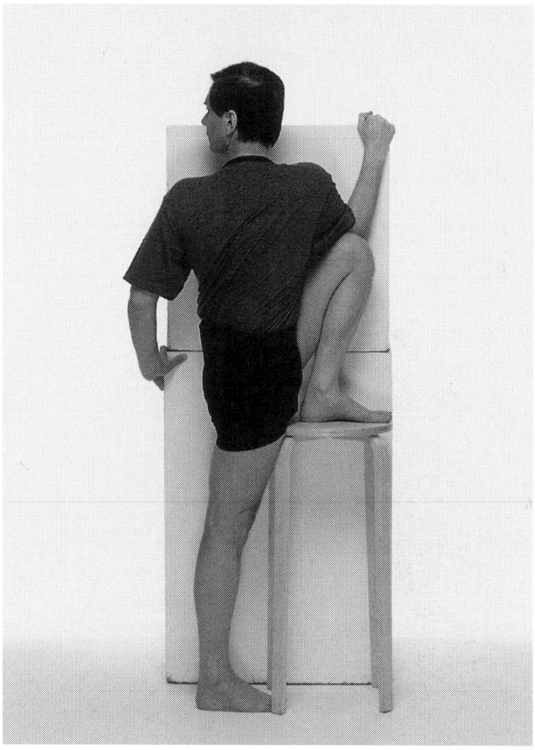

उत्थित-मरीच्यासन

Utthita-Marīcyāsana
Marīci's Pose (standing)

Method

Place a high stool against a wall with a ledge. Stand in *Tāḍāsana* in front of the stool with the right side against the wall. Place the right foot on the stool, with the knee pointing upwards and the hip and thigh resting against the wall. Keep the left leg vertical and stretching up strongly.

Exhale and turn towards the wall, holding onto the ledge. Press the left hip in. Turn the head and neck. Relax the face and breathe normally.

Stay for 20 to 30 seconds. Inhale and come to the centre. Repeat on the left.

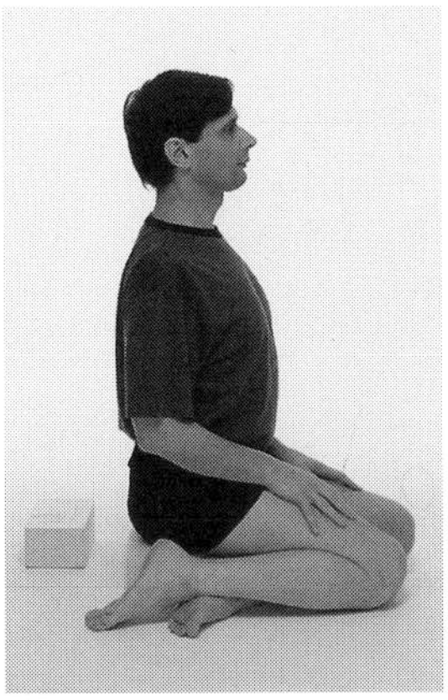

1

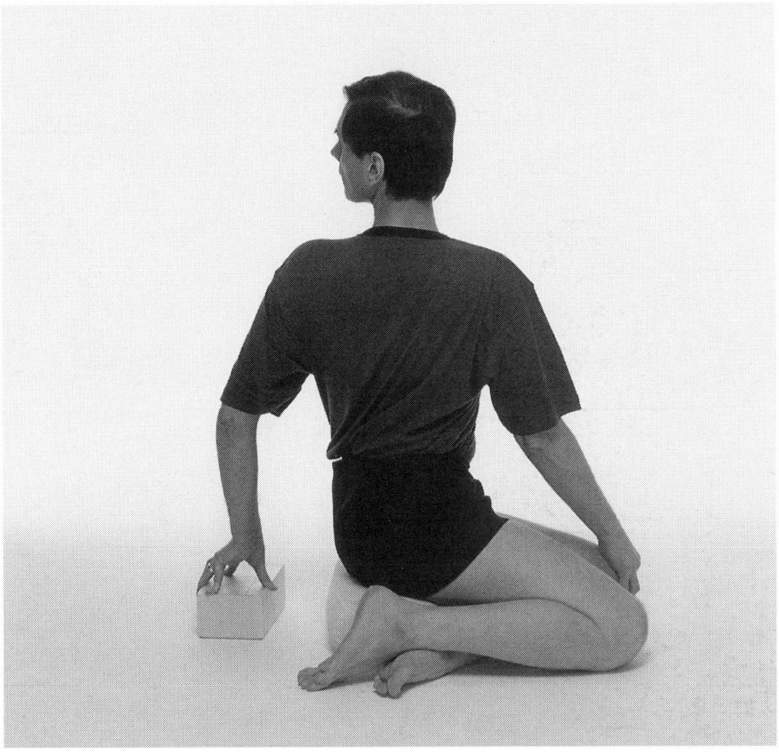

2

थरद्वाजासन

Bharadvājāsana Bharadvāja's Pose

Method

Sit on two folded blankets with the legs stretched out in front. Bend the knees and take the legs to the left, feet beside the left hip. Place the right foot on top of the left arch. Place the hands on the thighs and sit erect (1).

Turn to the right, placing the left hand on the right knee and the right hand on a brick placed behind the back. Draw the left thigh back into the socket and press it down. Exhale and turn the whole trunk strongly from the hips, using the leverage of the arms. Lift the chest, roll the shoulders back and press the back ribs and kidneys in. Breathe evenly and relax the face (2).

Stay for 20 to 30 seconds. Inhale and come to the centre.

Repeat on the left.

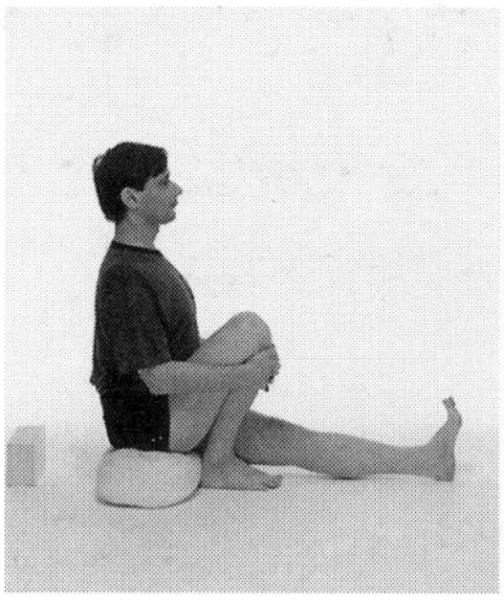

1

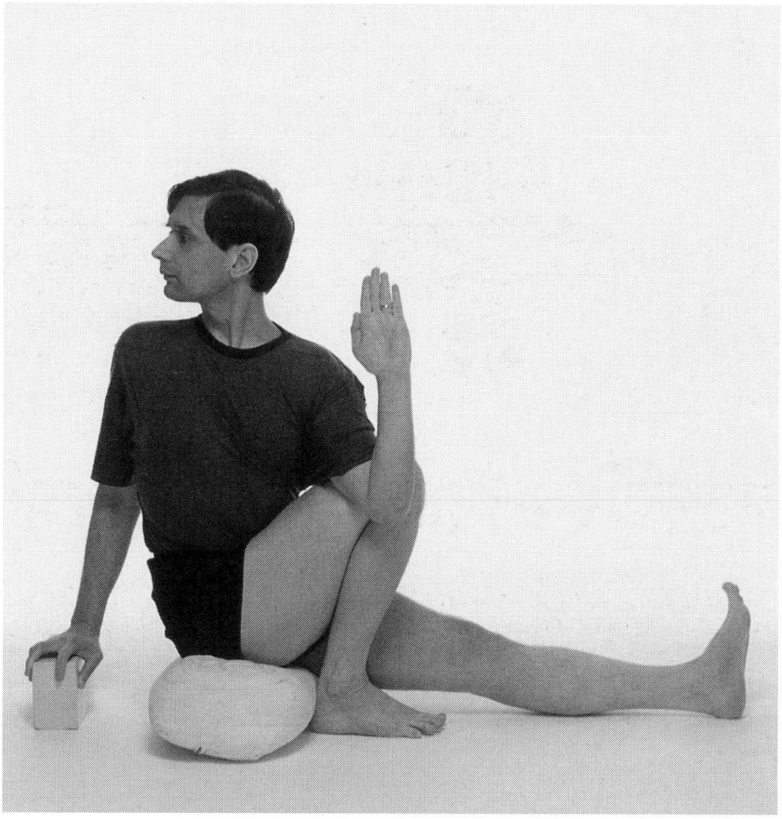

2

मरीच्यासन

Marīcyāsana Marīci's Pose

Method

Sit on a bolster with the legs stretched out in front. Lift the trunk. Bend the right knee and bring the foot towards the thigh. Let it touch the bolster and the left thigh. Hold the shin and stretch up (1).

Turn to the right, bend the left elbow and hook the arm against the outer right thigh. Keep the forearm vertical and the left hand facing away. Place the right hand on a brick behind the back. Lift the trunk. Exhale and turn further to the right. Roll the shoulders back. Press the back ribs and kidneys in, to make the back concave. Turn the head and neck. Breathe evenly and stay relaxed (2).

Stay for 20 to 30 seconds. Inhale, release the arm and come to the centre. Repeat on the left.

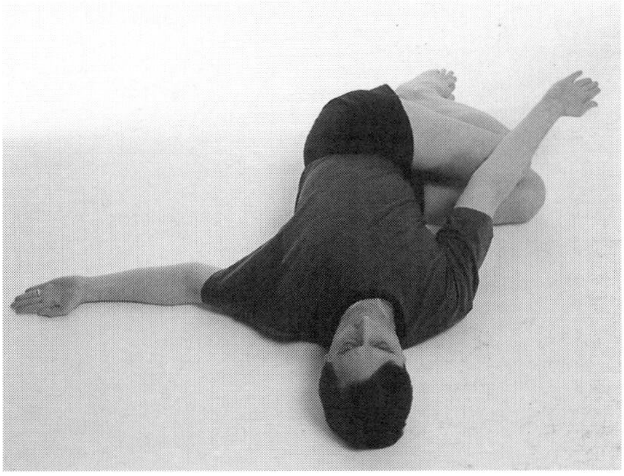

जठरपरिवर्तनासन १

Jaṭhara-Parivartanāsana I
Stomach Rolling Pose I

jaṭhara = stomach, abdomen; parivartana = revolving

Method

Lie on the floor in a straight line. Extend the arms sideways in line with the shoulders, keeping the shoulders down and shoulder blades in. Turn the palms to face up. Bend the knees over the abdomen.

Exhale and take the legs down to the right, at the same time revolving the abdomen to the left. Press the back of the right arm against the left thigh to increase the turn. Keep the head straight.

Stay for 20 to 30 seconds. Inhale, release the arm and come to the centre. Repeat on the left.

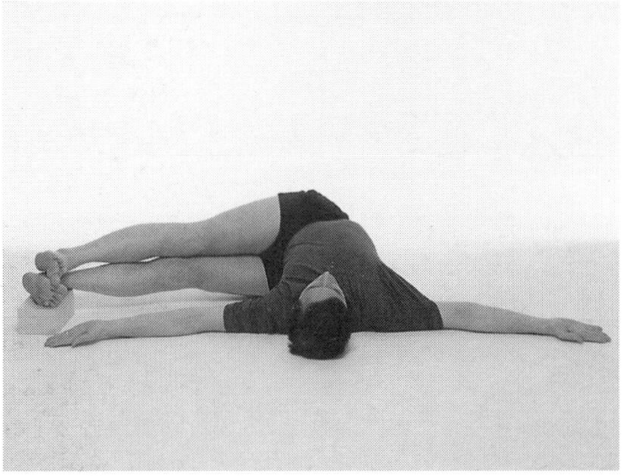

जठरपरिवर्तनासन २

Jaṭhara-Parivartanāsana II
Stomach Rolling Pose II

Method

Lie on the floor in a straight line. Extend the arms sideways in line with the shoulders, keeping the shoulders down and shoulder blades in. Turn the palms to face up. Bend the knees over the abdomen, then raise them vertically up. Straighten the knees.

Exhale and take the legs down to the right, towards the right shoulder. At the same time revolve the abdomen to the left. Press the left hip down to stop the lower trunk rolling to the side. Rest the feet on a brick or higher support. Keep the legs straight. Press the left shoulder down. Keep the head straight. Do not hold the breath.

Alternatively, rest the feet against the wall.

Stay for 20 to 30 seconds. Inhale, raise the legs and come to the centre. Repeat on the left.

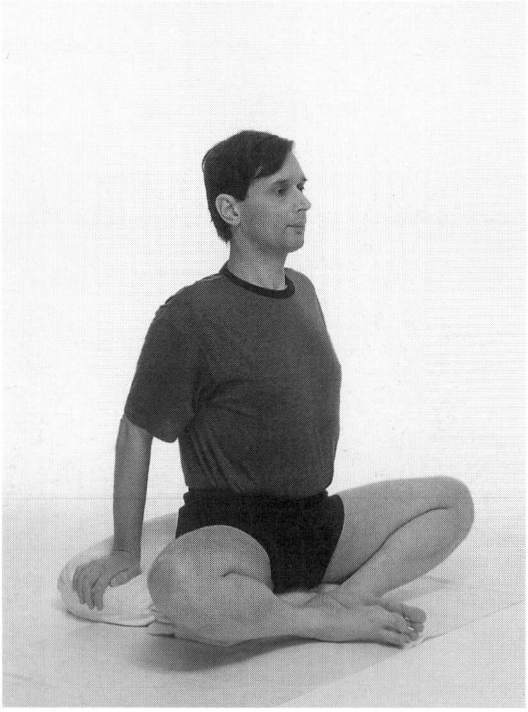

बद्धकोणासन

Baddhakoṇāsana Cobbler's Pose

baddha = bound; koṇa = angle

Method

Sit on a bolster with the legs stretched out in front. Bend the knees outwards and join the soles of the feet. Draw the feet close to the body. Place the hands on the bolster and stretch the trunk up. Take the shoulders down and back and lift the chest.

Stay for 30 seconds to 1 minute. Release the legs.

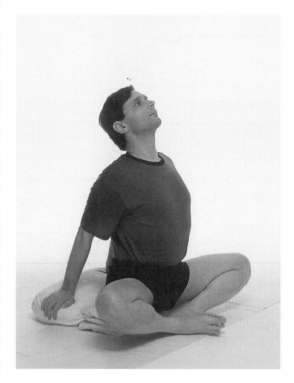

बद्धकोणासन

Baddhakoṇāsana Cobbler's Pose (concave)

Method

Sit in *Baddhakoṇāsana* . Extend the sides of the trunk, exhale and curve the trunk backwards. Press the back ribs and kidneys in. Take the head back and look up. Keep the eyes relaxed.

Stay for 30 seconds to 1 minute. Inhale and bring the trunk and head upright. Release the legs.

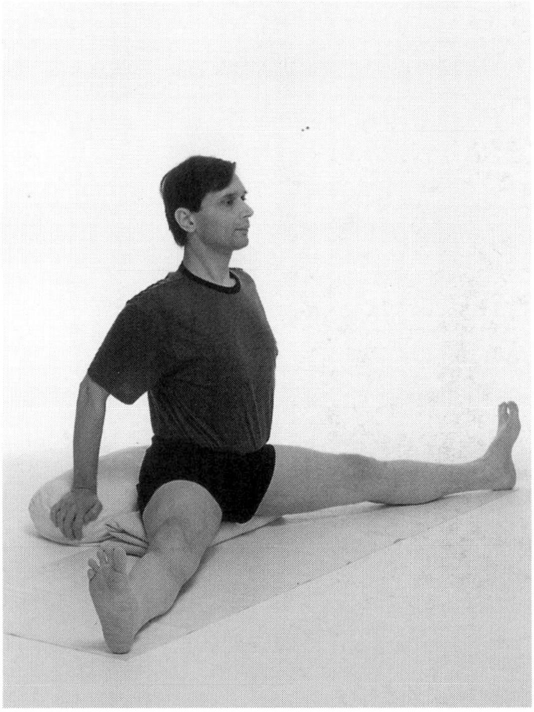

उपविष्टकोणासन

Upaviṣṭakoṇāsana Seated Angle Pose

upaviṣṭa = seated; koṇa = angle

Method

Sit on a bolster with the legs stretched out in front. Spread the legs to the sides, with the fronts of the legs facing up. Keep the knees straight and stretch the legs, feet and toes. Holding the bolster, take the shoulders back and extend the trunk upwards.

Stay for 30 seconds to 1 minute. Slowly bring the legs together.

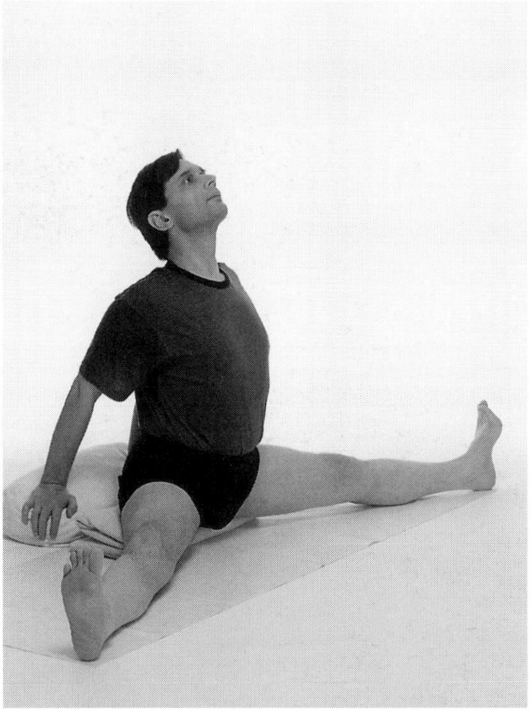

उपविष्टकोणासन

Upaviṣṭakoṇāsana Seated Angle Pose (concave)

Method

Sit in *Upaviṣṭakoṇāsana*. Lift the sides of the trunk, exhale and curve the trunk backwards. Press the back ribs and kidneys in. Take the head back and look up.

Stay for 30 seconds to 1 minute. Inhale and bring the trunk and head upright. Bring the legs together.

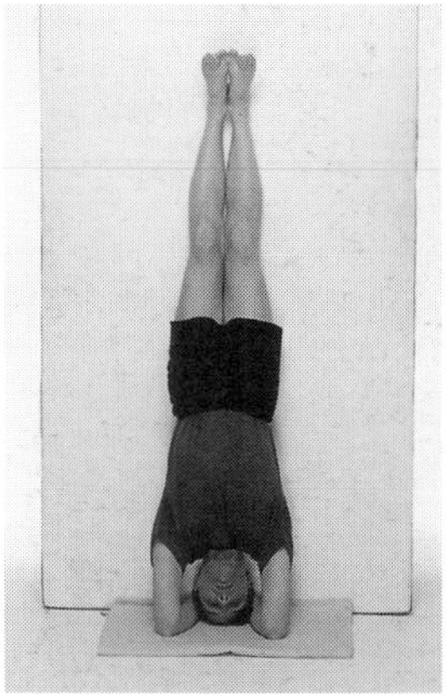
1

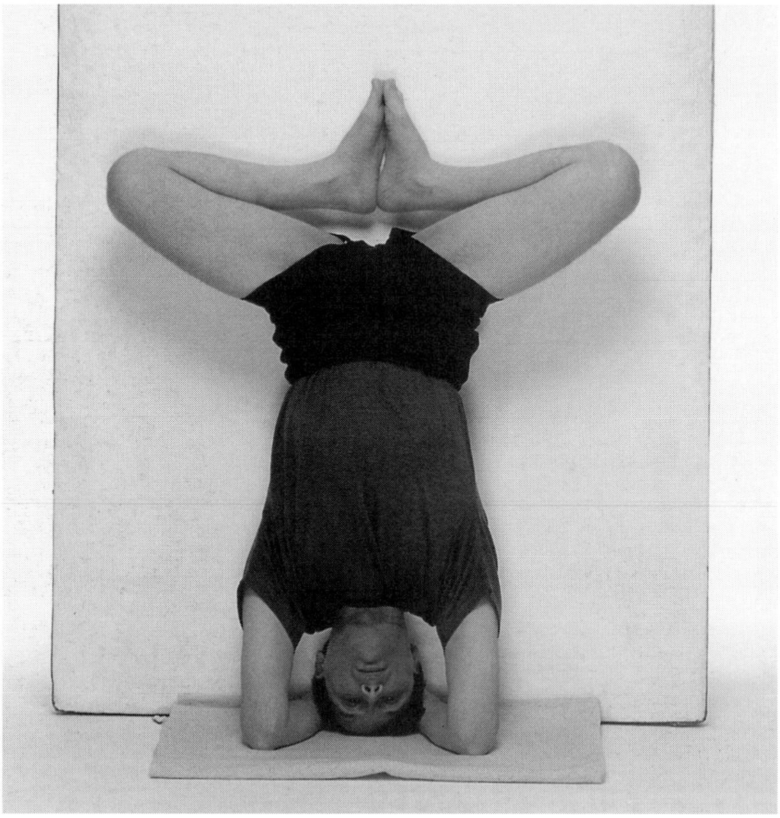
2

शीर्षासन स-बद्धकोणासन

Śīrṣāsana with Baddhakoṇāsana Head Balance with Cobbler's Pose

sa- = with

Method

Place a folded blanket against the wall, the neat edge inwards. Go up into *Śīrṣāsana*, following the method given on pages 100–101 (1). Stay for a minute or so.

Exhale, bend the knees outwards and join the soles of the feet. Bring the feet as close to the trunk as possible, resting them on the wall. Press the knees back. Lift the shoulders and hips (2).

Stay for 30 seconds to 1 minute. Inhale and straighten the legs. Stay in *Śīrṣāsana* a little longer or exhale and come down.

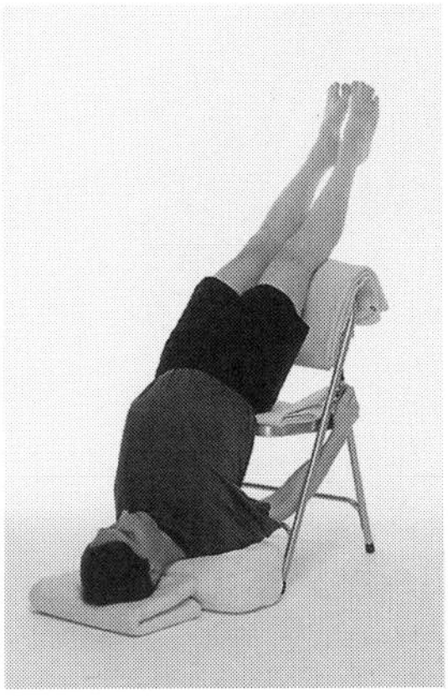

1

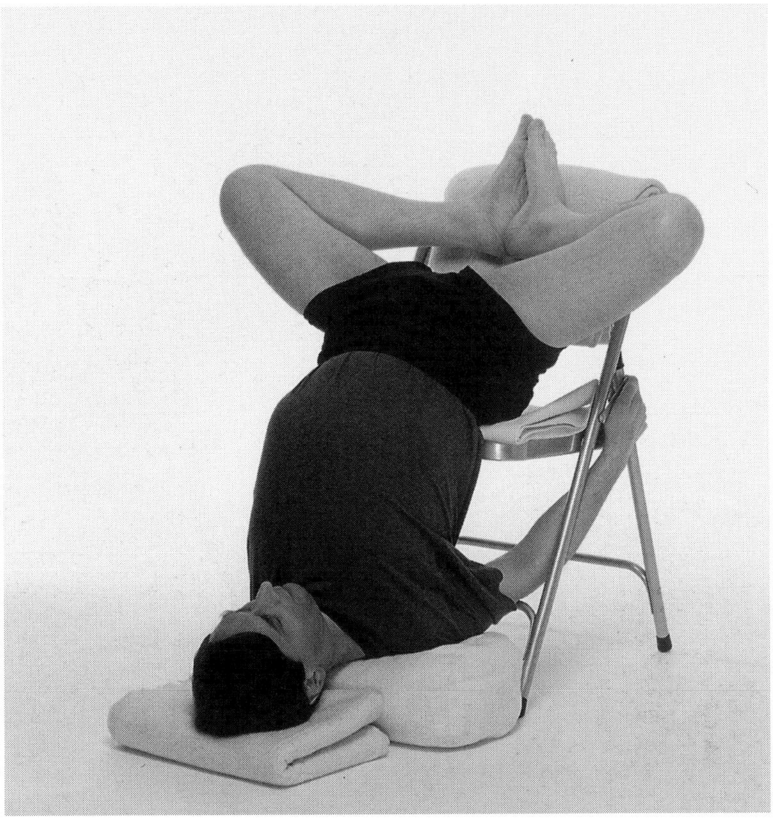

2

सर्वाङ्गासन स-बद्धकोणासन

Sarvāṇgāsana with Baddhakoṇāsana Shoulder Balance with Cobbler's Pose (on chair)

Method

Do *Sarvāṇgāsana* with a chair, following the method given on page 93. Before going into the pose place a blanket on the chair back. Stay for a few minutes (1).

Bend the knees outwards and join the soles of the feet. Rest the feet on the chair back (2).

Stay for 1 minute or longer. Straighten the legs. Stay in *Sarvāṇgāsana* a little longer or exhale and come down.

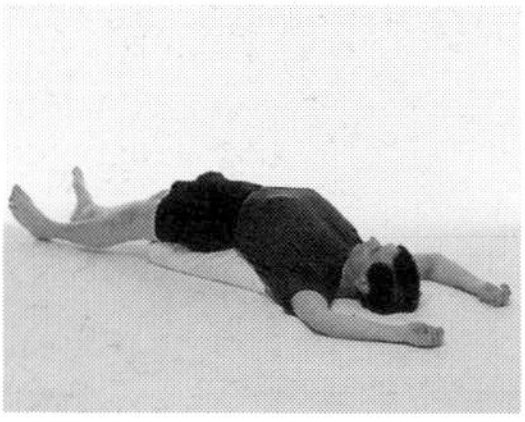

1

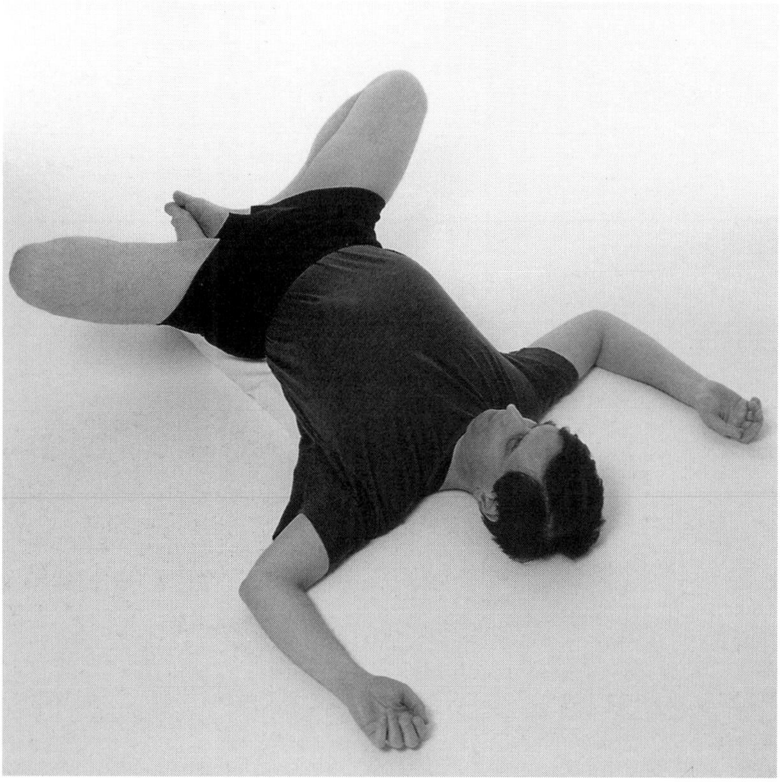

2

सेतुबन्ध-सर्वाङ्गासन स-बद्धकोणासन

Setubandha-Sarvāṅgāsana with *Baddhakoṇāsana* Shoulder Balance Bridge with Cobbler's Pose

sa- = with

Method

Place a bolster on the floor and sit on the narrow end of the bolster.

Lie back so that the waist curves over the other end and the shoulders and head rest on the floor. Stretch out the legs and take the arms over the head. Relax the arms and legs. Stay for a few minutes (1). Bend the knees outwards and join the soles of the feet. Bring the feet close to the body and rest them on the bolster (2).

Stay for 1 minute or longer. Straighten the legs. Stay in *Setubandha-Sarvāṅgāsana* a little longer or exhale and slide backwards to come down. Sit in simple cross-legs, or kneel, and bend forward, resting the head on the bolster.

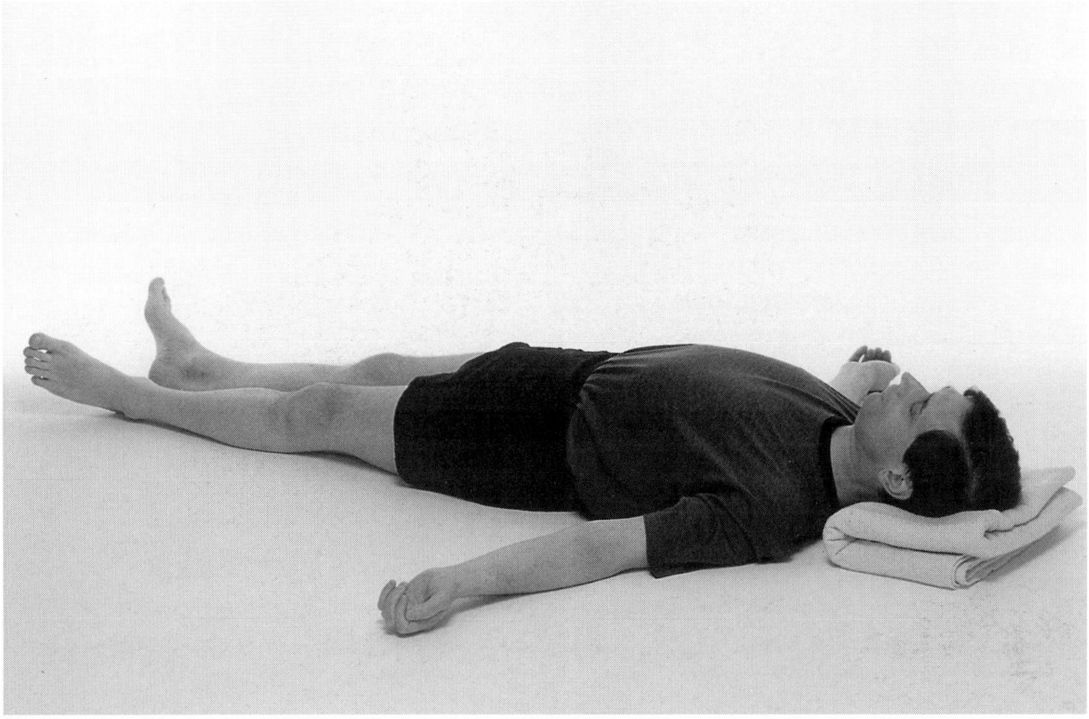

शवासन

Śavāsana Corpse Pose

Method

Lie on the back in a straight line. Place a folded blanket under the head and neck. Stretch the legs and arms before relaxing them. Close the eyes and let go completely.

Stay for 5 minutes or longer. Open the eyes gently, turn to the side and get up.

The Lungs and Heart

The Respiratory System

The air taken into the body becomes the life-breath (*prāṇa*). The mechanism of breathing determines the quantity and quality of breath, and thereby the quality of life. The natural capacity of the lungs is considerable, as is evidenced by the vocal power of babies and children. With age the upper ribs become narrow and the top lungs are used less and less. Air pollution is another hazard. Yoga practice encourages the rib cage and lungs to open well and restores the facility of breathing deeply. Weak and diseased lungs become stronger.

The Cardiovascular System

The heart is the sustainer of all the body's activities and is never allowed any respite. In order to remain unflagging it has to be free from pressure from the structures that surround it. When the thoracic spine supports the sternum (breast bone) in a lifted position, and the back ribs support the front ribs by a slight concave action, the heart has plenty of space to function. When the sternum and rib cage collapse inwards the heart area is constricted. Yoga practice gives space to the heart and alleviates pressure and pain even where there is the additional problem of the thickening of arteries due to faulty diet and lifestyle. With continued practice the heart becomes strengthened.

HOW THE *ĀSANAS* WORK

This programme consists mainly of supported supine poses and backbends that help to expand the chest area. *Pitta*, i.e. physiological energy, is increased and *vāta* is channelled and increased. Supported inverted poses continue the optimization of *vāta*, restoring its proper function. Supported relaxation promotes the same efficiency of respiration.

Supine Poses (*kapha* +, *pitta* +, *vāta* =)

The supine poses are done with a high support under the chest. This creates freedom in the heart region, removing stress. The heart is able to perform its function restfully.

Backbends (*kapha* –, *pitta* +, *vāta* +)

Supported backbends expand the chest and heart area further. The length of time in these positions gives sustained relief from stress.

Inverted Poses (*kapha* –, *pitta* +, *vāta* =)

Inverted poses alter the direction of the body and give relief from the pressure of gravity. The chest expands, giving space to the heart region.

Relaxation (*kapha* +, *pitta* –, *vāta* =)

With the chest comfortable on a high support strain is removed.

Props

Table, chair, stool, bench, bolster, blankets, belt

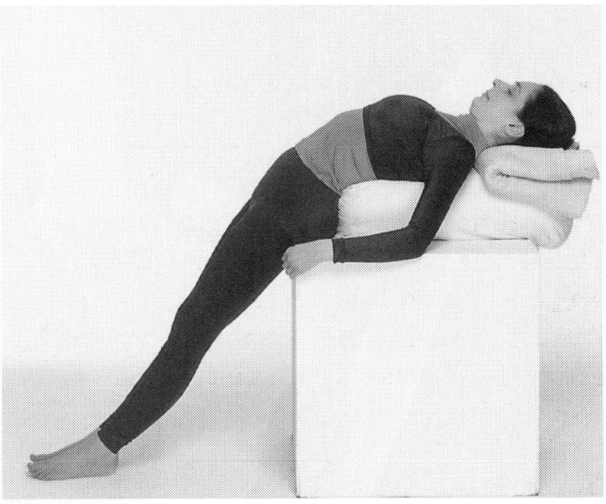

पूर्वोत्तासन १

Pūrvottānāsana I Anterior Stretching Pose I (on table)

pūrva = anterior, east; uttāna = stretching

Method

Place a bolster on a low table or high bed, with its narrow end a few inches from the edge. Place a folded blanket on top of the bolster at its far end. Sit in front of the bolster and lie back on it. Rest the head on the blanket. Stretch out the legs. Rest the arms beside the bolster.

Stay for 2 to 5 minutes. Bend the knees and turn to the side to get up.

Note

Adjusting the Props

Depending on the height of the table, more support may be required. Use a second bolster or folded blankets. The pose should be very comfortable and the chest able to open well.

Comfort in the Poses

These poses should be comfortable, so that it is possible to stay in them for some time. Different body shapes require different heights and numbers of bolsters and blankets. Experiment to get the best support. As a general rule, if part of the body feels strain, more support is needed.

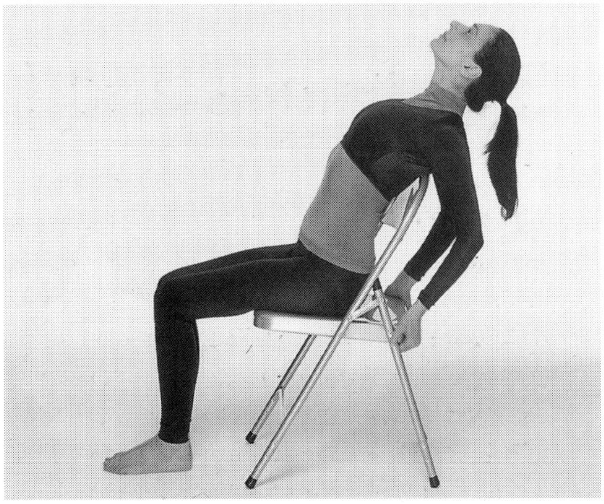

पूर्वोत्तानासन २

Pūrvottānāsana II Anterior Stretching Pose II

Method

Sit on a chair and stretch up. Exhale and lean back, curving the upper trunk over the chair back. For comfort, place a blanket over the back of a chair. Take the arms behind the chair and catch the seat. Take the head back.

Stay for 30 seconds to 1 minute. To stay longer, rest the head on the wall. Inhale and come up.

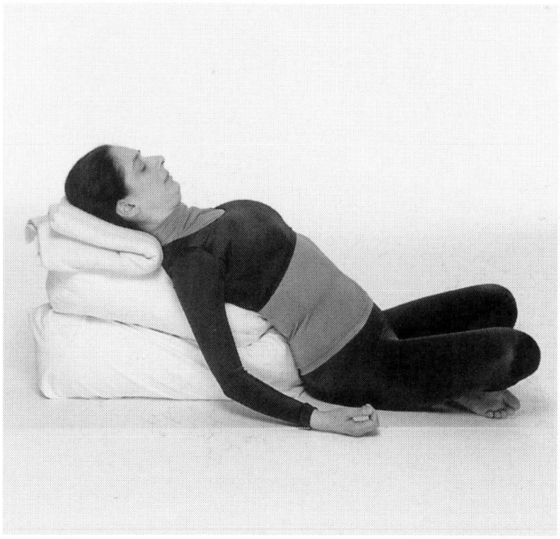

मत्स्यासन

Matsyāsana Fish Pose (simple)

Method

Place two bolsters on the floor, one on top of the other, with the end of the top bolster a few inches behind the end of the first. Sit in front of the bolsters in simple cross-legs. Hold the bolsters and lie back on them. The lumbar should rest on the lower bolster. Support the head with one or more folded blankets. Let the arms relax at the sides of the trunk.

Stay for 5 minutes or longer. Come up and change the cross-legs. Repeat on the other side.

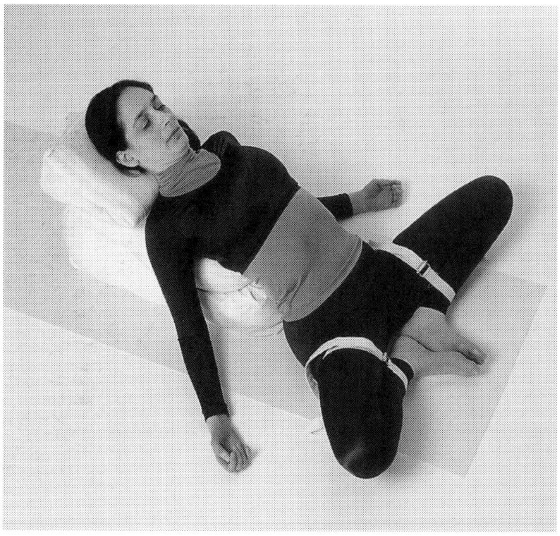

सुप्त-बद्धकोणासन

Supta-Baddhakoṇāsana Supine Cobbler's Pose

Method

Arrange two bolsters as above, one on top of the other. Sit on the lower bolster, bend the knees and bring the soles of the feet together. Draw the feet close to the body. Pass a belt around the lower back, over the thighs and under the ankles and feet, then tie it tightly to keep the thighs and calves together. Slide down off the bolster onto the floor. Then lie back on the bolsters. Support the head and neck with a folded blanket. Rest the arms to the sides.

Stay for 5 minutes or longer. Come up and untie the belt.

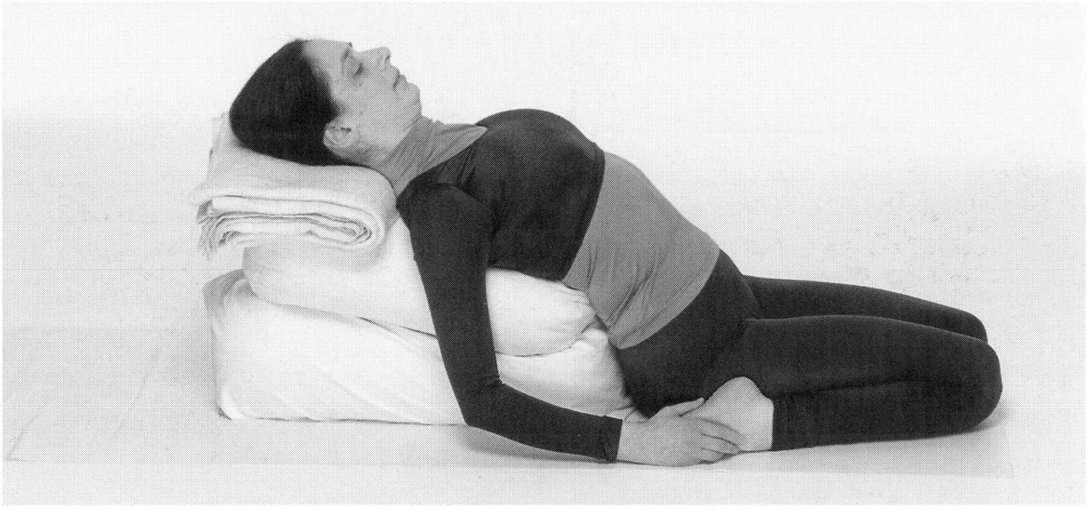

सुप्त-वीरासन

Supta-Vīrāsana Supine Hero Pose

Method

Arrange two bolsters as above, one on top of the other. Sit on the lower bolster and bend the legs back, with the feet on either side of the hips. (This is *Vīrāsana* – see page 60). Lie back, supporting the head and resting the arms beside the trunk. Use more height if necessary to make the pose comfortable.

Stay for 5 minutes or longer. Come up. Bend forward in *Adhomukha-Vīrāsana* with the toes together and knees apart.

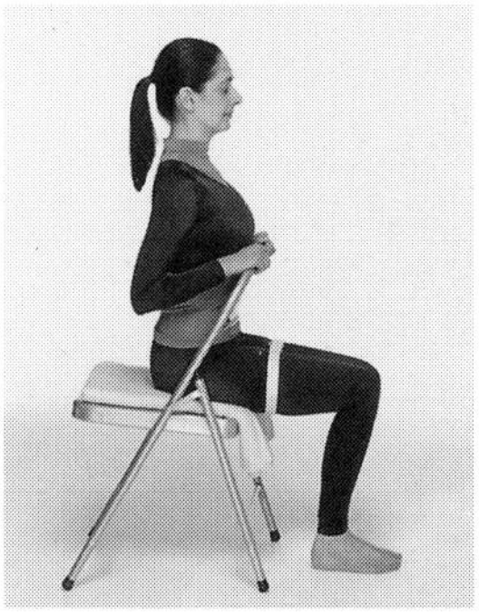

1

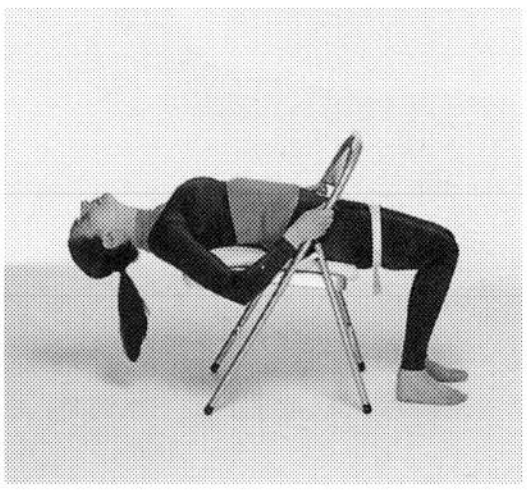

2

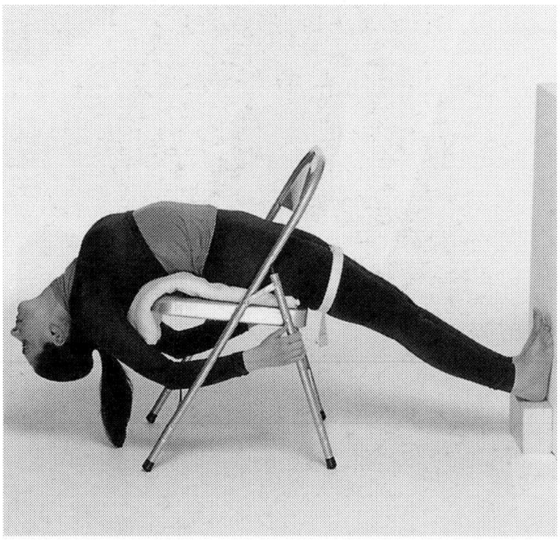

3

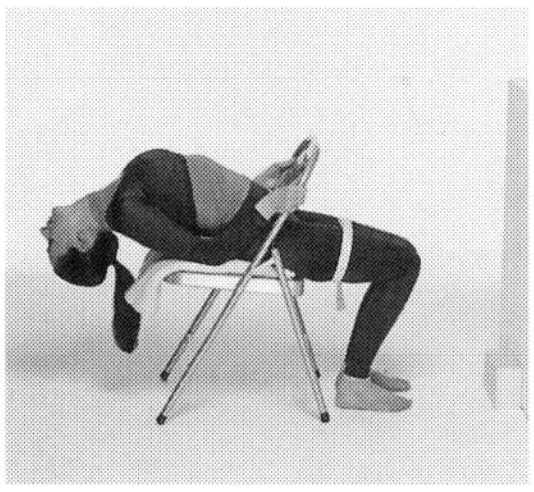

4

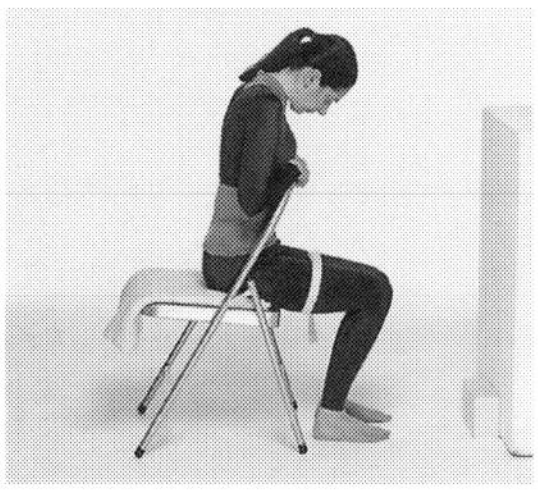

5

विपरीत-दण्डासन

Viparīta-Daṇḍāsana Inverted Staff Pose

Method

Place a chair 2 to 2½ feet way from the wall, with a mat and blanket on the seat. Place a brick against the wall centred with the chair. Sit backwards on the chair, inserting the legs in the gap between the seat and the back rest. Move as close to the back edge as possible. Tie a belt around the mid-thighs. Hold the chair back and sit straight (1).

Still holding the chair, exhale and curve back over the seat so that the back ribs touch the edge (2). Rest the back on the seat of the chair. Straighten the legs, raising the feet onto the brick. Take the arms inside the legs of the chair and hold the back legs. Relax the head (3).

Stay for 1 to 2 minutes. Breathe evenly. To come up, bend the legs and hold the chair at the top. Swing the trunk up, keeping it concave. Come up with the chest first, not the head (4).

Rest the trunk on the back of the chair (5).

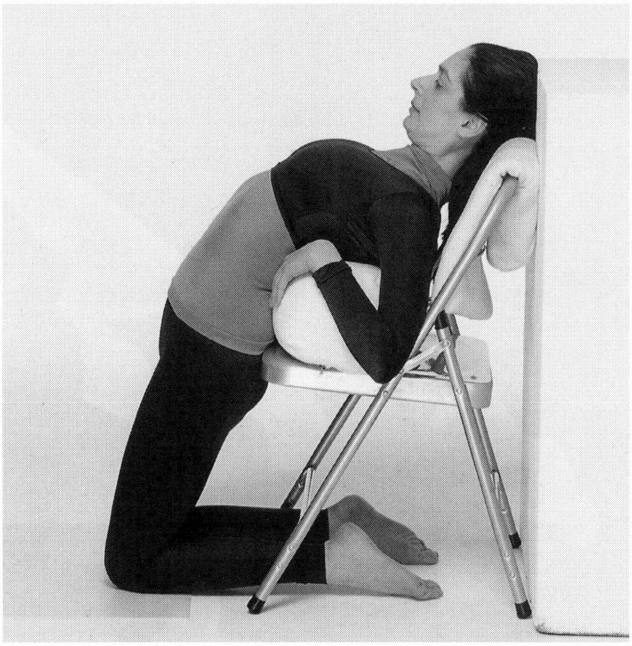

उष्ट्रासन

Uṣṭrāsana Camel Pose

Method

Place a chair against the wall. Place a bolster on the seat and a blanket on the back rest. Place a mat under the chair. Kneel with the back to the chair, taking the shins under the seat. Keep the knees and feet a little apart. Hold the bolster firmly against the lower back. Exhale, move the sacrum and coccyx (tailbone) forward and lean back onto the bolster, resting the head on the chair back. Continue holding the bolster so that it does not slip. Increase the height of the support if necessary to get a comfortable pose.

Stay for 1 to 2 minutes or longer. Breathe evenly. Come up with a concave action of the trunk, leading with the chest, not the head.

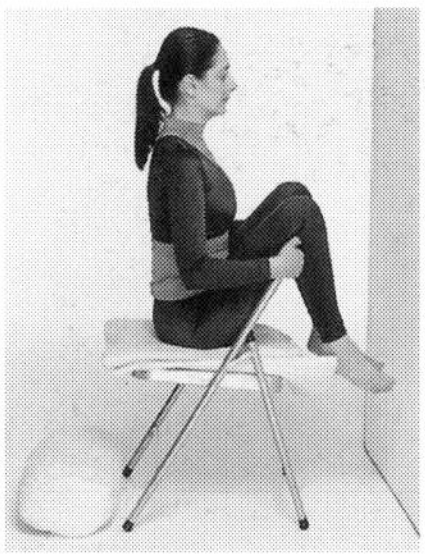

1

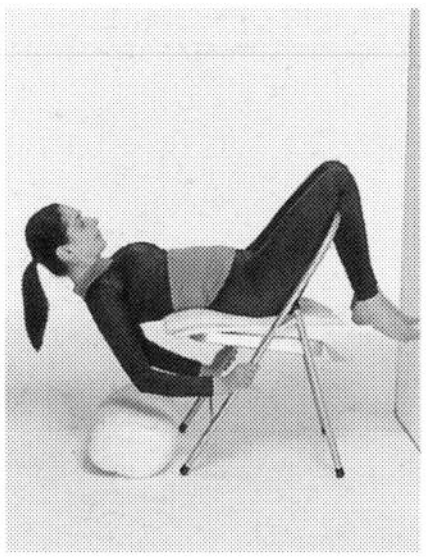

2

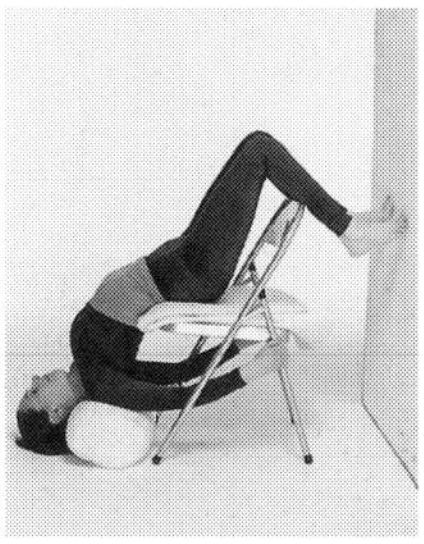

3

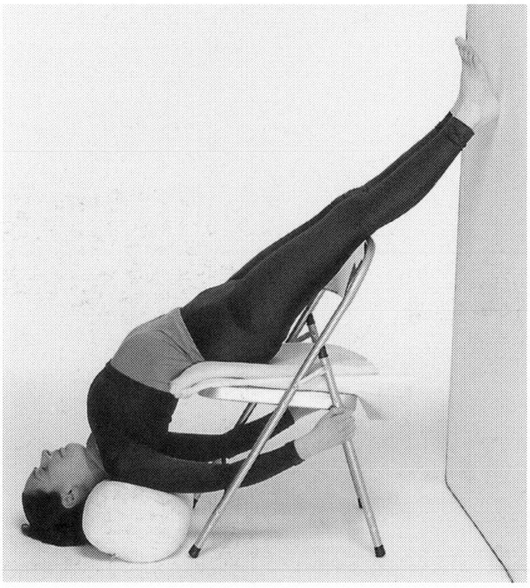

4

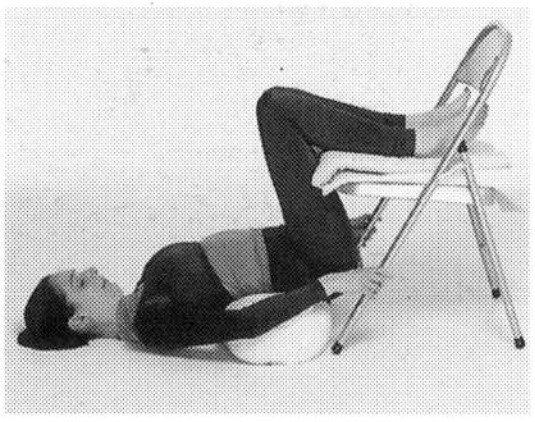

5

सर्वाङ्गासन

Sarvāṅgāsana Neck Balance (on chair)

Method

Place a chair 1 to 1½ feet away from the wall. Place a mat and blanket on the seat. Place a bolster crosswise on the floor in front of it. Sit backwards on the chair, bending the legs over the back. Hold the chair and move the buttocks closer to the back edge of the seat (1).

Lean back, simultaneously moving the hands to hold the front legs or seat of the chair. The waist should be over the front edge of the seat (2).

Immediately lower the trunk so that the shoulders rest on the bolster and the head on the floor. Take the arms inside the legs of the chair and hold the back legs (3).

Straighten the legs, resting the feet against the wall (4).

Stay for 5 minutes or longer.

To come down, ease the sacrum off the chair and slide backwards, with the back resting on the bolster and the calves on the chair (5). Turn to the side to get up.

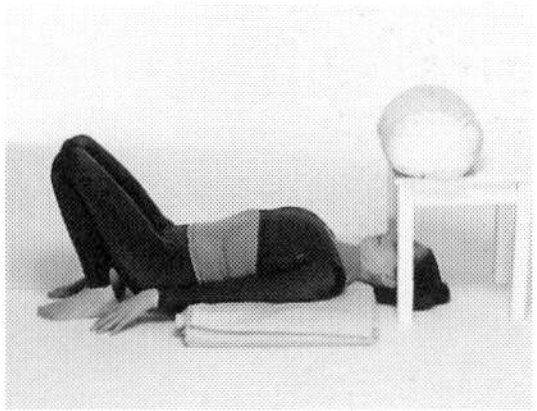

1

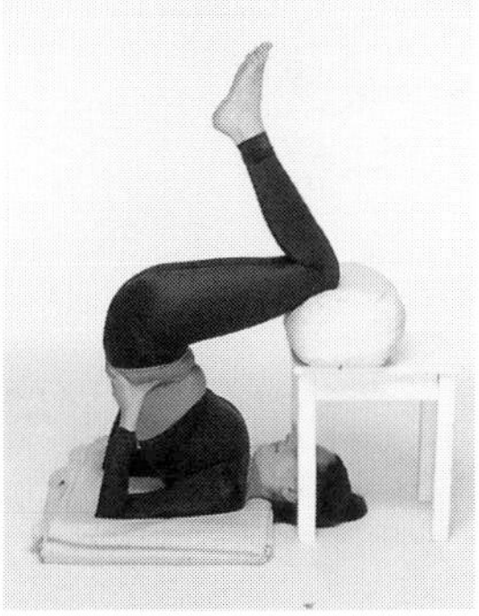

2

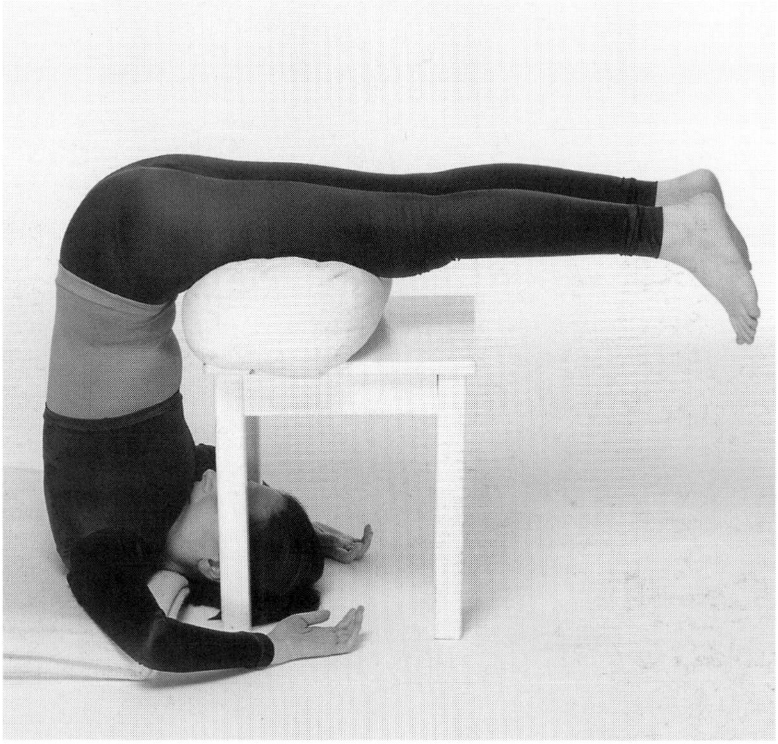

3

अर्ध-हलासन

Ardha-Halāsana Half-Plough Pose

Method

Place three or four folded blankets on the floor with the neat edges together. Place a stool in front of the blankets, and a bolster on the stool, for height. Lie down in a straight line with the shoulders on and the head off the blankets. Bring the stool over the head. Bend the knees. Press the shoulders down, move the shoulder blades in and turn the upper arms outwards (1).

Exhale and swing the trunk and legs up. Rest the knees on the bolster (2).

One at a time take the legs further over the bolster so that the top thighs are supported. Straighten the legs. Take the arms over the head. Relax (3).

Stay for 2 to 5 minutes. To come down, Hold the back or the stool, bend the legs and ease the thighs backwards off the bolster. Push the stool away and slide down. (Do not continue to hold the stool otherwise it will topple.)

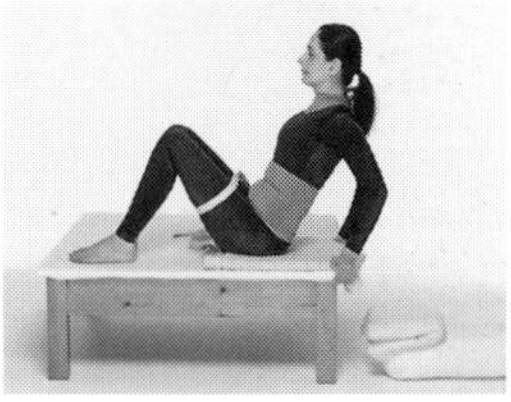

1

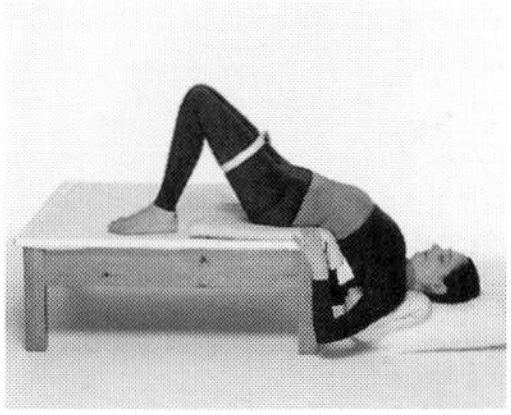

2

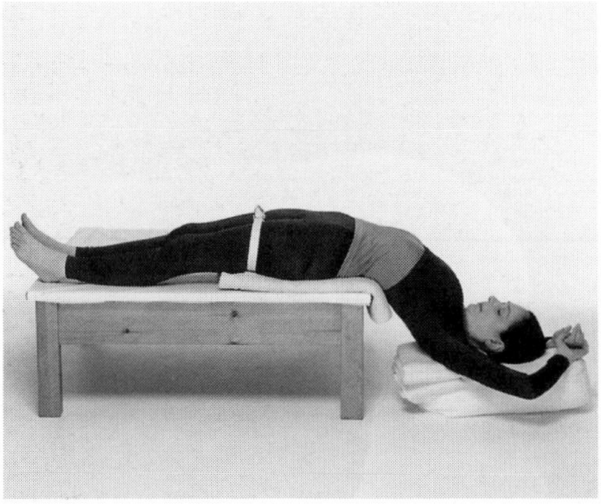

3

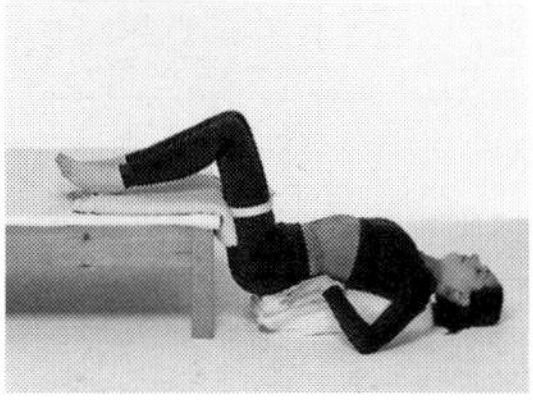

4

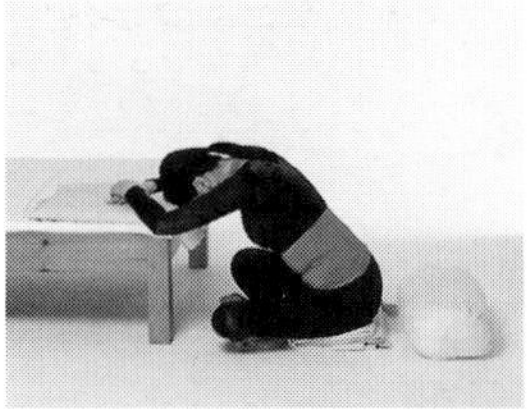

5

सेतुबन्ध-सर्वाङ्गासन

Setubandha-Sarvāṅgāsana Shoulder Balance Bridge (on bench)

Method

Place a blanket at one end of a bench. Place a bolster lengthwise on the floor in front of it, with a folded blanket on top of it near the bench. Sit on the bench, a little away from the edge. Tie the mid-thighs with a belt. Hold the bench and prepare to lie back. Measure to see that the waist will reach the edge of the bench (1).

Lean back, curving the waist over the edge of the bench, and lower the shoulders onto the folded blanket and the head onto the bolster (2).

Stretch out the legs. Take the arms over the head, resting them on the bolster (3).

Stay for 3 to 5 minutes. To come down, ease the back off the bench and slide backwards (4).

Remove the belt. Sit in simple cross-legs in front of the bench and rest the head on it (5).

Note

Back Pain

If the back hurts, raise the feet onto a support or add another blanket under the shoulders. Come down and redo the pose with the necessary supports.

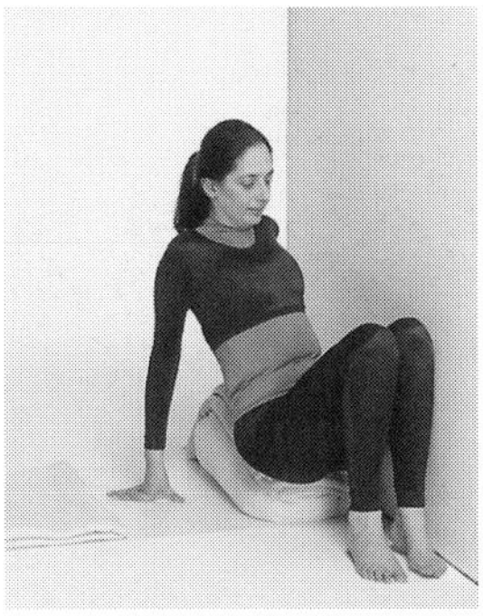

1

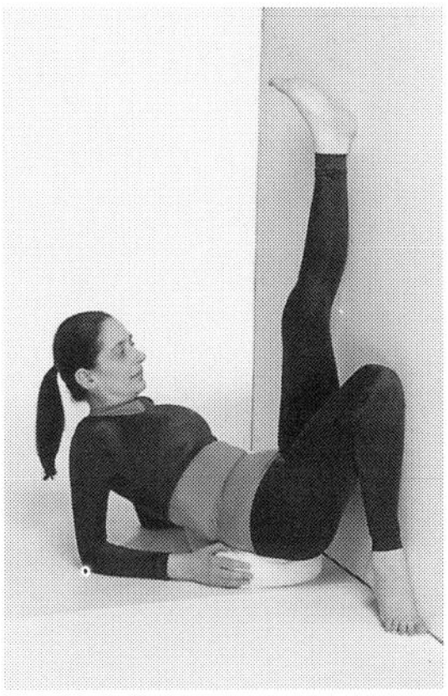

2

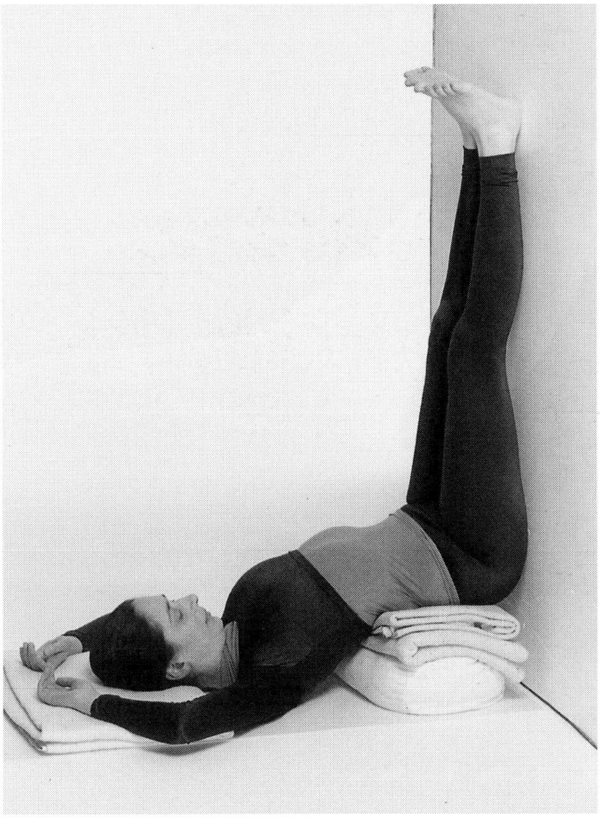

3

विपरीत-करणी मुद्रा

Viparīta-Karaṇī Mudrā Reverse Action Position

Method

Place a bolster lengthwise a little away from the wall, with one or two folded blankets on top. Keep another blanket nearby. Sit sideways on the bolster with one buttock lifted against the wall (1).

Lean back, at the same time turning the trunk towards the centre and lifting one leg up the wall. Lean on the elbows (2).

Lie down with the trunk perpendicular to the wall and both legs up. Move the bolster a little away from the wall so that the lower back is well supported and the base of the pelvis descends. Support the head and neck with the extra blanket. Take the arms over the head. Relax (3).

Stay for 5 minutes or longer. Slide backwards off the bolster, turn to the side and get up.

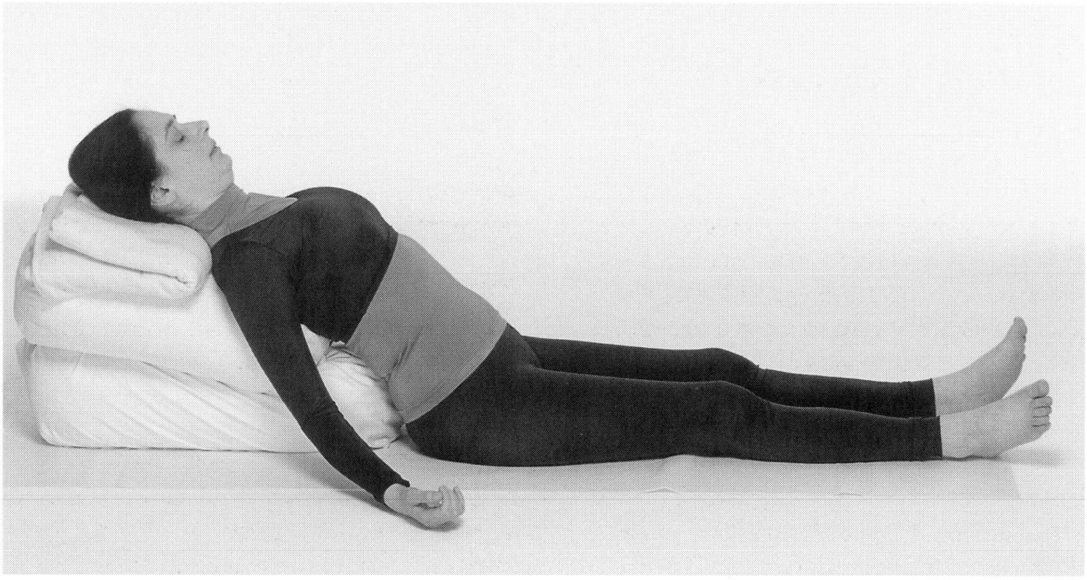

शवासन

Śavāsana Corpse Pose

Method

Place two bolsters lengthwise on the floor [as before], with the edge of the top one a little behind the edge of the bottom one. Sit in front of the bolsters and lie back. Place a folded blanket or blankets under the head and neck, so that the chin is lower than the forehead. Relax the arms by the side of the body. Relax the legs.

Stay for 5 minutes or longer. Breathe evenly. To come up, bend the legs, roll down off the bolsters and turn to the side.

Circulation

The Circulatory System

The circulation of blood to all parts of the body, including the extremities, allows the body to function well. Circulation is aided by movement. Poor circulation is aided by vigorous movement. A sedentary life style short of exercise risks the premature aging of tissues due to inadequate blood supply. Yoga practice emphasizes the stretching of muscles and joints, promoting circulation. While all active stretches are helpful, sequences of postures which are done fast and vigorously are particularly effective in combating sluggish circulation.

HOW THE *ĀSANAS* WORK

This programme incorporates fast movements which increase mobility (*vāta*) and physiological energy (*pitta*), and reduce heaviness and lethargy (*kapha*). To bring the body back to normal after exertion they are followed by supported inverted poses and relaxation, which equalize *vāta*.

Jumpings (*kapha* –, *pitta* +, *vāta* +)

These postures are done in quick succession, linked by jumps. They are a version of the traditional *Sūrya-Namaskāra*, Salute to the Sun. The fast movements invigorate the body and refresh the mind.

Rolls (*kapha* –, *pitta* +, *vāta* +)

These postures are done in quick succession, linked by rolls. The fast movements give impetus to the body and mind.

Inverted Poses (*kapha* –, *pitta* +, *vāta* =)

After vigorous exercise it is necessary to rest so that the heartbeat returns to normal. The inverted poses replenish the air which was used up during the previous exertion.

Relaxation (*kapha* +, *pitta* –, *vāta* =)

Relaxation calms and refreshes the body as well as the mind.

Props

Mat, chair, bench, blanket

Sequence A

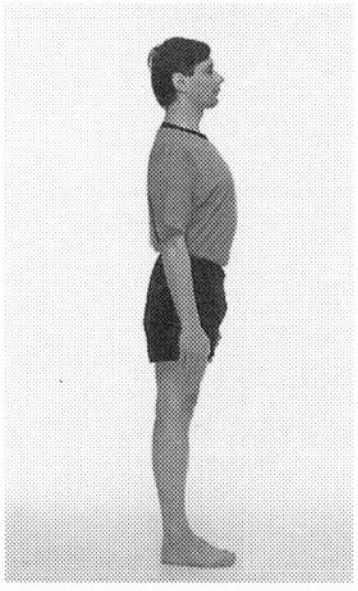
1
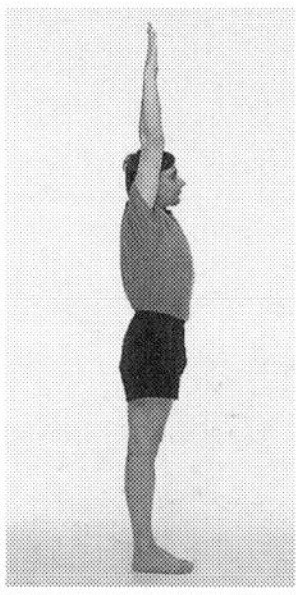
2
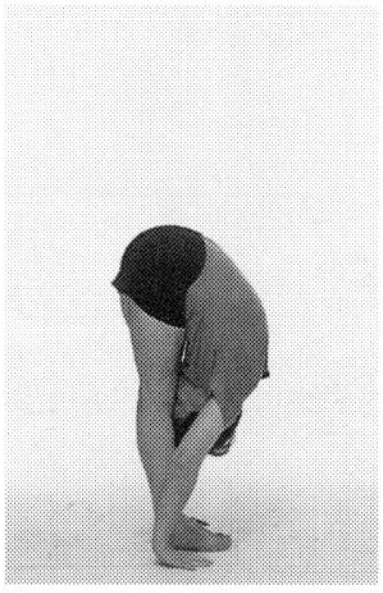
3
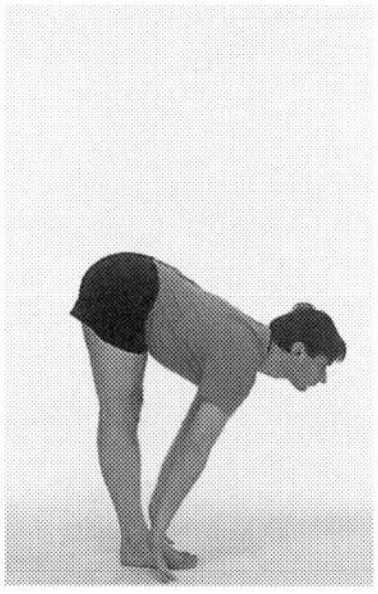
4
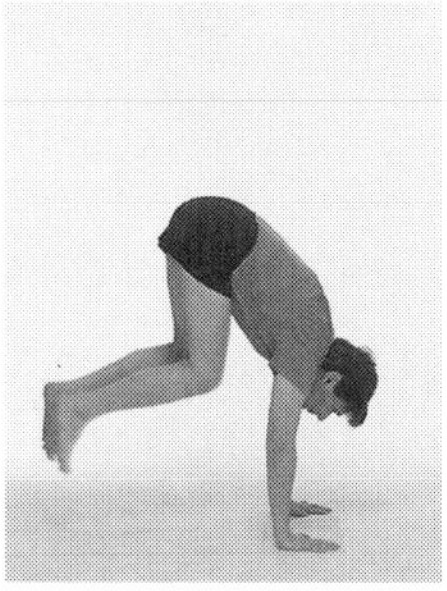
5
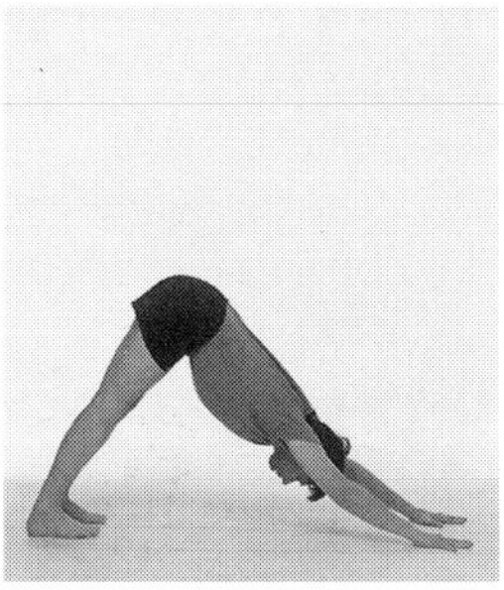
6
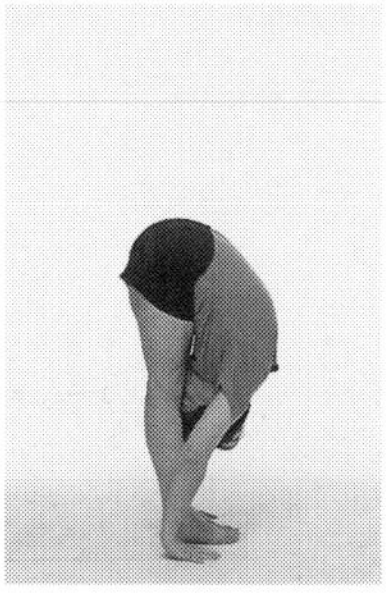
7
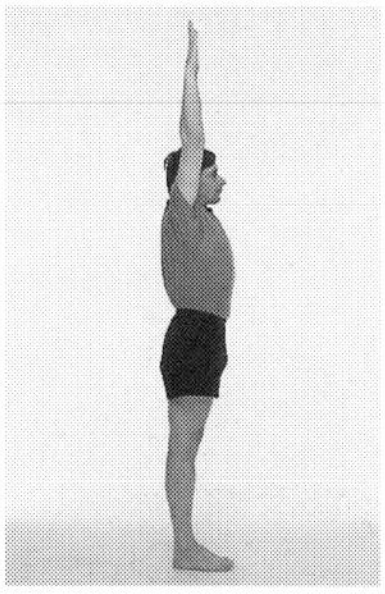
8

ताडासन

Tāḍāsana

Stand at the front edge of the mat in *Tāḍāsana* (see page 54) with the feet together, legs and trunk stretching up and the arms stretching down (1).

Inhale, raise the arms forward and up into

ऊर्ध्वहस्त-ताडासन

Ūrdhvahasta-Tāḍāsana

Keep the elbows tight, with the palms facing forward (2).

Exhale, swing down into

उत्तानासन

Uttānāsana Stretching Pose

ut = up, out; tāna = stretching

Keep the knees tight and the hands beside the feet (3).

Inhale, raise the head, make the back concave and look up (4).

Placing the palms flat on the floor, exhale, jump back (5) into

अधोमुख-श्वासन

Adhomukha-Śvāsana

Straighten the arms and legs and lift the hips (6).

Inhale, raise the head; exhale, jump forward into

उत्तानासन

Uttānāsana

Keep the knees tight and the hands (or fingertips) beside the feet (7).

Inhale, swing the trunk and arms up into

ऊर्ध्वहस्त-ताडासन

Ūrdhvahasta-Tāḍāsana

Stretch the legs, trunk and arms up (8).

Repeat the sequence 10 times, as fast as possible. Jump with both feet simultaneously (i.e. do not hop). Then rest in *Uttānāsana* with the feet one foot apart and catching the elbows.

Sequence B

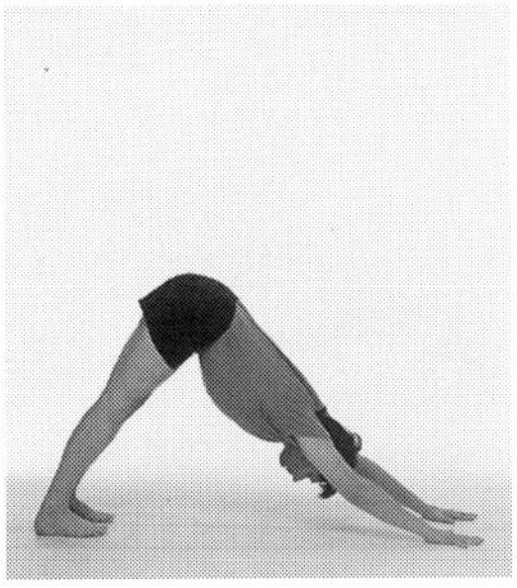
1

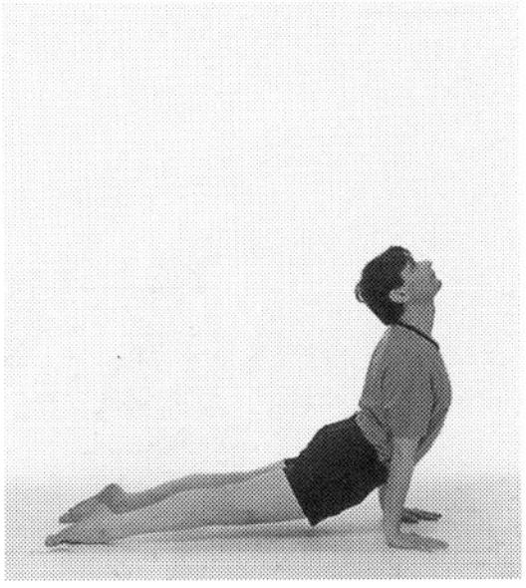
2

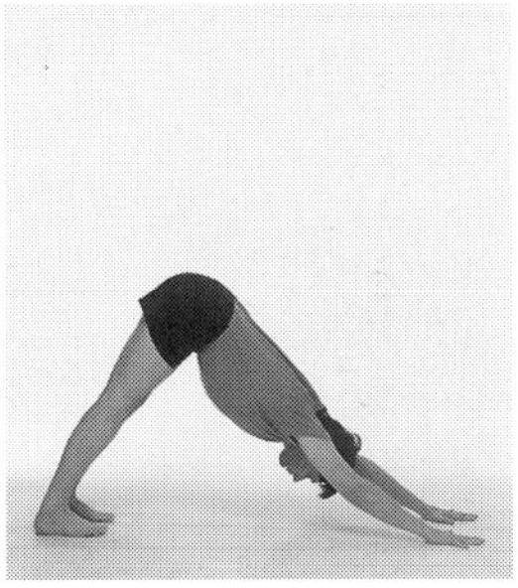
3

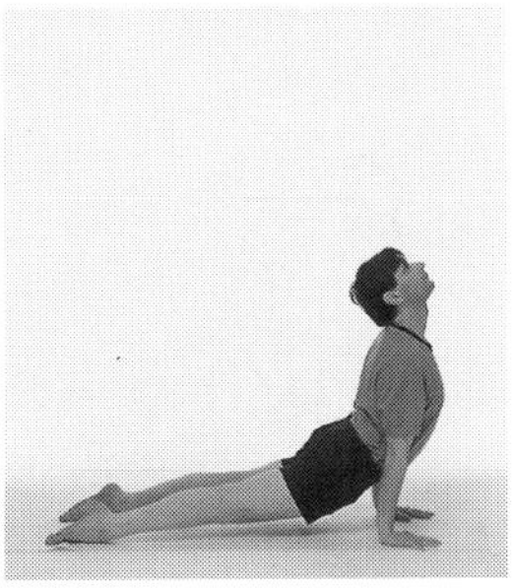
4

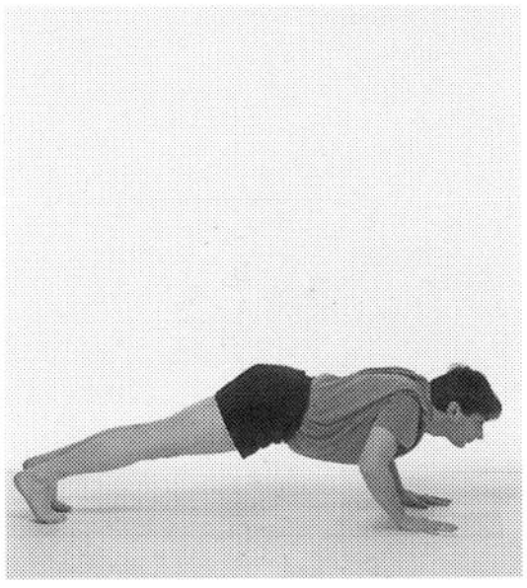
5

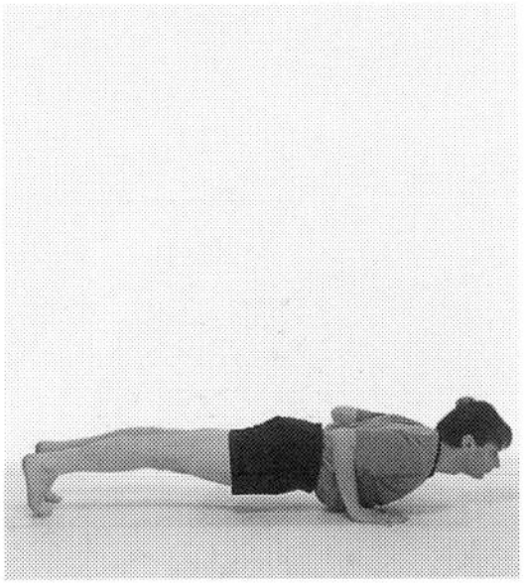
6

अधोमुख-श्वासन

Adhomukha-Śvāsana

Do *Adhomukha-Śvāsana.* Straighten the arms and legs and lift the hips (1).

Exhale, glide the body forward and roll onto the tops of the feet into

ऊर्ध्वमुख-श्वासन

Ūrdhvamukha-Śvāsana Dog Pose Head Up

ūrdhva = upwards; mukha = mouth, face; śva(n) = dog

Keep the legs parallel to the floor with the knees straight. Move the coccyx (tailbone) in. Keep the arms perpendicular to the floor with the elbows tight. Stretch the arms and trunk up. Open the chest (2).

Exhale, lift the hips, roll over the toes and go into

अधोमुख-श्वासन

Adhomukha-Śvāsana

Keep the arms and legs straight and lift the hips (3).

Repeat the sequence 10 times, as fast as possible. Then rest in *Uttānāsana* with the feet one foot apart and catching the elbows.

Later on, add

चतुरङ्गदण्डासन

Caturaṅga-Daṇḍāsana Four-Limbed Staff Pose

catur = four; aṅga = limb; daṇḍa = staff, rod

From *Ūrdhvamukha-Śvāsana (4)* curl the toes in, exhale and lower the body (5) so that the legs and trunk are in one plane, parallel to the floor. Keep the legs straight and take the shoulders back (6).

Go back into *Ūrdhvamukha-Śvāsana.*

Repeat these two poses several times. Then rest in *Uttānāsana* with the feet one foot apart and elbows folded.

When Sequences A and B are combined, this becomes *Sūrya Namaskāra,* the traditional Salute to the Sun.

Sequence C

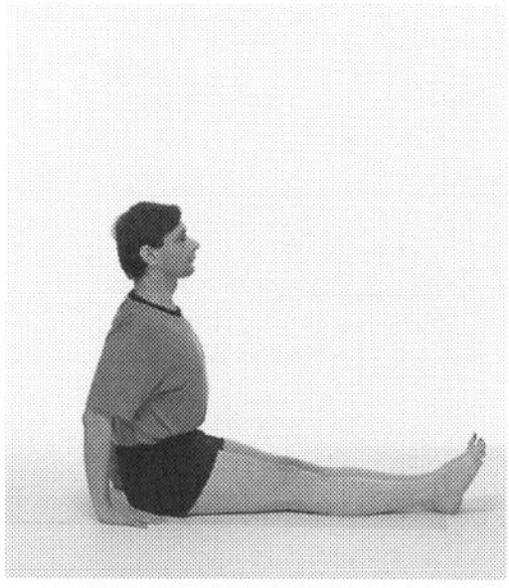
1

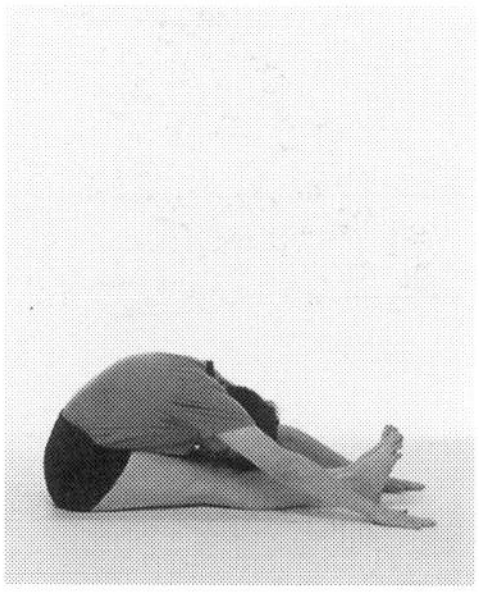
2

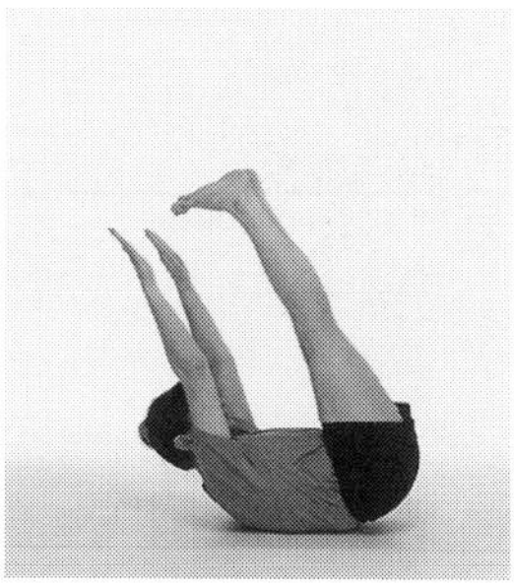
3

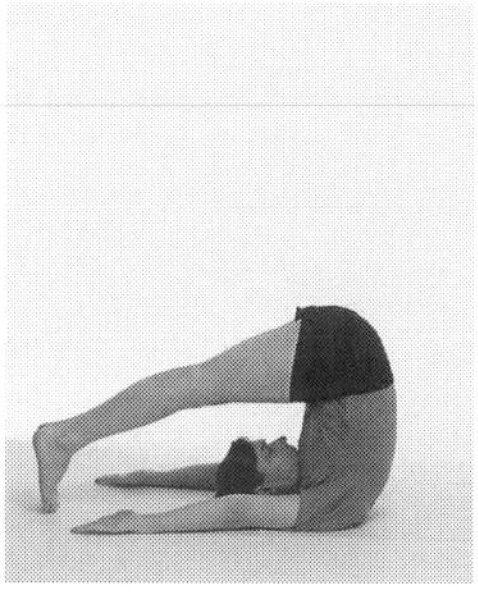
4

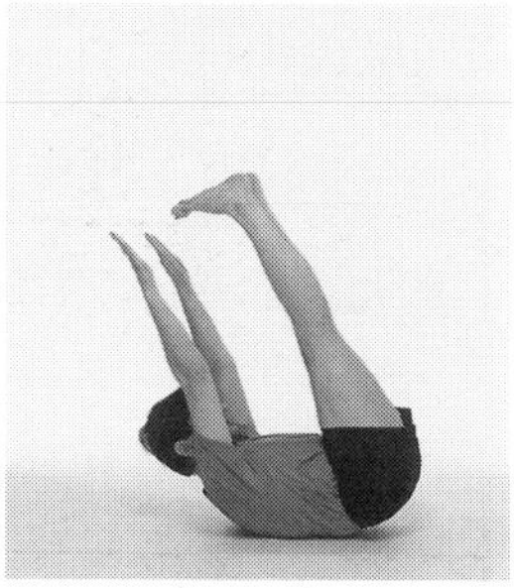
5

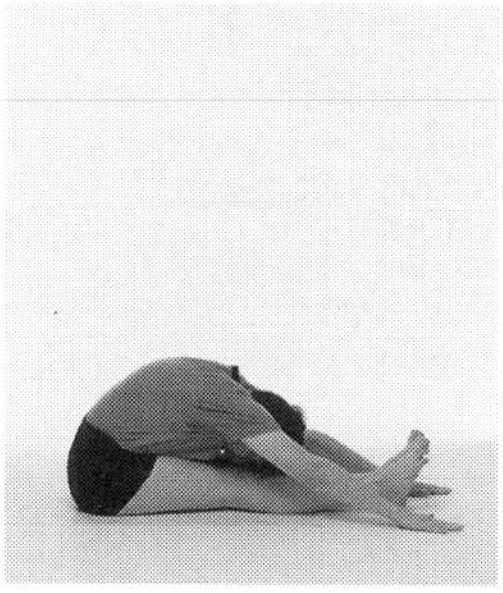
6

दण्डासन

Daṇḍāsana Staff Pose

daṇḍa = staff, rod

Sit with the legs stretched out in front. Place the hands beside the hips and stretch the trunk up. Roll the shoulders back and lift the chest (1).

Inhale, raise the arms, then exhale and bend forward into

पश्चिमोत्तानासन

Paśćimottānāsana

Fold the trunk over the legs. Keep the legs straight and stretch the arms forward (2).

Exhale, roll back (3) into

हलासन

Halāsana

Swing the legs and arms over the head, keeping the knees and elbows straight (4).

Exhale, roll forward (5) into

पश्चिमोत्तानासन

Paśćimottānāsana

Keep the legs and arms straight. Take the head down (6).

Repeat the sequence 10 times, as fast as possible. Then rest in *Paśćimottānāsana*.

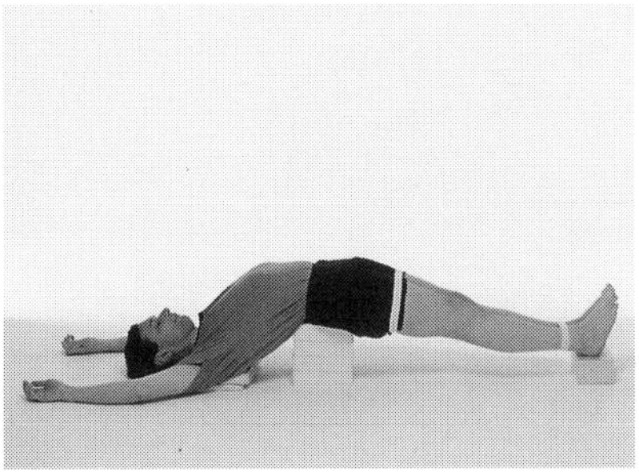

1

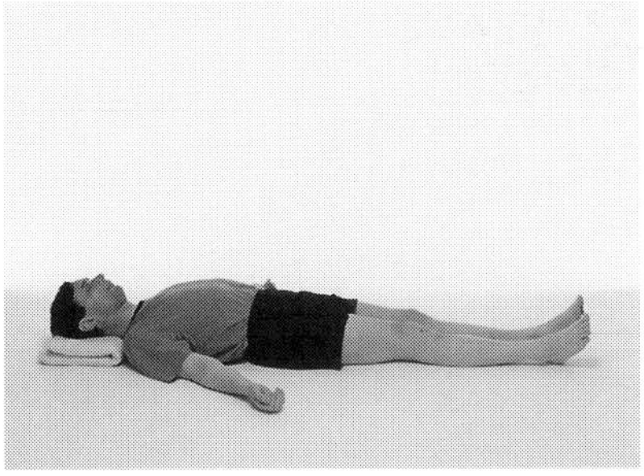

2

सर्वाङ्गासन

Sarvāṅgāsana Neck Balance (on chair)

Method

Follow the method given on page 93 (1).

Stay for 5 minutes or longer. Slide backwards off the chair to come down.

अर्ध-हलासन

Ardha-Halāsana Half-Plough Pose

Method

Follow the method given on page 85 (2).

Stay for 5 minutes or longer. Come down carefully, without a thump.

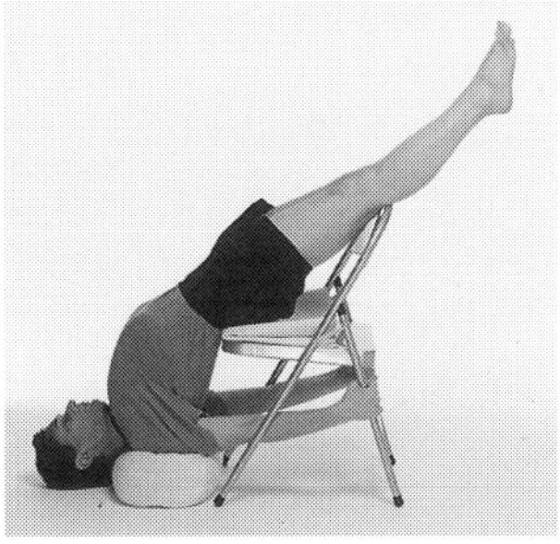

1

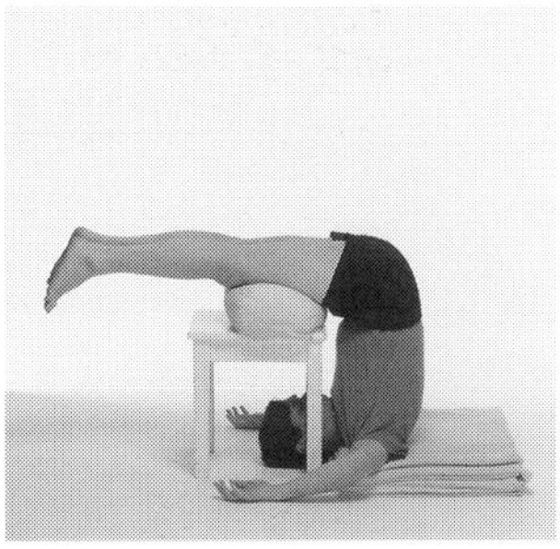

2

सेतुबन्ध-सर्वाङ्गासन

Setubandha-Sarvāṅgāsana Shoulder Balance Bridge (on blocks)

Method

Arrange blocks or cross-wise bolsters to a height of about one foot. Sit on one edge and tie the mid-thighs together with a belt. Lie back so that the waist curves over the other edge and the shoulders and head rest on the floor. Stretch out the legs, resting the feet on a support if necessary. Take the arms over the head (1).

Stay for 5 minutes or longer. Slide backwards to come down. Sit in simple cross-legs and bend forward, resting the head on the support.

शवासन

Śavāsana Corpse Pose

Method

Lie flat on the back with a folded blanket under the head and neck. Stretch the arms and legs, then relax them. Let the legs and feet drop further to the sides. Close the eyes and relax the face (2).

Stay for 5 minutes or longer. Open the eyes, turn to the side and get up.

The Female Organs

The female reproductive system is delicately tuned by hormones to monthly changes. Each month lining of the uterus breaks down and re-forms to provide the best condition for the egg which is released by the ovaries. Overarching this menstrual cycle are the life-cycle markers of menarche and menopause between which pregnancy may occur. It is not surprising that the continual fluctuation of body states is associated with irregularity, pain, tension and mood swings. So much change needs to be supported by stability. Yoga practice helps to achieve this. It can regularize the menstrual cycle, alleviate aches and cramps, and steady the mind.

Although the following programme is aimed at women, it is in fact also beneficial for men as it tones the pelvic organs.

HOW THE *ĀSANAS* WORK

This programme comprises a variety of poses giving different effects. It begins with poses involving making the lower back concave, which increases physiological energy in the pelvis (*pitta*) and decompressing *vāta*, balancing it. It continues with an inverted pose which reinforce these benefits. Supine poses then bring stability by increasing *kapha* while at the same time increasing *pitta*. Forward bends continue to increase *pitta*, simultaneously quieting *vāta*. Groin-opening poses further enhance the functioning of *pitta* in the pelvic organs and induce the proper channelling of *vāta*. The programme ends with more inverted poses which consolidate all of these actions.

Poses with a Concave Action (*kapha* –, *pitta* +, *vāta* =)

The concave action of the lower back and extension of the front of the body stretches the uterus, giving relief from pain/cramps.

Inverted Poses (*kapha* –, *pitta* +, *vāta* =)

The inversion of the female organs relieves the pressure of gravity on them. The abdomen rests against the back, becoming soft. Tension is removed from the organs. The inverted poses have a regulatory effect on the hormonal system. They also nourish the nerves. In this way irregular menses can improve. **Inverted poses should not be done during menstruation so as not to impede the exit of toxic waste material from the body.**

Supine Poses (*kapha* +, *pitta* +, *vāta* =)

When the chest is supported on a height the abdomen relaxes and the space inside the abdominal cavity increases. This removes compression of the organs and relieves pain.

Forward Bends (*kapha* +, *pitta* +, *vāta* –)

The abdomen becomes soft when the spine is horizontal. This allows the physiological processes to continue without strain. With the head resting on a support, the mind becomes calm.

Groin-opening Poses (*kapha* –, *pitta* +, *vāta* =)

The wide opening of the legs lifts the pelvis and creates space in the abdominal cavity. The reproductive organs are supported by the lift and relax in the extra space. The leg positions relieve heaviness in the thighs.

Props

Wall, chair, bench, bolster, mat, blankets, brick

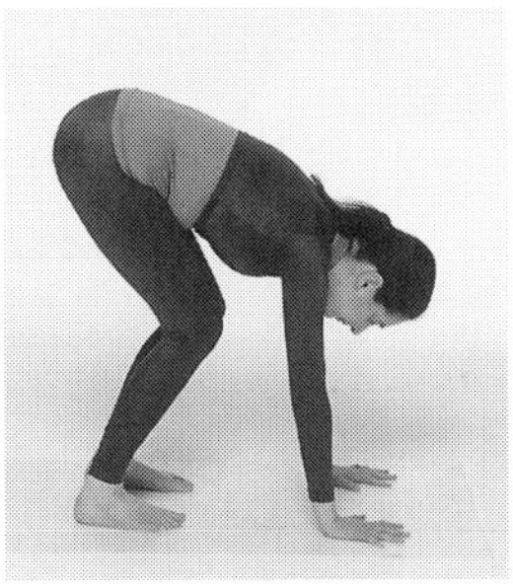

1

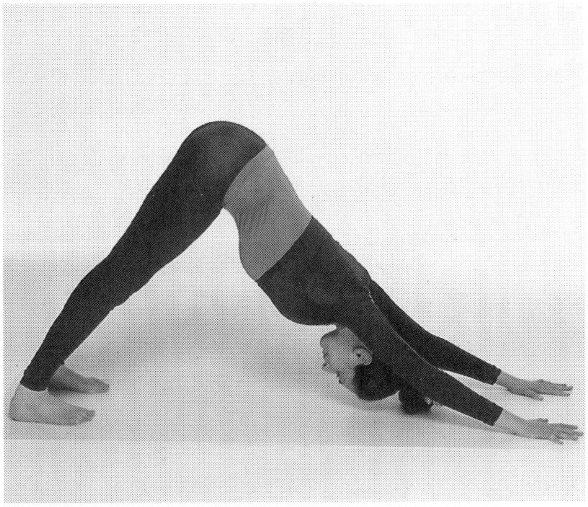

2

अधोमुख-श्वासन

Adhomukha-Śvāsana Dog Pose, Head Down

Method

Stand in *Tāḍāsana* (see page 54). Take the feet hip-width apart. Exhale, bend down and place the hands on the floor in front of the feet, shoulder-width apart. Spread the fingers (1).

Step 2 or 3 feet back. Align the feet and hands. Tighten the knees and elbows, stretch the trunk up and lift the hips. Move the trunk towards the legs and press the legs back, away from the trunk. Make the thoracic spine concave. Relax the head and neck (2).

Stay for 20 to 30 seconds. Inhale and stand straight.

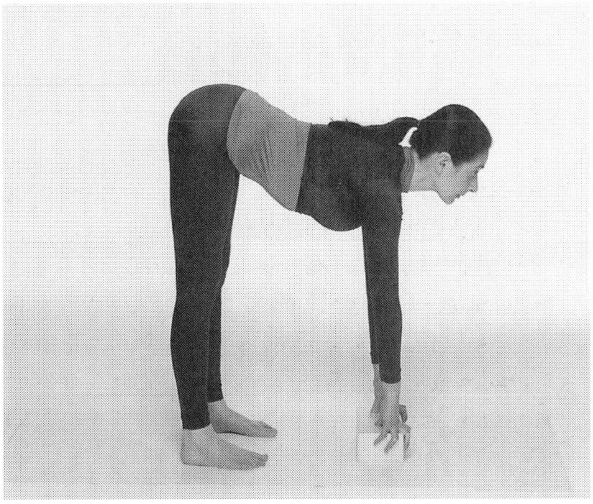

उत्तानासन

Uttānāsana Stretching Pose (concave)

Method

Stand in *Tāḍāsana* (see page 54). Take the feet hip-width apart. Exhale, bend down and place the hands on a brick in front of the feet. Tighten the elbows and knees and stretch the arms and legs up. Press the sacrum and thoracic spine in to make the back concave. Inhale and extend the front of the body forward. Extend the chin forward and look up. Relax the eyes and throat.

Stay for 20 to 30 seconds. Inhale and stand straight. Join the feet.

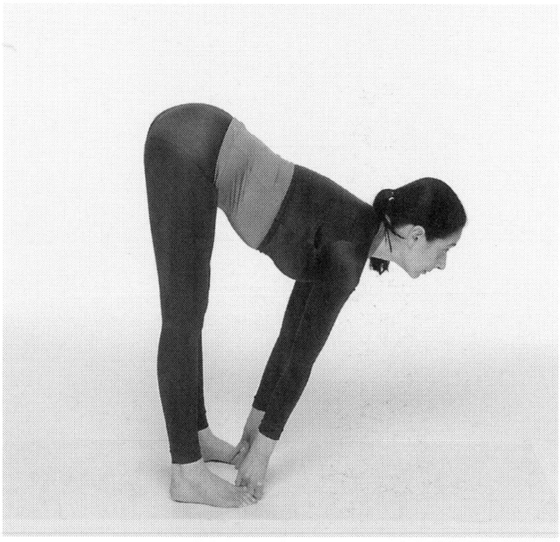

पादाङ्गुष्ठासन

Pādāṅguṣṭhāsana Thumb-to-Foot Pose (concave)

pāda = foot; aṅguṣṭha= thumb, big toe

Method

Stand in *Tāḍāsana* (see page 54). Take the feet hip-width apart. Exhale, bend down and catch the big toes with the index fingers and thumbs. Press the big toes down. Stretch the arms and legs up. Move the sacrum and thoracic spine in to make the back concave. Inhale and extend the front of the body forward. Extend the chin forward and look up. Do not strain the neck.

Stay for 20 to 30 seconds. Inhale and stand straight. Bring the feet together.

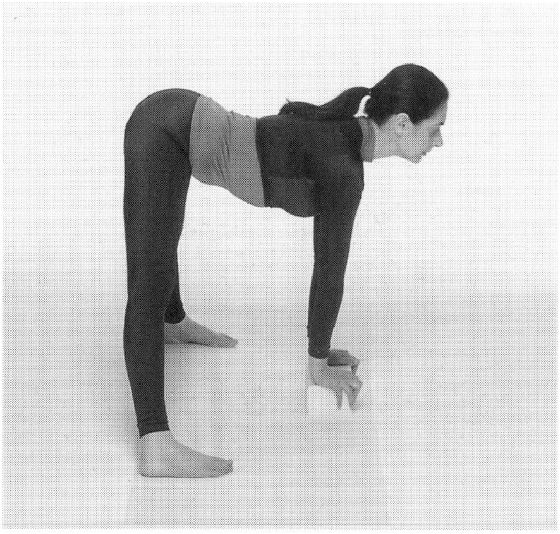

प्रसारितपादोत्तानासन

Prasāritapādottānāsana Wide-Legged Stretching Pose (concave)

prasārita = spread out; pāda = foot, leg; uttāna = stretching

Method

Stand in *Tāḍāsana* (see page 54). Place the hands on the hips. Take the feet five feet apart. Turn the feet a little in and press the outer feet down. Exhale, bend down and place the hands on a brick in front of the feet. Stretch the arms and legs up. Press the sacrum and thoracic spine in to make the back concave. Inhale and extend the front of the body forward. Extend the chin forward and look up. Do not strain the neck.

Stay for 20 to 30 seconds. Bring the feet in a little, then inhale and stand straight.

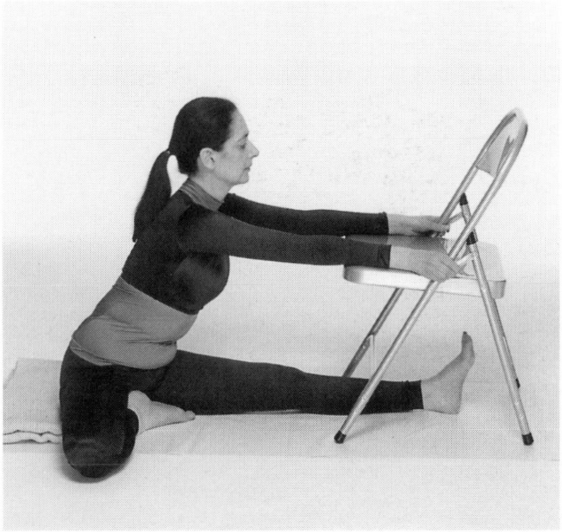

जानुशीर्षासन

Jānuśīrṣāsana Head-to-Knee Pose (concave)

Method

Sit on one or two folded blankets with the legs stretched out in front.

Pressing the hands down, stretch the trunk up, take the shoulders back and lift the chest. Bend the right leg to the side, taking the heel into its own groin. Place a chair over the left leg. Hold the chair, resting the forearms on the seat. Move the lower back in and up and make the thoracic spine concave. Inhale and lift the front of the body.

Stay for 20 to 30 seconds. Straighten the right leg. Repeat on the left.

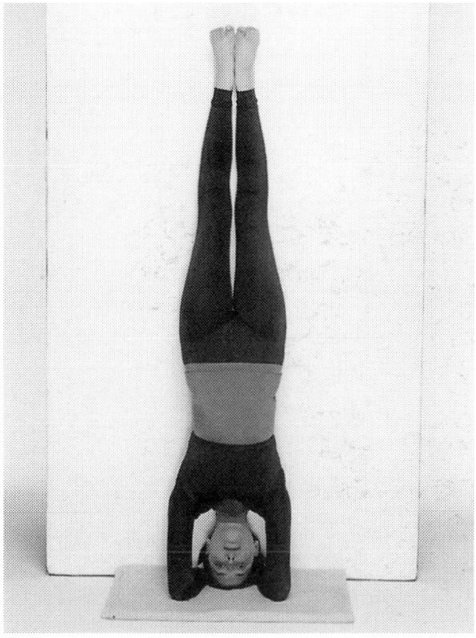

शीर्षासन

Śīrṣāsana Head Balance

Method

Follow the method given on pages 100–101.

Stay for a few minutes. Exhale and come down or do:

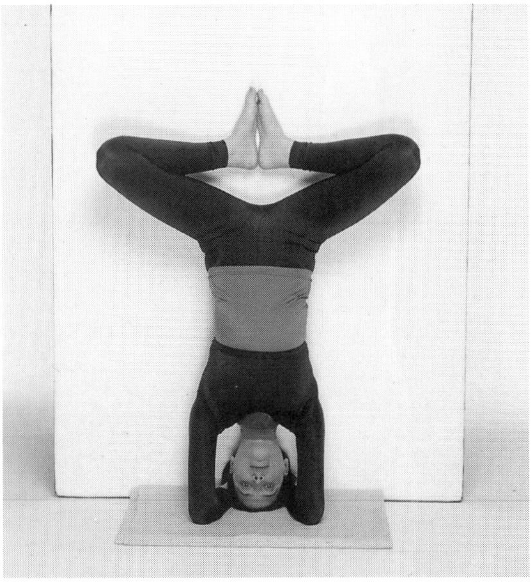

शीर्षासन स-बद्धकोणासन

Śīrṣāsana with *Baddhakoṇāsana* Head Balance with Cobbler's Pose

Method

Be in *Śīrṣāsana*. Lift the shoulders. Bend the knees outwards and join the soles of the feet. Bring the feet close to the body. Lift the hips, open the groins and press the knees back. Move the coccyx (tailbone) in.

Stay for 20 to 30 seconds. Straighten the legs. Exhale and come down or do:

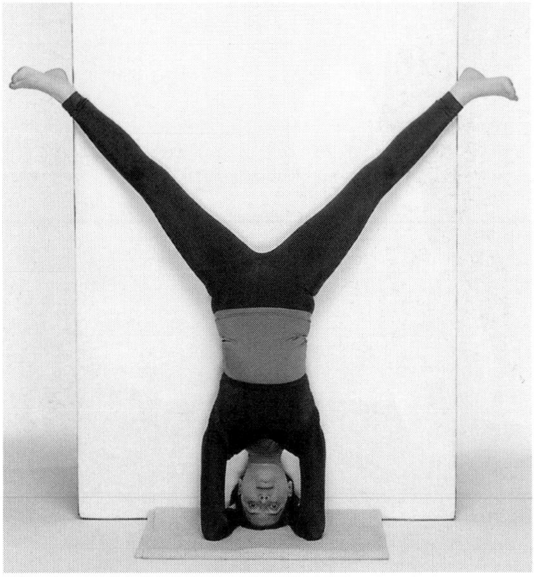

शीर्षासन स-उपविष्टकोणासन

Śīrṣāsana with *Upaviṣṭakoṇāsana* Head Balance with Seated-Angle Pose

Method

Be in *Śīrṣāsana*. Lift the shoulders. Spread the legs apart, turning them outwards. Tighten the knees and stretch the soles of the feet. Extend from the groins to the inner heels. Move the coccyx (tailbone) in.

Stay for 20 to 30 seconds. Join the legs. Exhale and come down.

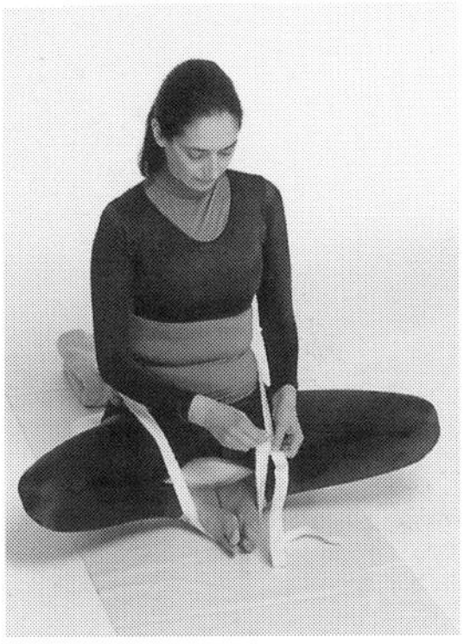

1

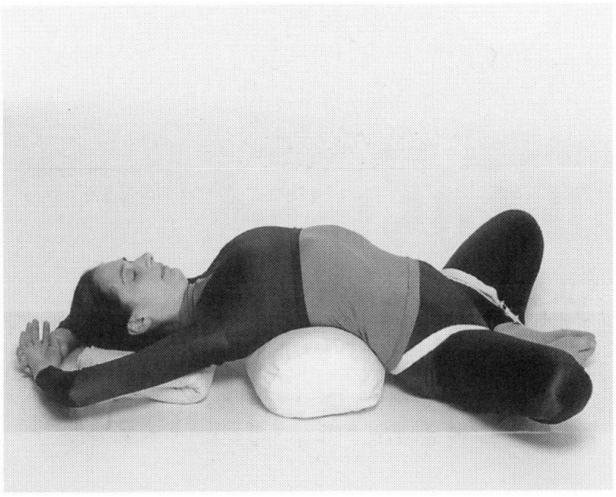

2

सुप्त-बद्धकोणासन

Supta-Baddhakoṇāsana Supine Cobbler's Pose (on bolster)

Method

Sit on a bolster placed crosswise. Bend the knees outwards and join the soles of the feet. Bring the feet close to the body. Pass a belt round the base of the pelvis, over the thighs and under the feet. Tie it tight, so that the thighs and calves touch (1).

Slide forward off the bolster, hold it against the body and lie back over it. The shoulders should reach the floor. If they do not, place a folded blanket under the shoulders and head. Take the arms over the head (2).

Stay for 5 minutes or longer. Inhale and come up. Untie the belt.

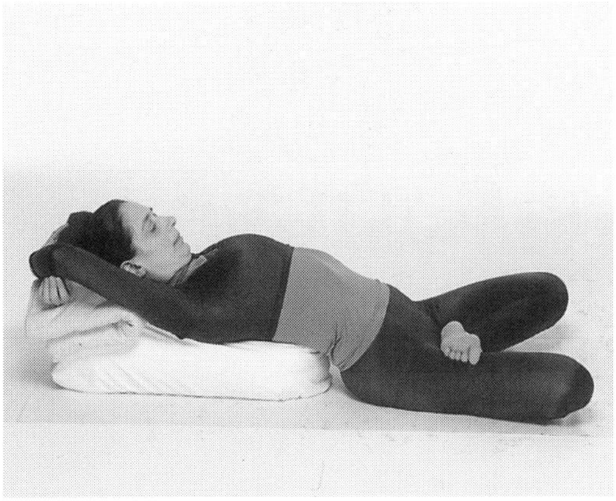

मत्स्यासन

Matsyāsana Fish Pose (on bolster)

Method

Sit in simple cross-legs in front of a bolster placed lengthwise. Lie back on it, making sure the sacrum (lower black) is supported. Support the head with a folded blanket. Take the arms over the head .

Stay for 3 to 5 minutes. Inhale and come up. Change the cross-legs and repeat.

Later on, lie back in *Ardha-Padmāsana*, Half Lotus Pose. Place the right foot on top of the left thigh, in the groin. Fold the left leg underneath. Stay for 3 to 5 minutes. Repeat with the left leg on top.

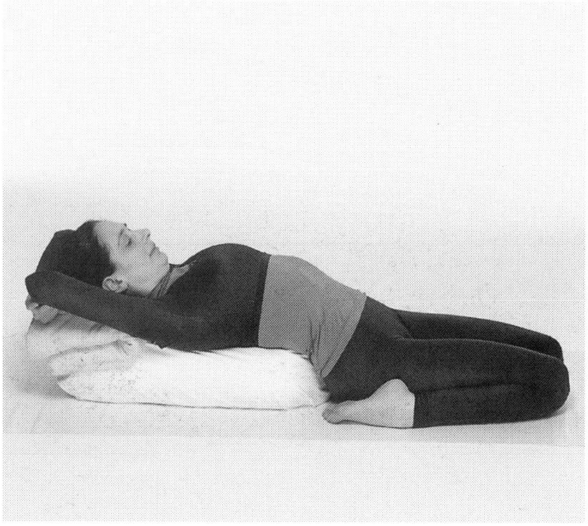

सुप्त-वीरासन

Supta-Vīrāsana Supine Hero Pose (on bolster)

Method

Follow the method given on page 125. Sit in *Vīrāsana* and lie back on a bolster placed lengthwise. Support the head on a folded blanket. Take the arms over the head.

Stay for 3 to 5 minutes. Inhale and come up. Bend forward in *Adhomukha-Vīrāsana*, with the toes together and the knees apart (see page 59).

Note

If it is difficult to go down, raise the height of the supports, both for sitting and lying.

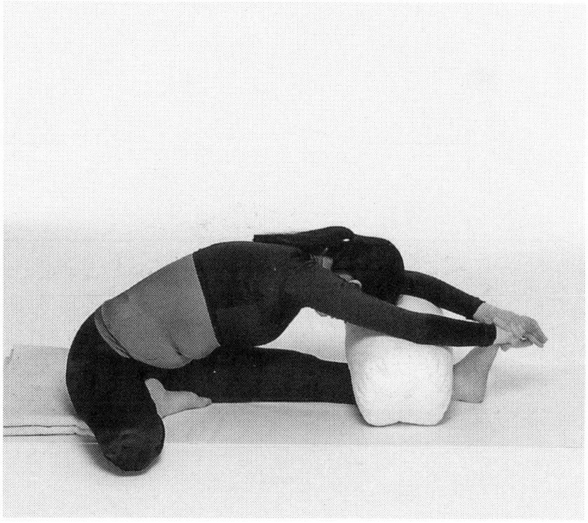

जानुशीर्षासन

Jānuśīrṣāsana Head-to-Knee Pose (on bolster)

Method

Sit on one or two folded blankets with the legs stretched out in front.

Stretch the trunk up, take the shoulders back and lift the chest. Bend the right leg to the side, taking the heel into its own groin. Keep the left leg straight and the right leg relaxed. Place a bolster on the left shin. Exhale and bend forward, resting the forehead on the bolster. Rest the arms on the bolster.

Stay for 1 to 2 minutes. Inhale and come up. Straighten the right leg. Repeat on the left.

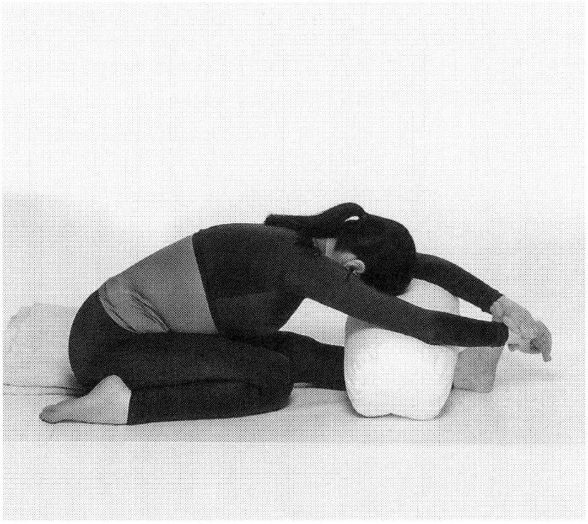

एकपाद-वीर-पश्चिमोत्तानासन

Ekapāda-Vīra-Paśćimottānāsana Posterior Stretch with One Leg in Hero Pose (on bolster)

Method

Sit on two folded blankets with the legs stretched out in front.

Stretch the trunk up, take the shoulders back and lift the chest. Bend the right leg back, placing the foot beside the hip. Move the blanket under the left buttock. If the body tilts, add another blanket. Place a bolster on the extended shin. Exhale and bend forward, resting the forehead and arms on the bolster.

Stay for 1 to 2 minutes. Inhale and come up. Straighten the right leg. Repeat on the left.

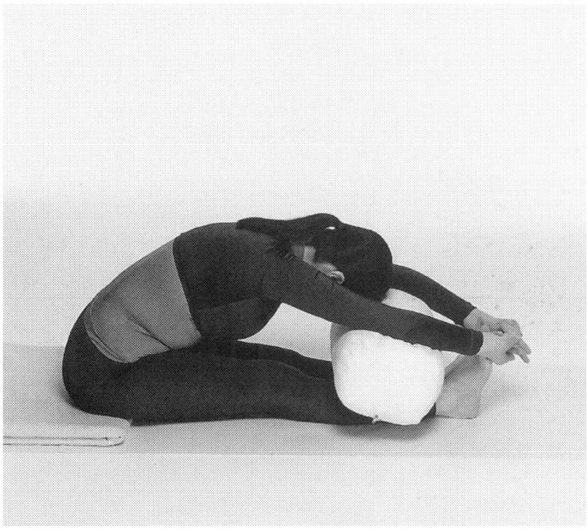

पश्चिमोत्तानासन

Paśćimottānāsana Posterior Stretching Pose (on bolster)

Method

Sit on one or two folded blankets with the legs stretched out in front.

Stretch the trunk up, take the shoulders back and lift the chest. Place a bolster on the shins. Exhale and bend forward, resting the forehead and arms on the bolster. Relax the throat.

Stay for 2 to 3 minutes. Inhale and come up.

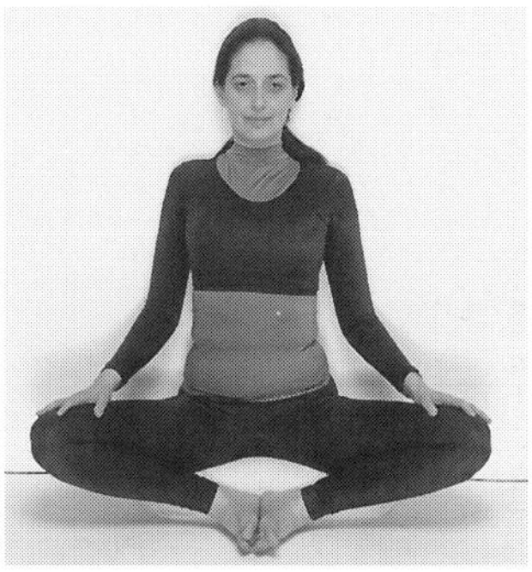

1

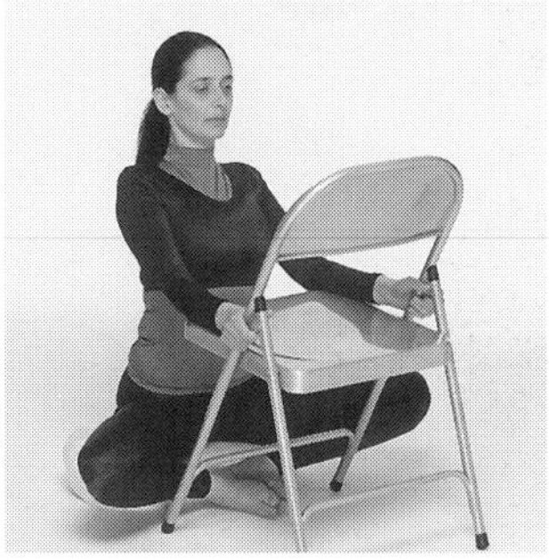

2

बद्धकोणासन

Baddhakoṇāsana
Cobbler's Pose

Method I (using a wall)

Sit on a bolster placed lengthwise against the wall. Bend the knees outwards and join the soles of the feet. Bring the feet close to the body. Rest the back against the wall. Take the shoulders back and lift the chest. Place the hands on the knees. Lift the lower back, open the groins and press the knees down. Keep the head straight (1).

Stay for 3 to 5 minutes. Release the legs.

Method II (using a chair)

Sit on a bolster placed lengthwise. Bend the knees outwards and join the soles of the feet. Bring the feet close to the body. Place a chair in front and hold it, resting the forearms on the seat. Do not lean forward but keep the trunk upright. Take the shoulders back and lift the chest. Lift the lower back, open the groins and press the knees down (2).

Stay for 3 to 5 minutes. Release the legs.

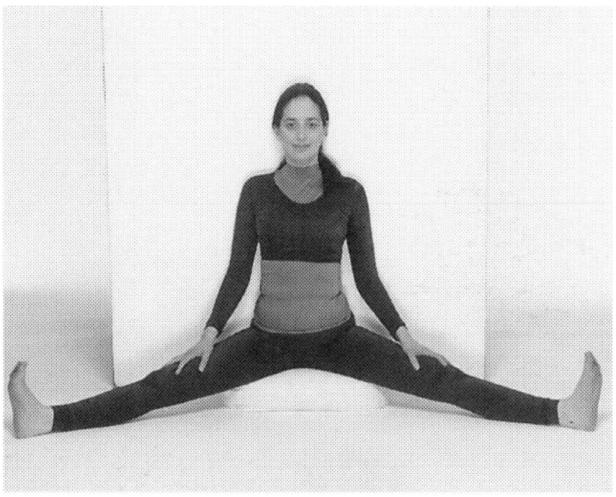

1

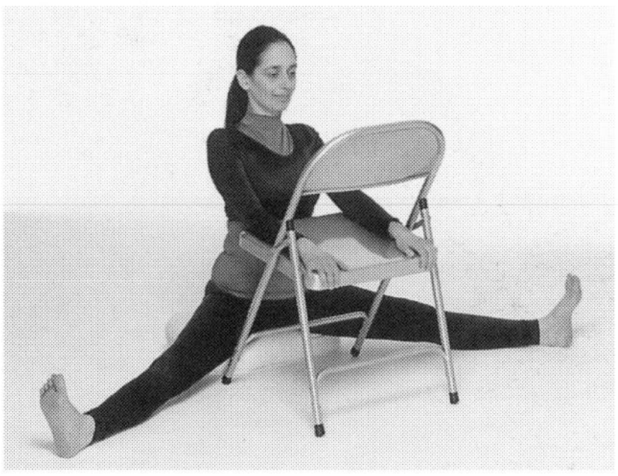

2

उपविष्टकोणासन

Upaviṣṭakoṇāsana
Seated Angle Pose

Method I (using a wall)

Sit on a bolster placed lengthwise against the wall. Spread the legs wide. Straighten the knees and stretch the soles of the feet up. Do not let the legs roll outwards. Rest the back against the wall. Take the shoulders back and lift the chest. Place the hands on the knees. Lift the lower back, open the groins and stretch from the groins to the inner heels (1).

Stay for 3 to 5 minutes. Bring the legs together.

Method II (using a chair)

Sit on a bolster placed lengthwise. Spread the legs wide. Straighten the knees and stretch the soles of the feet. Do not let the legs roll outwards. Place a chair in front and hold it, resting the forearms on the seat. Keep the trunk upright. Take the shoulders back and lift the chest. Lift the lower back and stretch from the groins to the inner heels (2).

Stay for 3 to 5 minutes. Join the legs.

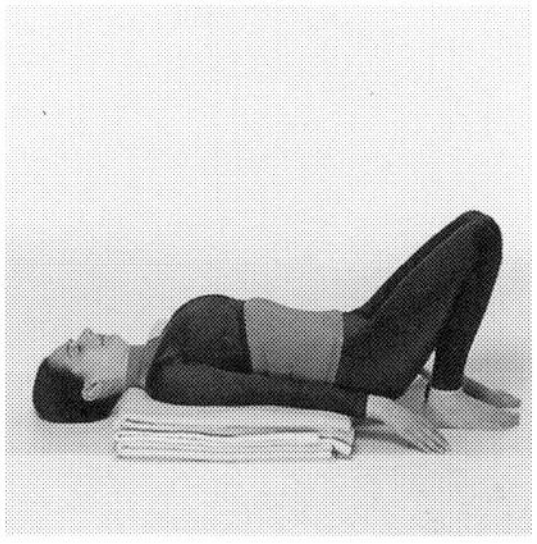
1

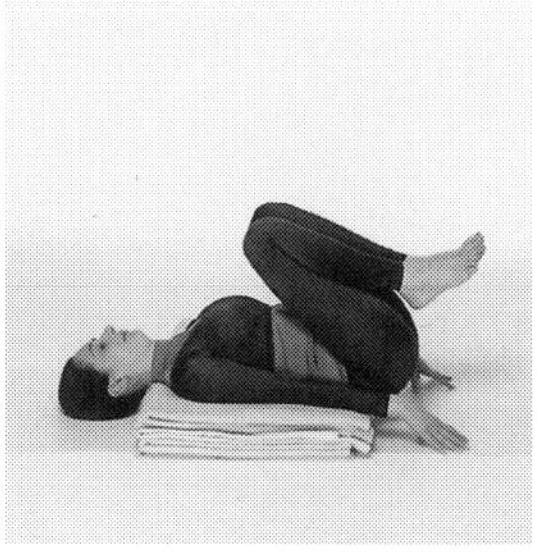
2

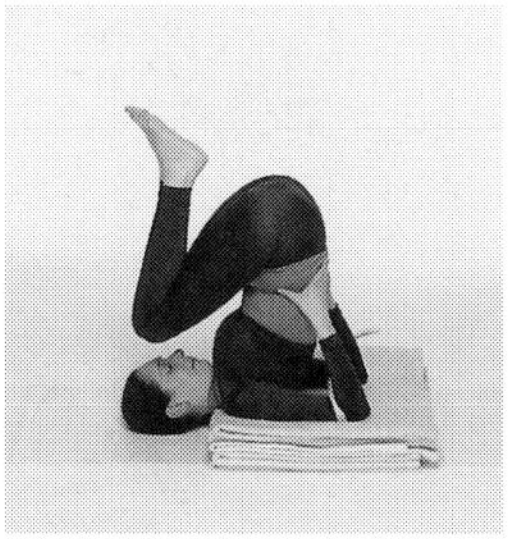
3

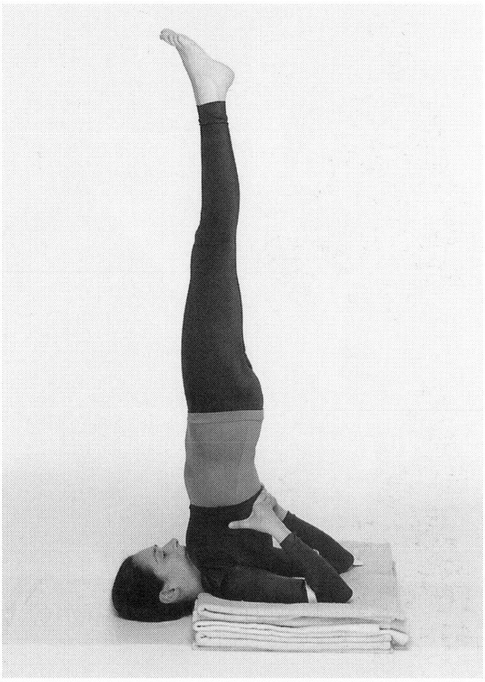
4

सर्वाङ्गासन

Sarvāṅgāsana Shoulder Balance

Method

Place three or four folded blankets on the floor with the neat edges together. Lie down with the shoulders on the blankets and the head on the floor. Move the shoulders away from the neck and press them down. Press the shoulder blades in and lift the sternum (breast bone). Lengthen the arms and turn the palms to face down. Bend the knees (1).

Exhale and bend the knees over the abdomen. If this is difficult, place a bolster or support under the hips (2).

Exhale and raise the trunk. Immediately support the back with the hands (3).

Straighten the trunk and legs up. Keep the feet together. Bring the elbows in. When confidence is gained in the pose, it is helpful to tie a belt round the upper arms, just above the elbows. This keeps the elbows in and gives a stronger support to the back (4).

Stay for 5 minutes or longer. Exhale, bend the legs and slide down gently or do:

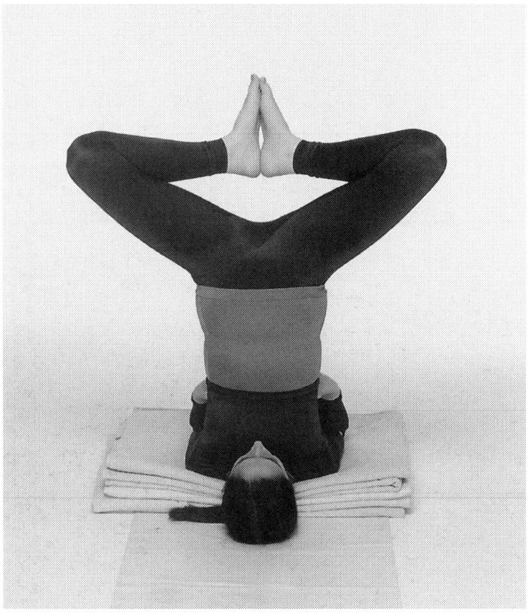

सर्वाङ्गासन स-बद्धकोणासन

Sarvāṅgāsana with *Baddhakoṇāsana* Shoulder Balance with Cobbler's Pose

Method

Be in *Sarvāṅgāsana*. Stretch the trunk and legs well. Exhale, bend the knees outwards and join the soles of the feet. Bring the feet close to the body. Lift the hips, open the groins and press the knees back.

Stay for 20 to 20 seconds. Straighten the legs. Exhale and go into:

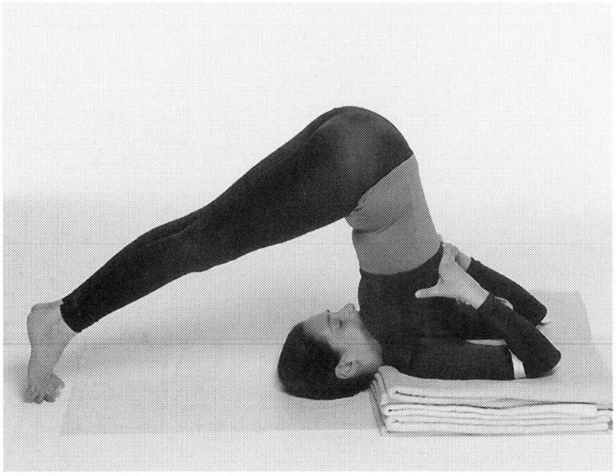

हलासन

Halāsana Plough Pose

Method

Be in *Sarvāṅgāsana*. Exhale and lower the feet to the floor. Go with bent or straight legs. Keep the feet together and rest on the tips of the toes. Lift the trunk and hips. Tighten the knees and lift the thighs, knees and shins.

Stay for 2 to 3 minutes. Exhale, bend the legs and slide down gently.

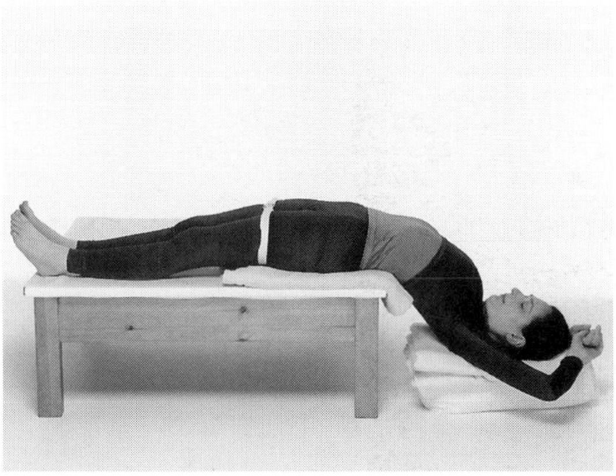

सेतुबन्ध-सर्वाङ्गासन

Setubandha-Sarvāṅgāsana Shoulder Balance Bridge (on bench)

Method

Follow the method given in on page 109.

Stay for 5 minutes or longer. Bend the legs, remove the belt and slide backwards off the bench. Sit in simple cross-legs and bend forward, resting the forehead on the bench.

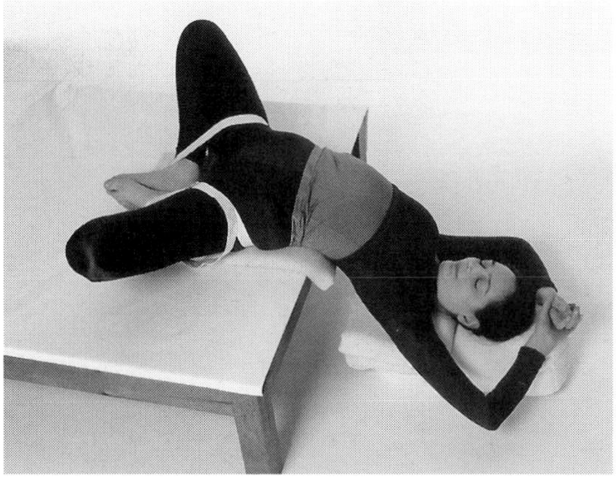

सेतुबन्ध-सर्वाङ्गासन स-बद्धकोणासन

Setubandha-Sarvāṅgāsana with *Baddhakoṇāsana* Shoulder Balance Bridge with Cobbler's Pose (on bench)

Method

Prepare the bench as before and sit on it. Before going into *Setubandha-Sarvāṅgāsana* bend the knees outwards and join the feet in *Baddhakoṇāsana*. Pass a belt round the base of the pelvis, over the thighs and under the feet. Tie the thighs and calves shins together tightly. Hold the bench and lie back, curving the waist over the edge and lowering the shoulders and head onto the bolster. Tighten the belt further. Take the arms over the head.

To come down, raise the feet and slip them out of the loop of the belt. Slide backwards off the bench. Bend forward in simple cross-legs, resting the forehead on the bench.

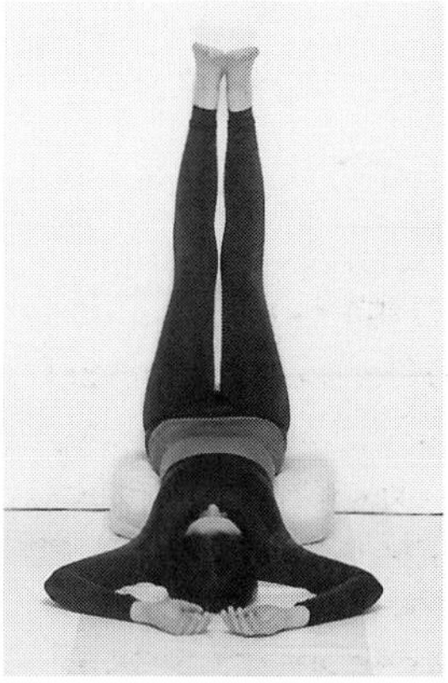
1

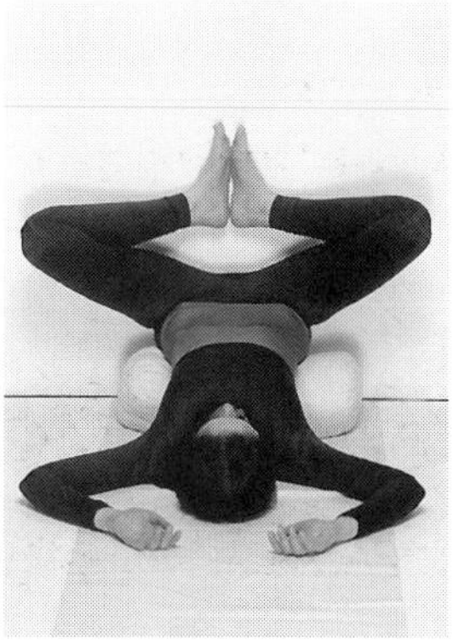
2

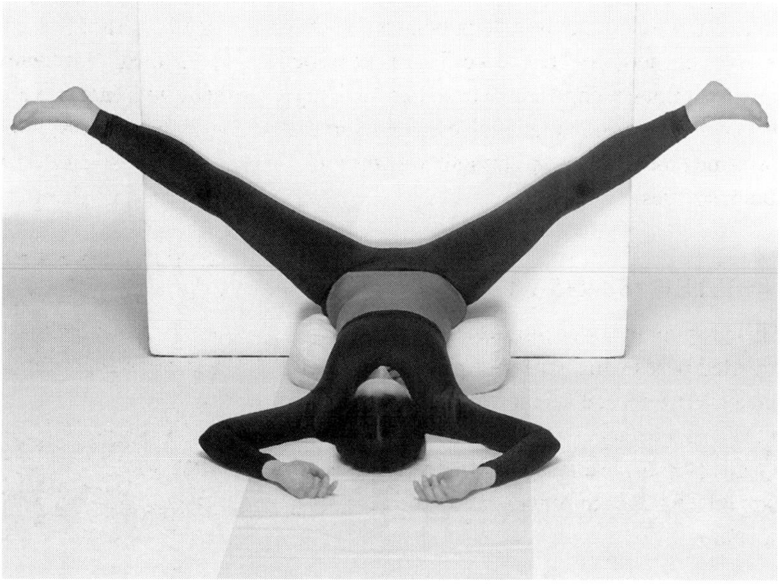
3

विपरीत-करणी मुद्रा स-बद्धकोणासना स-उपविष्टकोणासना

Viparīta-Karaṇī Mudrā with Baddhakoṇāsana and Upaviṣṭakoṇāsana Inverted Action Position with Cobbler's Pose and Seated-Angle Pose

Method

Follow the method given on page 131. Stay for a few minutes (1).

Then bend the knees outwards and join the feet in *Baddhakoṇāsana*. Bring the feet close to the body and rest them on the wall (2).

Stay for a few minutes.

Then spread the legs wide apart, resting them on the wall. Keep the knees straight (3).

Stay for a few minutes. Bring the legs together. Slide backwards off the bolster, turn to the side and get up.

Body Immunity

The body's resistance to and recovery from disease is nature's gift of healing. Overexertion, chronic illness, trauma and exposure to pollutants deplete its reserves of energy and resilience. These can be built up again through Yoga practice, so that the body recovers faster from fatigue, illness and injury. At the same time it builds up strength to withstand future stresses.

HOW THE *ĀSANAS* WORK

This programme concentrates on supported inverted poses which enhance physiological processes (*pitta*) and restore depleted *vāta*, bringing it back into balance. At the same time they reduce fatigue (*kapha*). Relaxation with the chest on a support continues the energization and balancing of *vāta*.

Inverted Poses (*kapha* –, *pitta* +, *vāta* =)

Supported inverted poses held for some time expand the ribcage and promote deep breathing from the top of the lungs. The increased oxygenation infuses the body with energy. Secondly, they act on the endocrine system. *Śīrṣāsana* brings blood to the all-important pituitary gland and *Sarvāṅgāsana* and its variations to the thyroid gland.

Relaxation (*kapha* +, *pitta* –, *vāta* =)

Relaxation with the chest supported similarly opens the chest and facilitates effortless deep breathing. The quietness of the pose refreshes the mind.

Props

Wall, chair, stool, bench, bolster, blankets

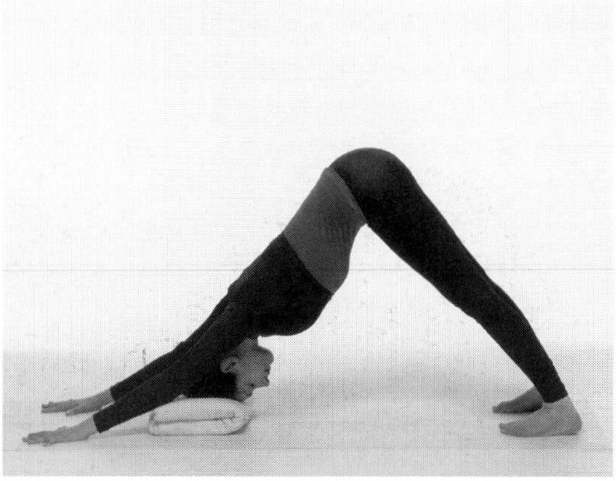

अधोमुख-श्वासन

Adhomukha-Śvāsana Dog Pose, Head Down (supported)

Method

Follow the method given on page 139, resting the head on a bolster and/or blankets. Stretch the arms and trunk up and keep the legs firm. Extend the heels downwards. Though the head presses down, there should be no discomfort. Lift the body upwards.

Stay for 30 seconds to 1 minute. Exhale and come down. Kneel and bend forward in *Adhomukha-Vīrāsana* (see page 59).

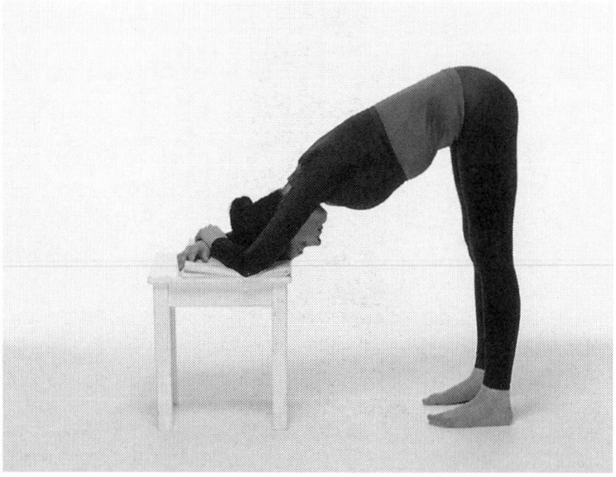

उत्तानासन

Uttānāsana Stretching Pose (on chair)

Method

Stand in *Tāḍāsana* (see page 54) and take the feet one foot apart. Exhale, bend forward and rest the head and arms on a stool or chair, with a blanket placed on top for comfort. Move the stool forward or backward so that the legs remain vertical. If the lower back is stiff, take the feet further apart.

Stay for 1 to 2 minutes. Inhale and come up.

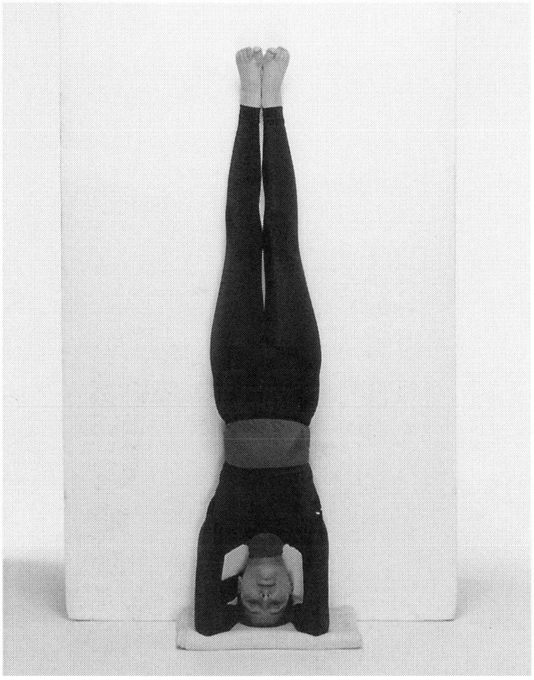

शीर्षासन

Śīrṣāsana Head Balance

Method

Follow the method given on pages 100–101.

Stay for 1 to 5 minutes. Exhale, bend the knees and come down. Rest with the head down for a short while.

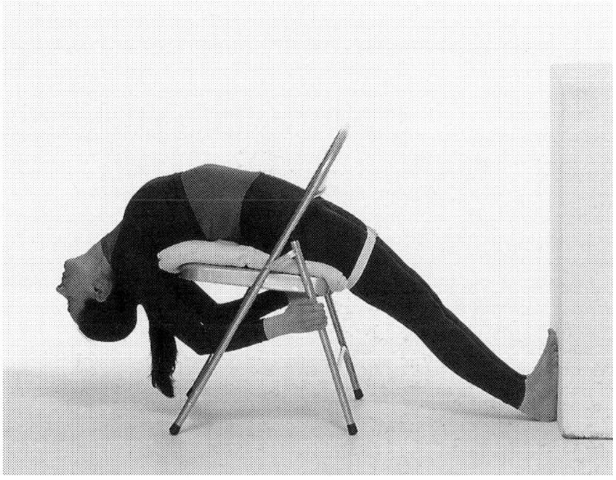

विपरीत-दण्डासन

Viparīta-Daṇḍāsana Inverted Staff Pose (on chair)

Method

Follow the method given on page 126.

Stay for 2 to 5 minutes. Bend the legs and hold the chair. Inhale and come up with a concave back.

सर्वाङ्गासन

Sarvāṅgāsana Shoulder Balance (on chair)

Method

Follow the method given on page 93.

Stay for 5 minutes or longer. Exhale and slide carefully backwards off the chair to come down.

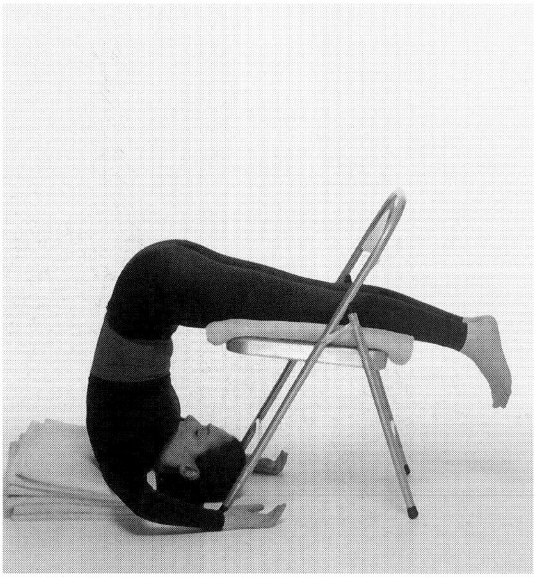

अर्ध-हलासन

Ardha-Halāsana Half-Plough Pose

Method

Follow the method given on page 85. Instead of a stool it is possible to use a chair, if the gap between the seat and back rest is wide enough for the legs to pass through.

Stay for 5 minutes or longer. Exhale and slide slowly down.

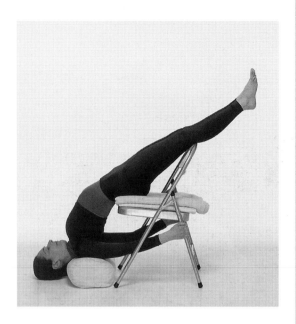

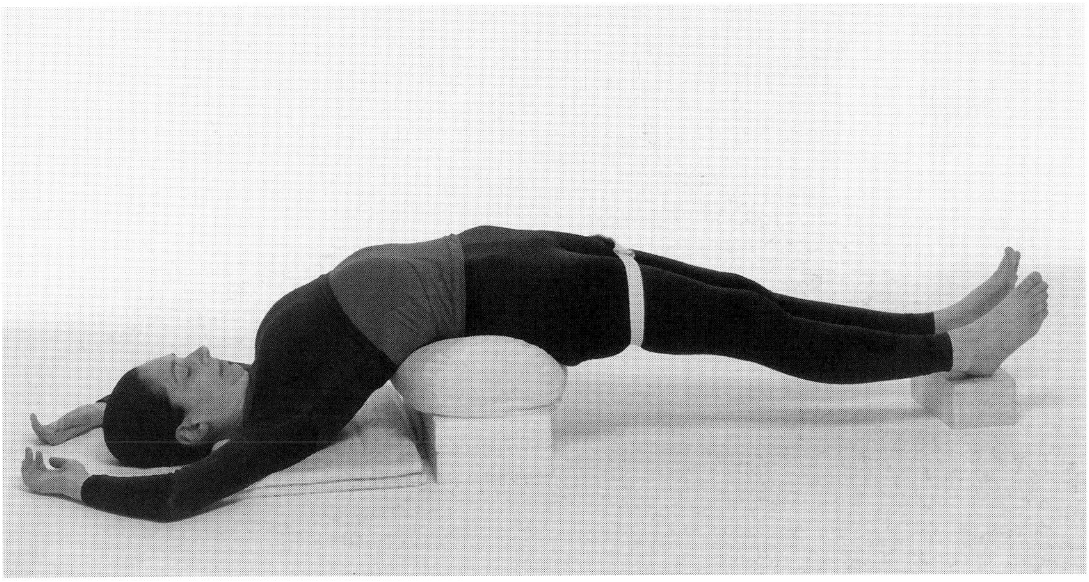

सेतुबन्ध-सर्वाङ्गासन

Setubandha-Sarvāṅgāsana Shoulder Balance Bridge (on bench)

Method

Follow any of the methods given so far. Another method is to use blocks and a bolster to support the lower back, and a brick for the feet.

Stay for 5 minutes or longer. Lift the hips, exhale and slide backwards. Sit in simple cross-legs and rest the head on the support.

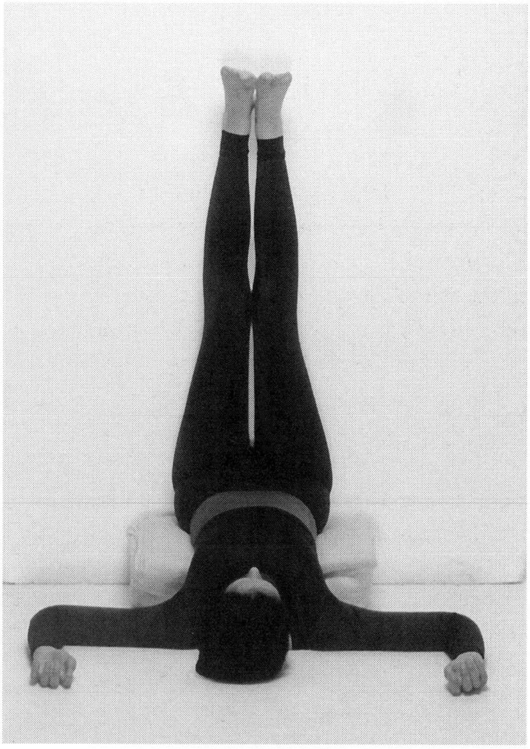

विपरीत-करणी मुद्रा

Viparīta-Karaṇī Mudrā Reverse Action Position

Method

Follow the method given on page 131.

Stay for 5 minutes or longer. Exhale and slide backwards. Turn to the side and get up.

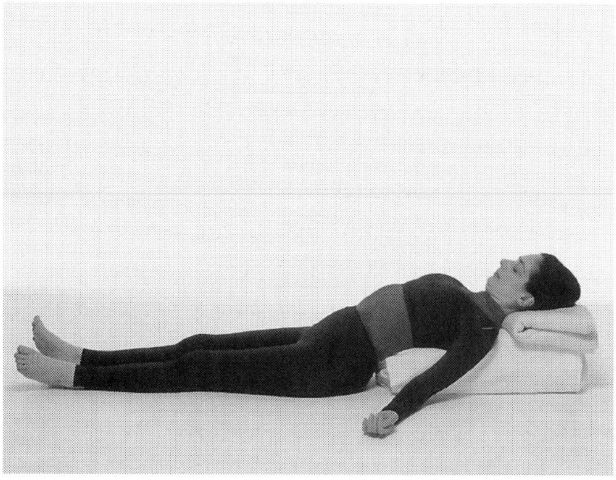

शवासन

Śavāsana Corpse Pose

Method

Follow the method given on page 74.

Stay for 5 to 10 minutes. Roll off the bolster to the side before getting up.

Mental and Emotional Well-being

The receiving and acting faculties together consist of ten components: the five organs of sense (eyes, ears, nose, tongue and skin), and the five organs of action (arms, legs, speech the generative organ and the excretory organ). Added to these is the eleventh, the mind or inner organ. Its function is to control the other organs, but in everyday life the reverse is often the case. The misuse of the sensory organs is deleterious both to physical health and to mental well-being. Through Yoga practice the senses as well as the mind can be trained to resist stimulation and to rest. This brings serenity.

One of the components of Yoga practice (the fifth of the eight limbs) is the non-excitation of the senses by their stimuli, called withdrawal from the objects of sense (PYS 2.54). When this is achieved the senses remain in their essential nature, which is a state of rest. The mind is the ruler of the senses, and when it is tranquil, so are the senses. This gives health to the mind.

Overuse of the Senses

There is a close link between the mind and the breath: "When the breath moves, the mind moves; when it is still, the mind is still" (HYP 4.23). This is the rationale behind the practice of *prāṇāyāma*, breath control. By following the breath with the mind's eye a quiet, introverted psychological state is brought about which is conducive to deep concentration and meditation. Deliberately training the rhythms of inhalation, exhalation and retention develops this quality of mind to a high degree.

Inhalation

Emphasis on inhalations increases the amount of oxygen taken in and energizes the mind.

Exhalation

Emphasis on exhalations quietens the senses and brain more and more deeply and brings about profound relaxation.

Retention

Retaining the breath for a period of time after inhalation or exhalation augments the effect of the breath. It slows down the cycle of breaths and allows a deeper experience. In retention after inhalation the energy is as if taken to a condenser to augment its active and kinetic output. In retention after exhalation the potential for passivity and relaxation is increased.

The Tension-free Mind

The mind is the instrument of knowledge, and as an instrument it processes and acts on the information it receives from the senses. The eye sees and transmits its vision; the mind evaluates the data and sends messages to the organs of action. Influencing the mind is each person's individualness (*ahaṃkāra*) which makes the decision of which act to perform, on the basis of "I want this" or "I do not want that."

The Senses

When the senses are tired there is fatigue, discomfort or worse. For example, too much reading, or reading in poor light causes eyestrain. Repeated subjection to loud noises affects hearing. Similarly, over-stimulation of the mind through intellectual activity or through emotional turbulence leads to mental tension and insomnia. Yoga practice relaxes and refreshes the senses and helps the mind to unwind. Over time it strengthens the senses and mind, promoting relaxed concentration and equilibrium of the emotions.

HOW THE *ĀSANAS* AND *PRĀṆĀYĀMA* WORK

This programme consists of poses which bring *vāta* into balance. Supported supine poses deepen shallow respiration and also promote stillness (*kapha*). Inverted poses similarly restore depleted respiratory energy. Supported forward bends and relaxation induce calm (*kapha*). When *vāta* is balanced, that is, not more or less than its optimum, the body can be transcended in *prāṇāyāma*. *Prāṇāyāma* goes beyond the *doṣas* to act on the mind, which is governed by *guṇas*. This technique reduces mental agitation (*rajas*) and induces lightness and stillness by the combined action of *sattva* and *tamas*.

Supine Poses (*kapha* +, *pitta* +, *vāta* =)

Supine poses with the chest supported allow the ribcage and lungs to expand. Deep breathing occurs naturally, replenishing the oxygen which has been depleted through overwork.

Inverted Poses (*kapha* –, *pitta* +, *vāta* =)

Inverted poses bring blood to the head and make air circulate in the upper lungs. This refreshes the sense organs and brain and re-oxygenates the body. *Śīrṣāsana* is not helpful for headaches because the body weight is taken on the head. *Ardha-Halāsana* is beneficial for headaches.

Forward bends (*kapha* +, *pitta* +, *vāta* –)

In forward bends the light pressure of the head on a support soothes the brain. The back brain rests on the front brain, quieting its normal state of activity. When a bandage is wrapped round the forehead the gentle circumferential pressure gives further relief from tension.

Relaxation (*kapha* +, *pitta* –, *vāta* =)

In *Śavāsana* the senses are trained to disengage themselves from their objects.

***Prāṇāyāma* (*rajas* –, *sattva* + [with the aid of *tamas*])**

In *prāṇāyāma* the mind is trained to follow the breath. This exchange of external for internal preoccupation makes the mind calm and steady. By concentrating on exhalations as in *Viloma Prāṇāyāma* II the mind relaxes more and more deeply. It is not suitable for those suffering from depression as it increases the introversion of the mind.

Props

Chair, bench, bolster, bandage

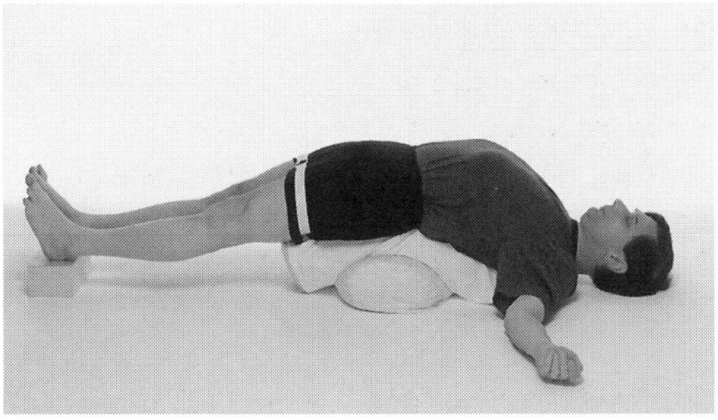

सेतुबन्ध-सर्वाङ्गासन

Setubandha-Sarvāṅgāsana Shoulder Balance Bridge (on bolsters)

Method

Place two bolsters on the floor in the shape of a cross, with the top one lengthwise. Sit on one end of the top bolster and tie the mid-thighs together with a belt. Slide a little forward, then lie back on the bolster, resting the shoulders and head on the floor. Raise the feet on a brick if necessary. Relax the arms by the sides of the body.

Stay for 5 minutes or longer. Bend the knees, untie the belt and slide backwards. Turn to the side to get up.

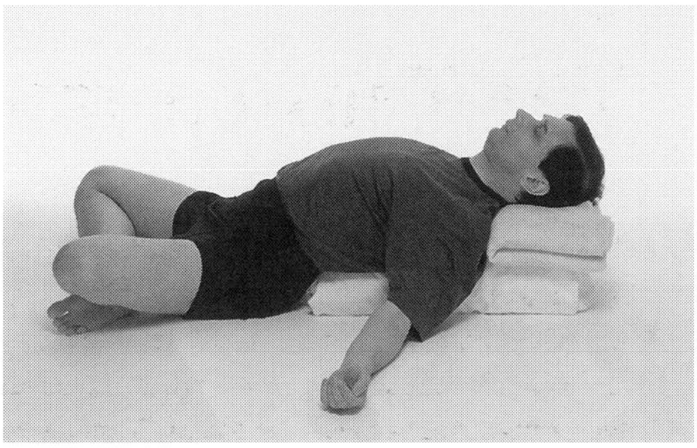

1

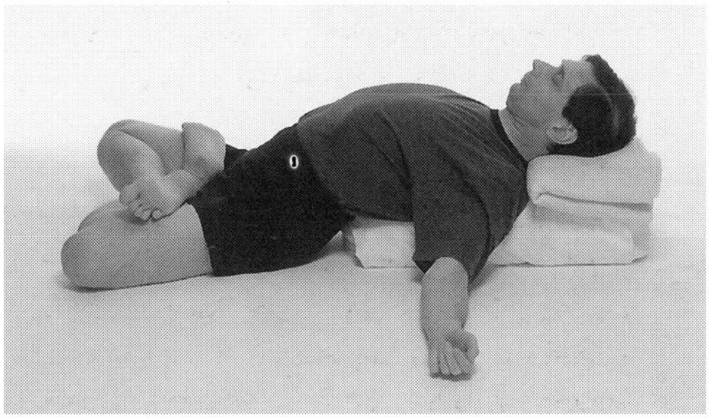

2

मत्स्यासन

Matsyāsana Fish Pose (simple)

Method

Lie back on a bolster placed lengthwise with the legs simple crossed. Support the head with a folded blanket (1).

Alternatively, do *Ardha-Padmāsana* (Half Lotus Pose) with the right foot on top of the left thigh and the left leg underneath (2).

Stay for 3 to 5 minutes, then change the cross-legs. Release the legs, turn to the side and get up.

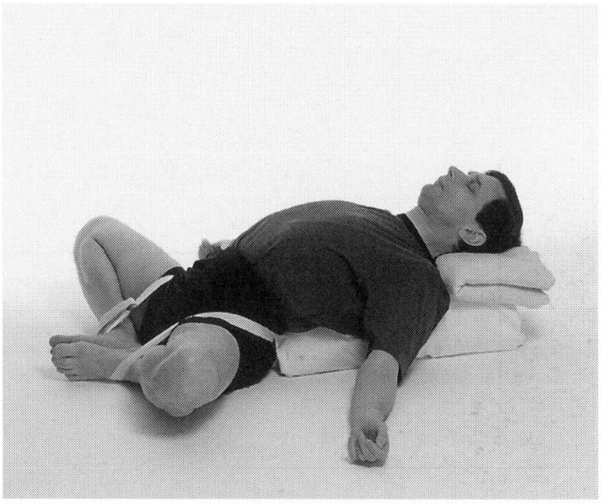

सुप्त-बद्धकोणासन

Supta-Baddhakoṇāsana Supine Cobbler's Pose (on bolster)

Method

Follow the method given on page 143.

Stay for 5 minutes or longer. Come up and untie the belt.

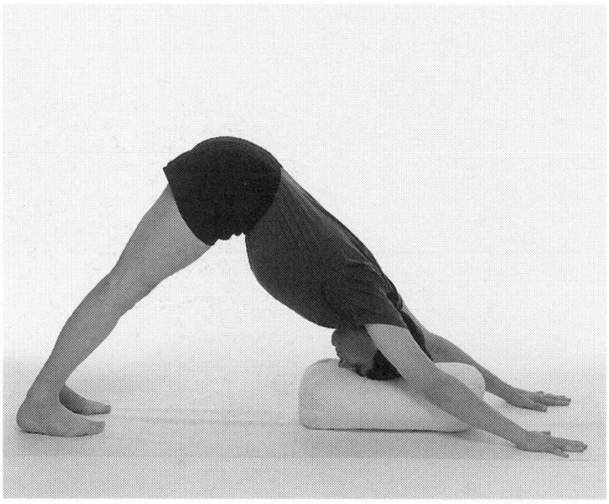

अधोमुख-श्वासन

Adhomukha-Śvāsana Dog Pose, Head Down (head supported)

Method

Follow the method given on page 152.

Stay for 1 to 2 minutes. Exhale and come down. Kneel and bend forward in *Adhomukha-Vīrāsana* (page 59).

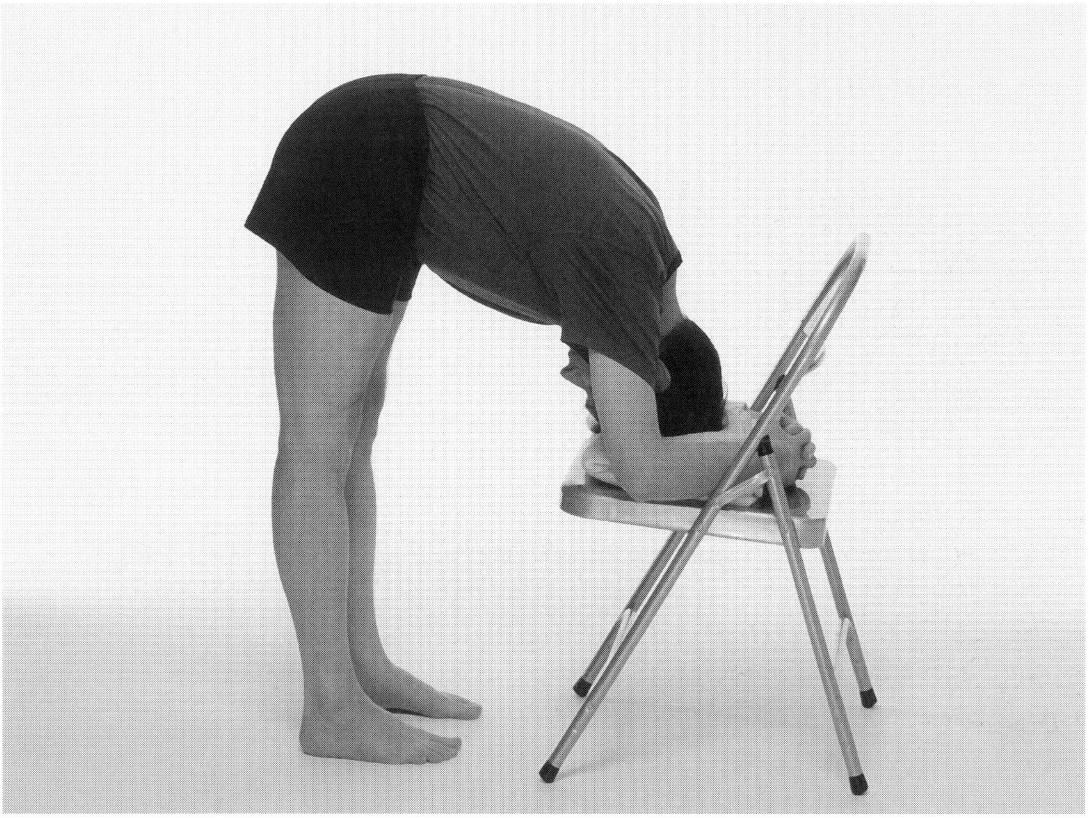

उत्तानासन

Uttānāsana Stretching Pose (on chair)

Method

Follow the method given on page 152.

Stay for 1 to 2 minutes. Inhale and stand straight.

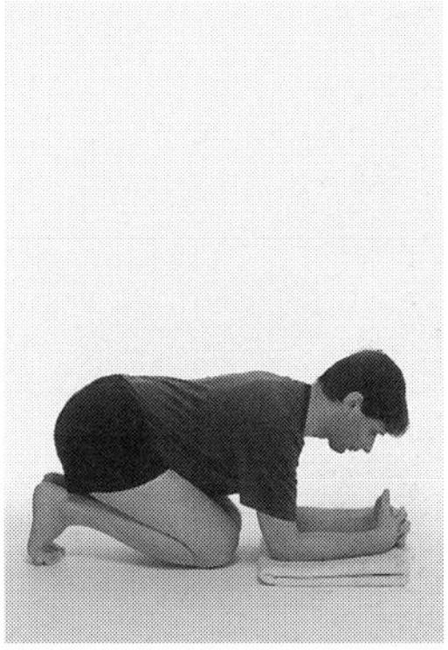

1

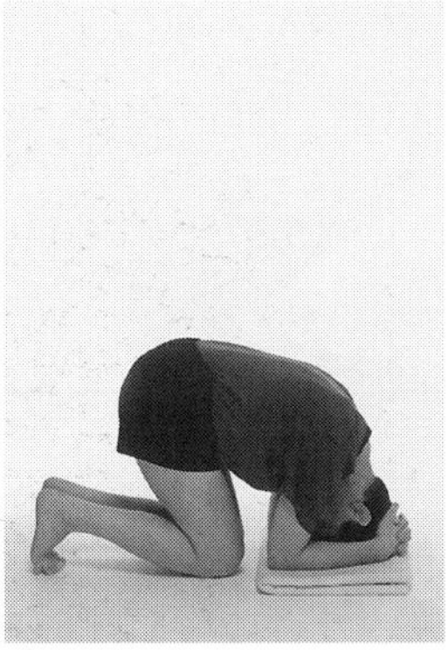

2

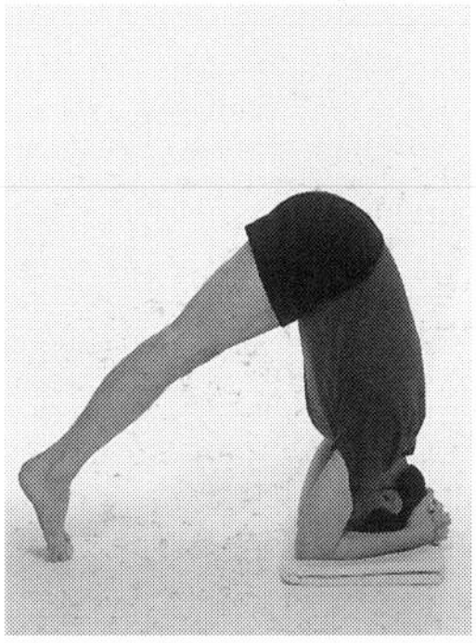

3

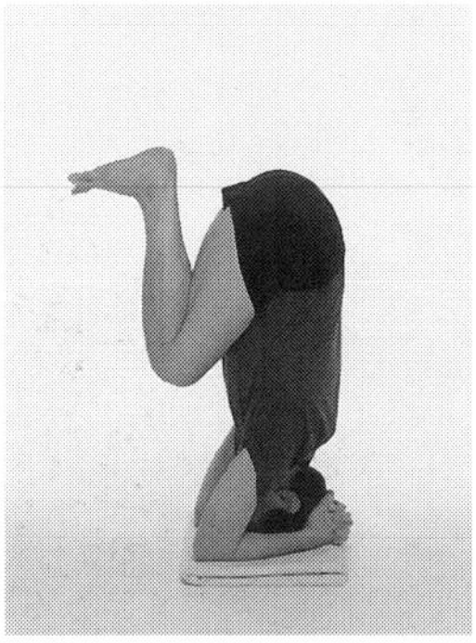

4

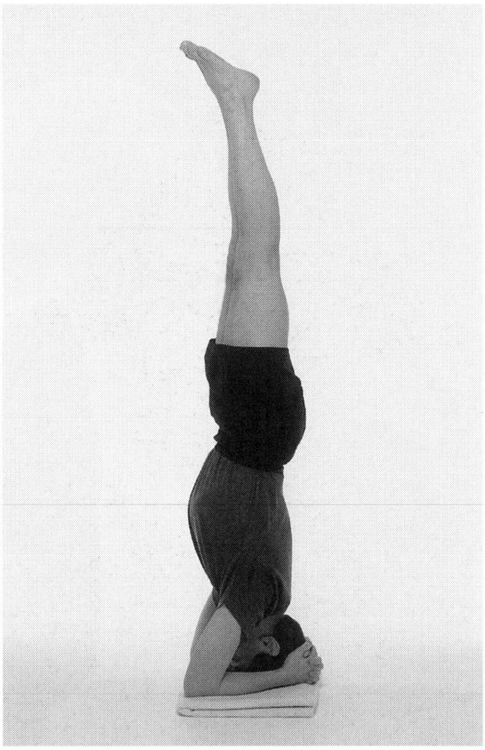

5

शीर्षासन

Śīrṣāsana Head Balance

Method

This method is for those who are confident about being able to balance independently. Otherwise, *Śīrṣāsana* should be done against the wall. To learn to balance, stay with the feet 2 or 3 inches away from the wall. When this is easy, do *Śīrṣāsana* with the hands a few inches away from the wall and stay in the pose without touching the wall. When this is easy, go into the middle of the room.

Place a folded blanket on the floor, away from the wall and any furniture, with the neat edge to the front. Kneel in front of it, interlock the fingers and place the forearms on the blanket. Keep the elbows in line with the shoulders and the shape of the two arms symmetrical. Move the shoulders back away from the neck (1).

Place the crown of the head on the floor, with the back of the head against the hands. Lift the shoulders again (2).

Raise the hips and straighten the knees. Walk in a little. Keep the shoulders lifted, the shoulder blades in and the chest forward (3).

Exhale, bend the legs and jump up, bringing the knees towards the abdomen (4).

Continue the upward swing of the legs till the thighs are vertical and the knees bent back. Lift the shoulders and stretch the trunk up.

Straighten the legs up. Tighten the knees. Move the tailbone into the body and tighten the buttocks. Stretch the trunk and legs up. Keep the shoulders lifted and the head relaxed. Breathe normally (5).

Stay for 1 to 5 minutes. Exhale, bend the knees and come down. Kneel and bend forward, resting the forehead.

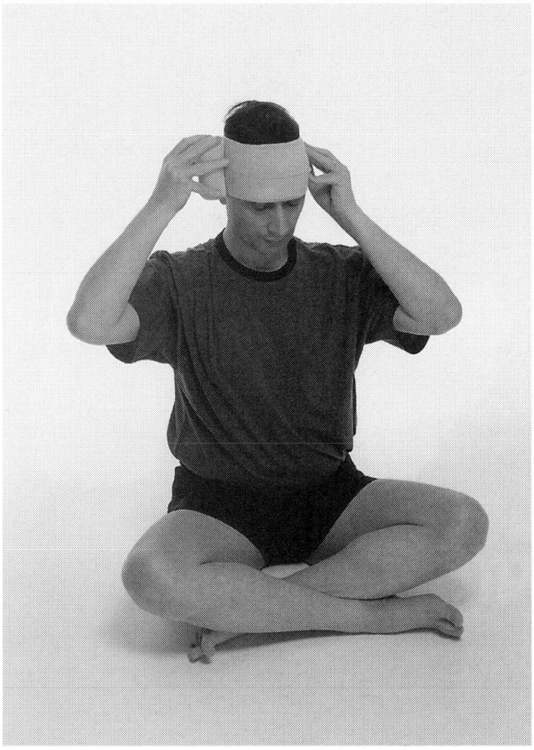

Tying a bandage

Method

Use a cotton crepe bandage. Wrap a bandage around the forehead and back of the head.

To undo it, unroll it slowly; do not pull it off.

Note
The Effect of the Bandage

The gentle pressure of the bandage soothes the mind and quietens the mind. It induces a feeling of coolness in the hand.

Many postures may be done with a bandage tied in this way: in particular, forward bends where the head rests on a support. This is very effective in relieving headaches.

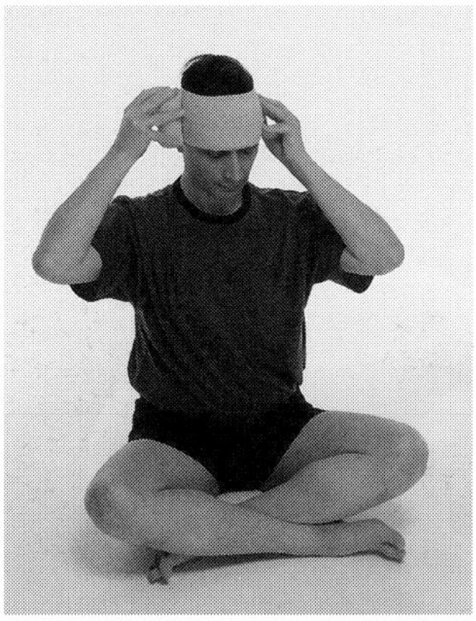

1

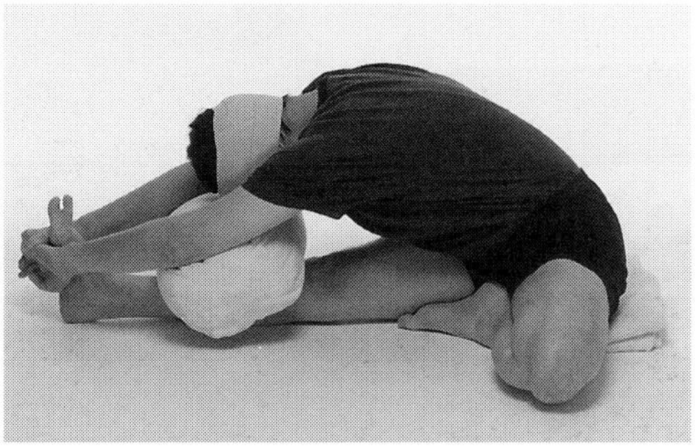

2

जानुशीर्षासन

Jānuśīrṣāsana Head-to-Knee Pose (supported)

Method

Wrap a bandage around the forehead (1).

Follow the method given on page 144 (2).

Stay for 1 to 2 minutes. Repeat on the left.

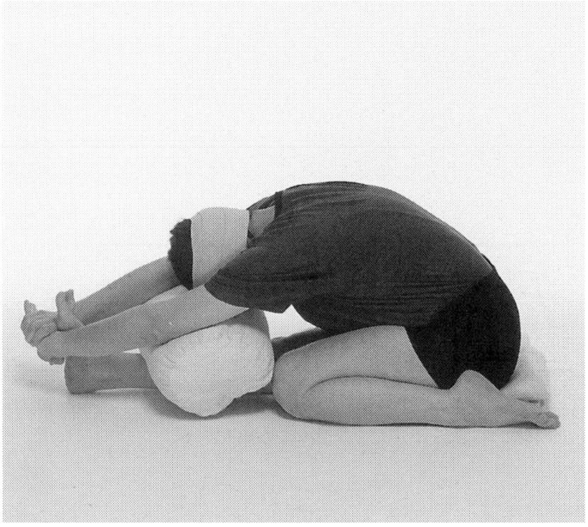

एकपाद-वीर-पश्चिमोत्तानासन

Ekapāda-Vīra-Paścimottānāsana Posterior Stretch with One Leg in Hero Pose (supported)

Method

Follow the method given on page 145.

Stay for 1 to 2 minutes. Repeat on the left.

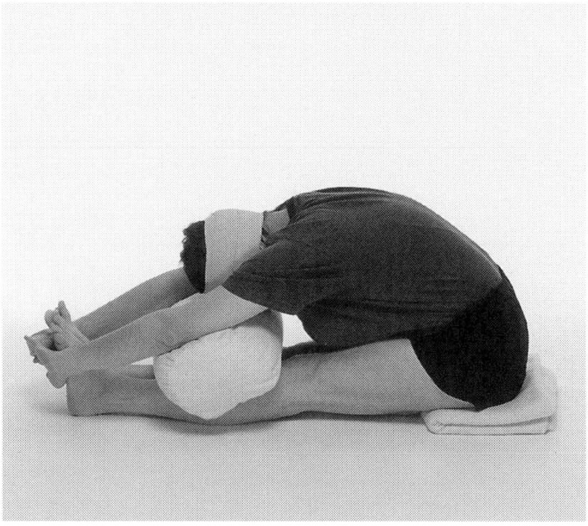

पश्चिमोत्तानासन

Paścimottānāsana Posterior Stretching Pose (supported)

Method

Follow the method given on page 145.

Stay for 2 to 3 minutes.

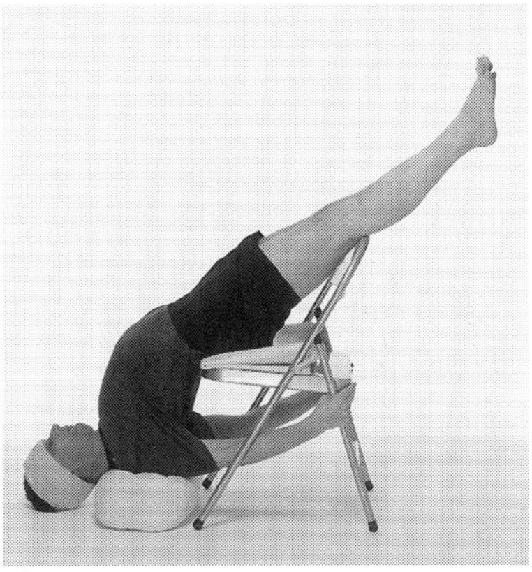

1

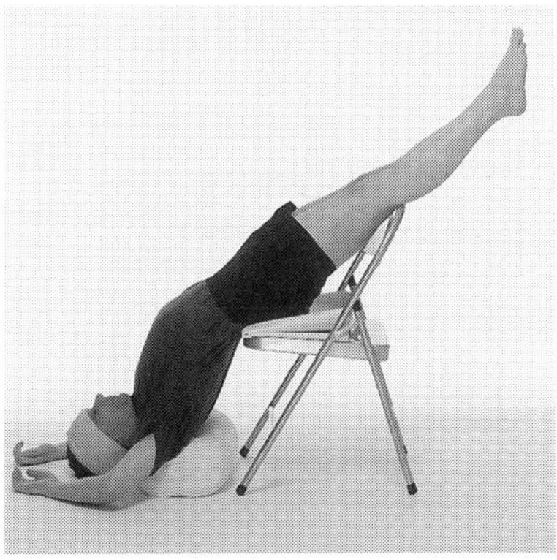

2

सर्वाङ्गासन

Sarvāṅgāsana Shoulder Balance (on chair)

Method

Follow the method given on page 93 (1). Stay for a little while.

Then, making sure the shoulders are securely on the bolster, take the arms over the head (2).

Stay for 5 minutes or longer. Exhale, slide backwards off the chair or go into:

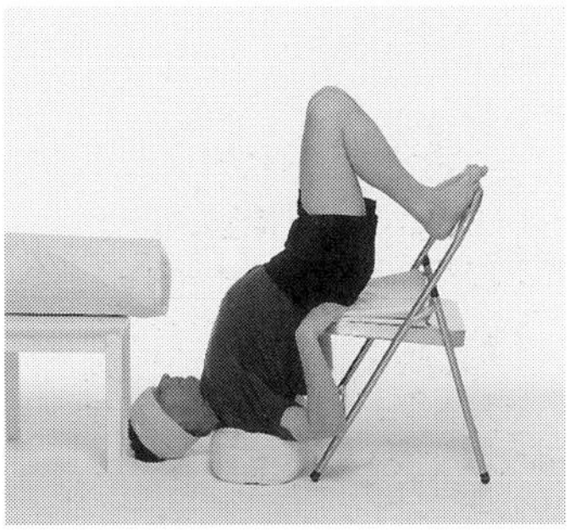

1

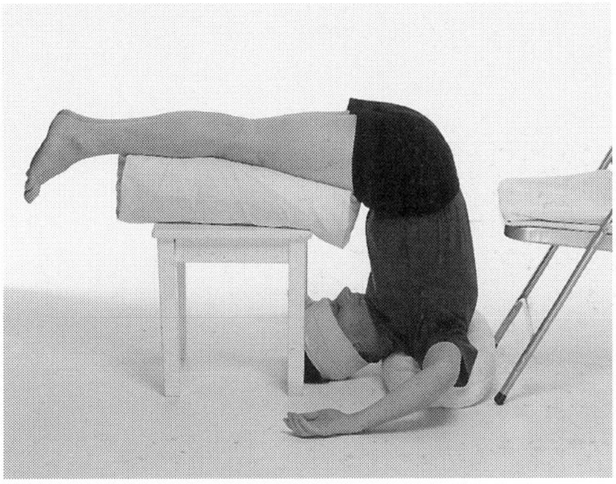

2

अर्ध-हलासन

Ardha-Halāsana Half-Plough Pose

Method

Follow the method given on page 85. Alternatively, before going into *Sarvāṅgāsana*, prepare the stool and bolster and place it near the head. In *Sarvāṅgāsana*, bend the legs and place the feet on the back of the chair. Hold the seat (1).

Carefully lift the sacrum off the seat. Take the legs over onto the stool. If necessary bring the stool closer. Support the thighs right to the tops. Make sure the shoulders are supported well on the blankets, then take the arms over the head (2).

To come down, hold the chair. Bend the knees and ease the hips backwards. Lift the legs and rest the feet on the back of the chair. Push the stool away. Then slide backwards off the chair.

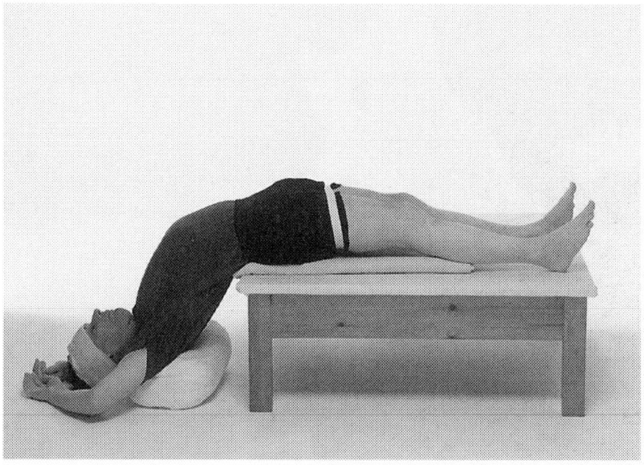

सेतुबन्ध-सर्वाङ्गासन

Setubandha-Sarvāṅgāsana
Shoulder Balance Bridge (on bench)

Method

Follow the method given on page 109.

Stay for 5 minutes or longer. Slide backwards off the bench to come down. Sit in front of it in simple cross-legs and bend forward.

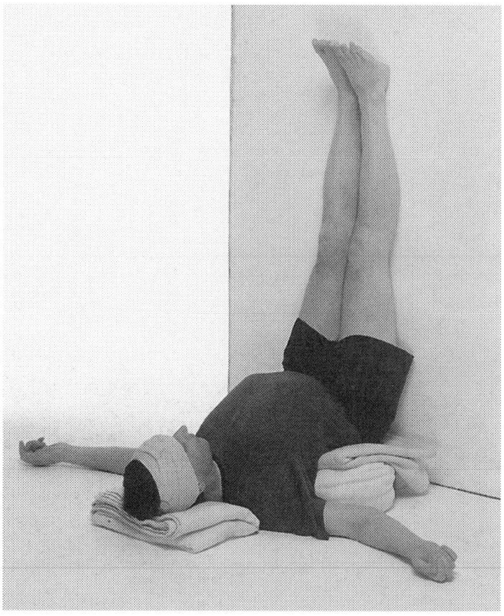

विपरीत-करणी मुद्रा

Viparīta-Karaṇī Mudrā
Reverse Action Position

Method

Follow the method given on page 131.

Stay for 5 minutes or longer. Slide backwards to come down.

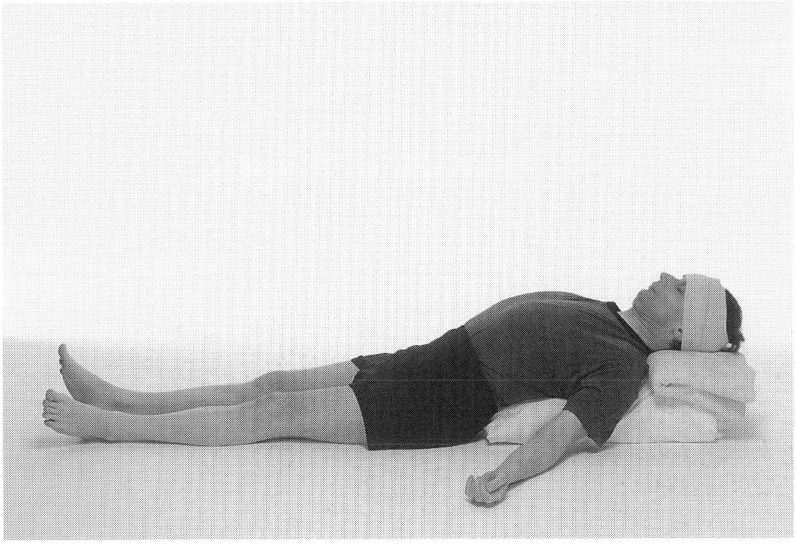

शवासन

Śavāsana Corpse Pose (on bolster)

Method

Lie with the back supported on a bolster placed lengthwise, the buttocks on the floor. Support the head and neck with a folded blanket. Move the shoulders away from the neck and press them down. Dispose the arms and legs symmetrically. Stretch and then relax them. Keep the palms facing up. If the abdomen is tense, take the legs a little further apart. Relax the thighs. Keep the sternum lifted. Close the eyes.

Relax the face. Let the eye-balls descend into the sockets. Relax the forehead, temples and area around the eyes. Widen the space between the eyebrows. Gently draw the outer corners of the eyes to the sides. Relax the cheeks. Relax the jaws; let the lower jaw fall slightly away from the upper jaw. To do this, open the mouth slightly, then close it so that the lips are barely touching. Relax the lips; draw the lip corners slightly away from each other. Let the tongue rest on the floor of the mouth and descend further back into the throat. Relax the throat; let it rest on the back of the neck. Relax the chin. Relax the ears; let them hear sounds passively, without straining. Relax the nose and nostrils; let air pass in and out without distorting their shape. Let the brain shrink inside the skull. Relax the scalp.

Spend a few minutes relaxing the body and senses deliberately in this way.

After a while begin to follow the breath with the mind's eye. Watch the inhalations and exhalations; make them smooth and rhythmic. Breathe evenly with the right and left nostrils and lungs. Gradually prolong the breaths, but be careful not to strain. The air should enter the lungs without disturbing the head. Breathe softly, slowly and deeply. (This is *Ujjāyi-Prāṇāyāma* Conquest-Helping Breath.) After a few minutes cease the deep breathing and revert to normal breathing.

When *Śavāsana* and *Ujjāyi-Prāṇāyāma* become familiar, add the pose overleaf:

विलोम-प्राणायाम २

Bāhya-Viloma-Prāṇāyāma Exhalation in Stages

bāhya = external; *viloma* = against the grain; *prāṇa* = breath, life-breath, vital air; *āyāma* = restraint, control

Method

Exhale completely, to empty the lungs of stale air.

Take a deep inhalation, drawing the breath in from the sides of the pubis. Keep the abdomen deflated towards the spine, widen the floating ribs and open the rib cage outwards and upwards. Inhale till the breath reaches the collar bones, if possible, but do not strain to do this. After inhaling fully, press the shoulders down and move the shoulder blades in. Maintain the lift of the upper trunk and exhale in three stages as follows:

Exhale partially, pause, exhale partially, pause, complete the exhalation. Make the partial exhalations smooth and unhurried. Enjoy the stillness of the pauses. Towards the end of the exhalation allow the abdomen to recede further towards the spine. Do not allow the sternum to collapse. Keep the head relaxed throughout.

After the interrupted exhalation take two or three normal breaths so that the lungs recover. If strain is still felt, make the partial exhalations and pauses shorter. ##

Repeat from # to ## 6 times.

Revert to normal breathing and lie quietly. Open the eyes. Turn to the right, coming down off the bolster. Stay on the side, with the blanket still supporting the head. Roll to the other side and get up.

Remove the bandage by unrolling it carefully. Do not pull it off the head, as this will spoil the soothing effect of the bandage.

The Affirmative Mind

The mind is constructed to learn and to apply its learning to all situations in life. This makes it so resourceful that it is predisposed to overcome obstacles. This natural gift becomes tarnished when negative feelings and experiences overwhelm positive mental attitudes and will-power. Yoga practice helps the mind to regain the courage to face difficulties and to remain cheerful.

HOW THE *ĀSANAS* AND *PRĀṆĀYĀMA* WORK

This programme consists of supported supine poses which stimulate physiological functioning in the chest (*pitta*) and brings *vāta* to an ideal state of plenty. Inverted poses continue these effects while at the same time refreshing the mind, reducing dullness (*kapha*). Supported backbends increase *vāta* by increasing the oxygen intake, enhance physiological functioning (*pitta*) and combat lethargy (*kapha*). Relaxation brings *vāta* into balance. The *prāṇāyāma* technique energizes the mind directly, increasing initiative (*rajas*) and brightness (*sattva*) and dispelling dullness (*tamas*).

Supine Poses (*kapha* +, *pitta* +, *vāta* =)

Supine poses on a support lift and expand the chest. This increases the intake of oxygen, energizing the body and mind. The sternum (breast bone) remains raised rather than sinking towards the heart and the diaphragm is expanded rather than constricted. These open positions discourage fear and depression.

Inverted Poses (*kapha* –, *pitta* +, *vāta* =)

Inverted poses increase the flow of blood to the brain and the flow of air into the top lungs. The effort required in jumping up into the arm- and elbow-balance creates exhilaration. The energy pumped into the body in large quantities banishes apathy.

Backbends (*kapha* –, *pitta* +, *vāta* +)

Backbends expand and lift the chest to a great degree, flushing the body with oxygen. The curving of the spine backwards lengthens the anterior spine and increases the flow of blood to it and to the nerves of the spinal cord. As a result the nervous system is strengthened, building stamina and will-power. Backbends are extremely invigorating and create positive mental energy. They are the key to youthfulness.

Relaxation (*kapha* +, *pitta* –, *vāta* =)

Relaxation settles the mind and body prior to *prāṇāyāma*.

***Prāṇāyāma* (*sattva* +, *rajas* +, *tamas* –)**

Concentrating on inhalations energizes the mind by increasing the oxygen intake. *Viloma Prāṇāyāma* I is not suitable for those suffering from hypertension.

Props

Wall, table, chair, bench, bolster, blankets, brick, belt

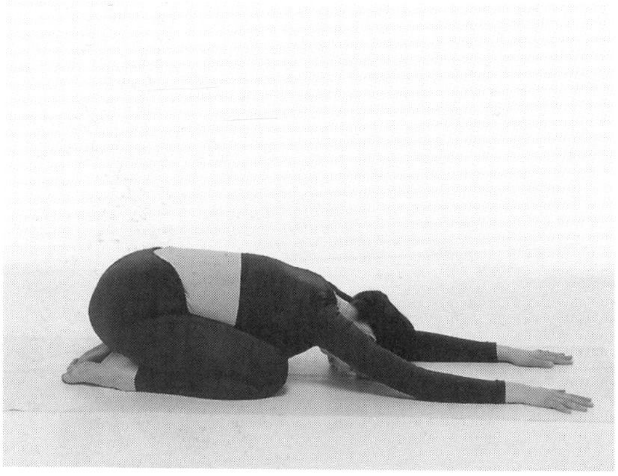

अधोमुख-वीरासन

Adhomukha-Vīrāsana Hero Pose, Head Down

Method

Follow on from previous pose.

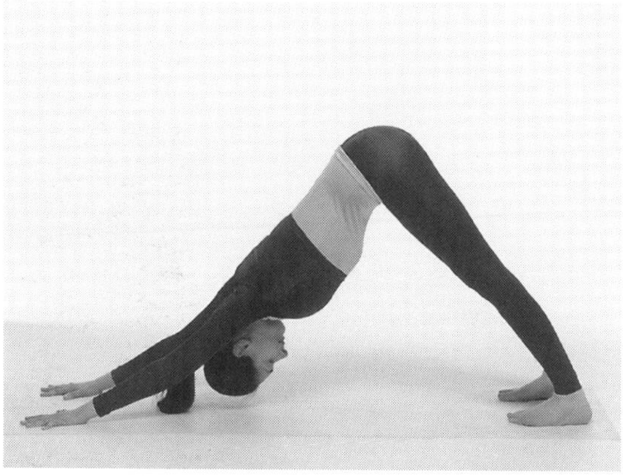

अधोमुख-श्वासन

Adhomukha-Śvāsana Dog Pose, Head Down

Method

Follow the method given on page 139.

Stay for 1 to 2 minutes. Exhale, kneel and bend forward.

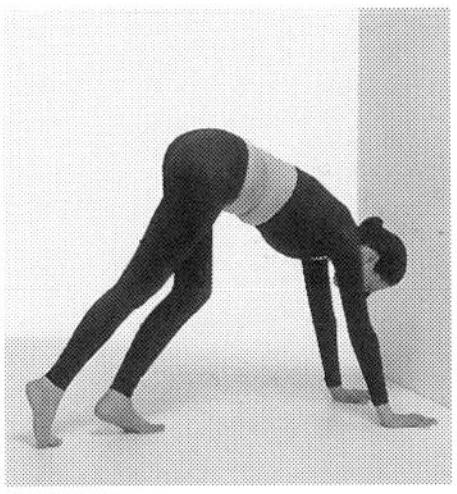

1

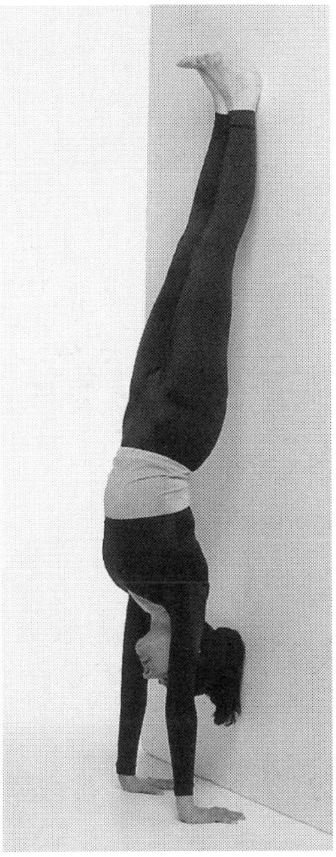

2

अधोमुख-वृक्षासन

Adhomukha-Vṛkṣāsana Full-Arm Balance or Hand Stand

adho = downward; mukha = face, mouth; vṛkṣa = tree

Method

Go near the wall. Bend down and place the palms down 4 to 6 inches away from it, shoulder-width apart. Align the hands and spread the fingers. Step back, as if preparing to do *Adhomukha-Śvāsana* (Dog Pose). Bend one leg and keep the other straight (1).

Kick the straight leg upwards to the wall. With a strong kick the other one follows suit. **Do not bend the elbows**. Join the legs. Press the heels firmly against the wall. Lift the shoulders and stretch the trunk and legs up. Move the coccyx (tailbone) in. Keep the head relaxed (2).

Stay for 10 to 30 seconds. Exhale and come down, one leg at a time.

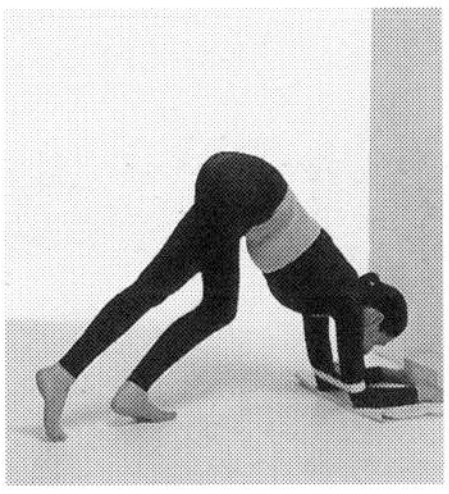

1

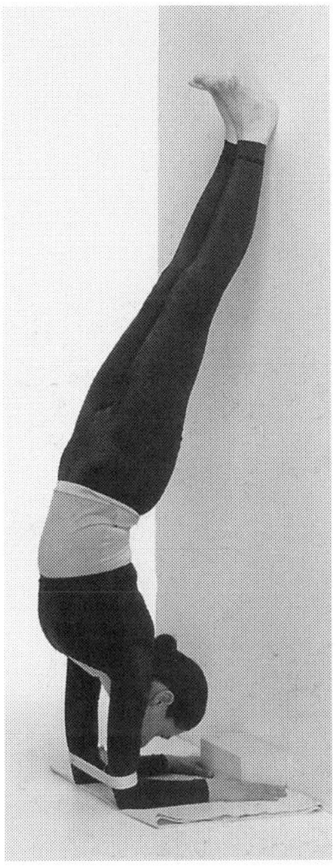

2

पिच्छ-मयूरासन

Piccha-Mayūrāsana Elbow-Balance (Peacock Tail Pose)

piccha = feather, tail-feather; mayūra = peacock

Method

Go near the wall. Kneel and tie a belt round the upper arms just above the elbows, shoulder-width apart. Place the forearms down and hold a brick between the index fingers and thumbs, with the palms down. The brick support stops the hands moving inwards and, together with the belt, gives the arms strength. Touch the wall with the middle finger. Lift the hips and straighten the legs. Step back and prepare to jump up. Bend one leg and keep the other straight. **Keep the head up (1).**

Kick the straight leg upwards to the wall. With a strong kick the other one follows suit. Join the legs. Press the heels firmly against the wall. Lift the shoulders and stretch the trunk and legs up. Move the chest forwards and take the coccyx (tailbone) in (2).

Stay for 10 to 30 seconds. Exhale and come down, one leg at a time.

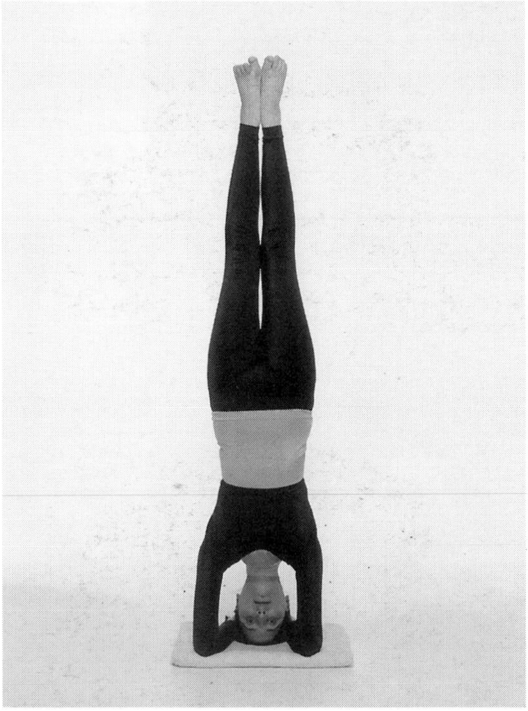

शीर्षासन

Śirṣāsana Head Balance

Method

Follow the method given on page 162 for doing *Śirṣāsana* independently.

Alternatively, do it against the wall as shown previously (see pages 100–101).

Stay for 2 to 5 minutes. Exhale and come down. Kneel and bend forward till the head comes back to normal.

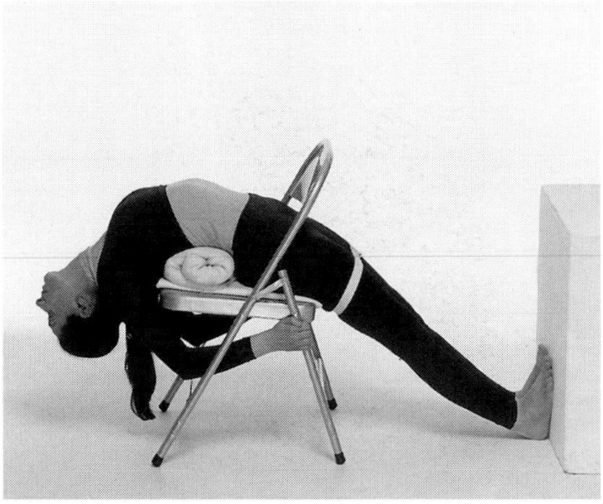

विपरीत-दण्डासन

Viparīta-Daṇḍāsana Inverted Staff Pose (on chair)

Method

Follow the method given on page 126. Roll an extra blanket and place it across the chair seat before going down. This opens the chest further.

Stay for 2 to 5 minutes. Bend the legs and hold the top of the chair. Inhale and come up with the back concave. Lean forward over the back of the chair.

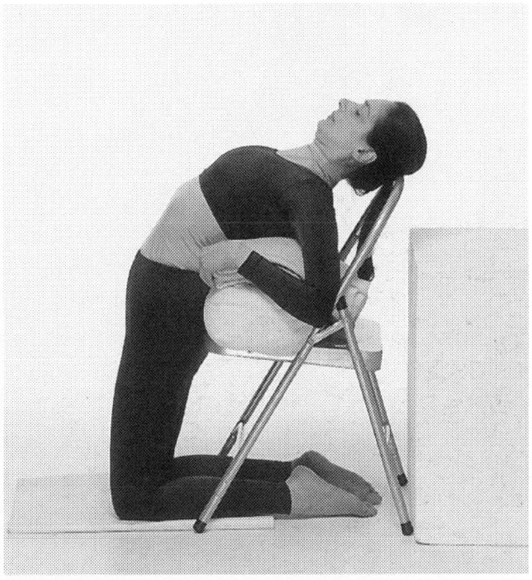

उष्ट्रासन

Uṣṭrāsana Camel Pose (on chair)

Method

Follow the method given on page 100.

Stay for 2 to 5 minutes. Inhale and come up.

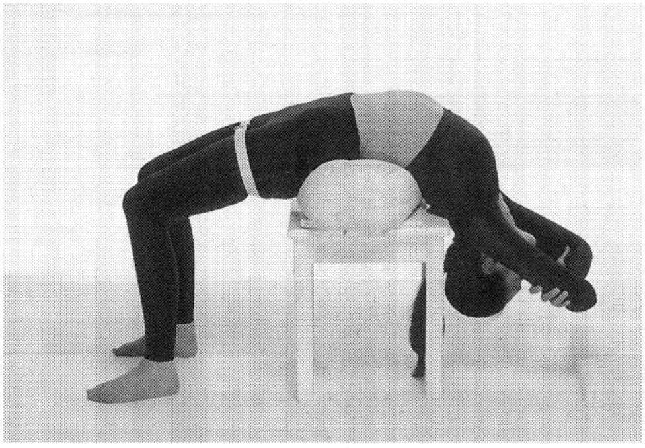

1

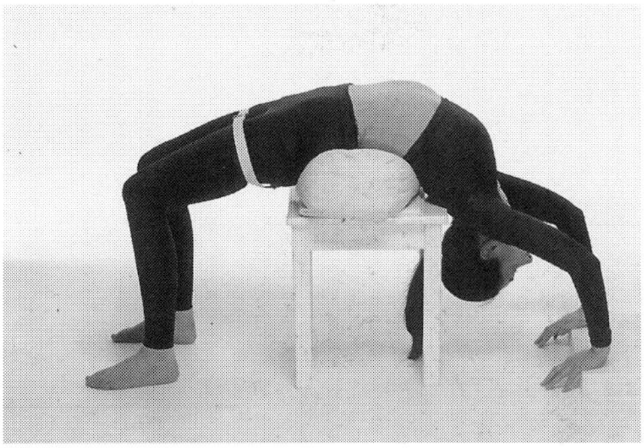

2

ऊर्ध्व-धनुरासन

Ūrdhva-Dhanurāsana Upward Bow Pose (from chair)

ūrdhva = upwards; dhanus (dhanur) = bow

Method

Place a stool 1½ to 2 feet away from the wall. On it place a mat and bolster. Place two bricks against the wall, shoulder-width apart. Sit on the bolster with the back to the wall. Optionally tie the legs together at mid-thigh with a belt.

Slide a little forward so that the tailbone is off the bolster. Lie back over the bolster. Take the arms over the head and fold the elbows (1).

Stay for a little while, then place the hands on the bricks. Keep the legs firm (2).

Stay for 20 to 30 seconds. Bring the arms back and hold the stool. Inhale and swing the body up.

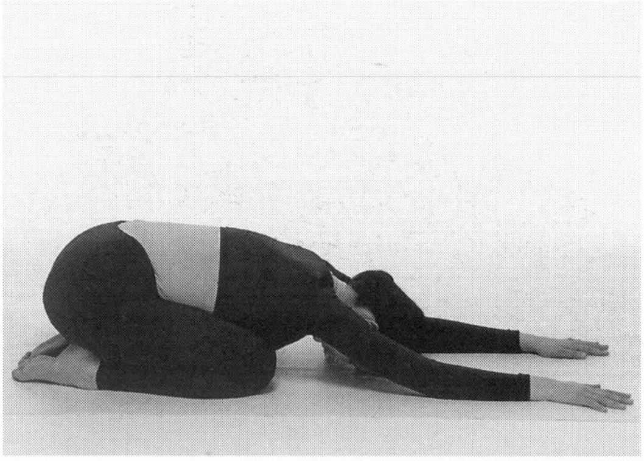

अधोमुरव-वीरासन

Adhomukha-Vīrāsana
Hero Pose, Head Down

Method

Kneel and bend forward for 30 seconds to 1 minute.

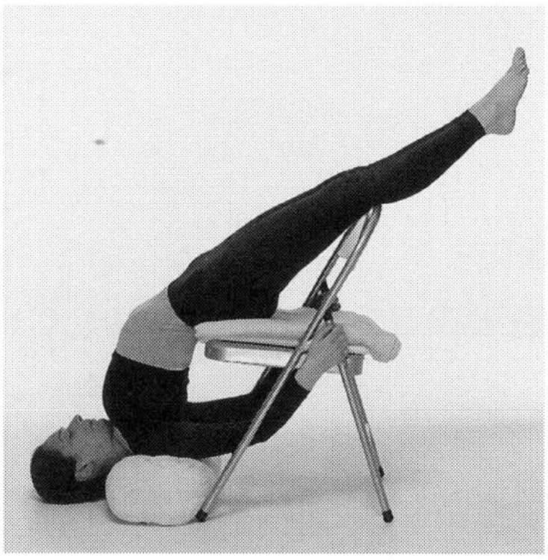

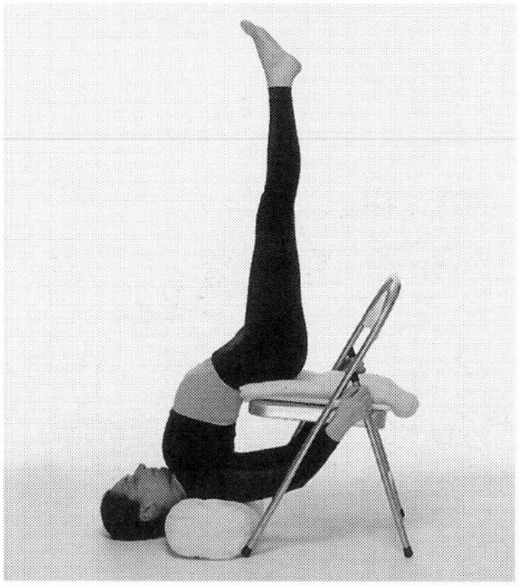

सर्वाङ्गासन

Sarvāṅgāsana Shoulder Balance (on chair)

Method

Follow the method given on page 93 (1).

Bend the legs and place the feet on the back of the chair. Then take the legs vertically up. Press the outer hips down and stretch the legs (2).

Stay for 5 minutes or longer. Alternate between the two positions. Slide backwards off the chair to come down.

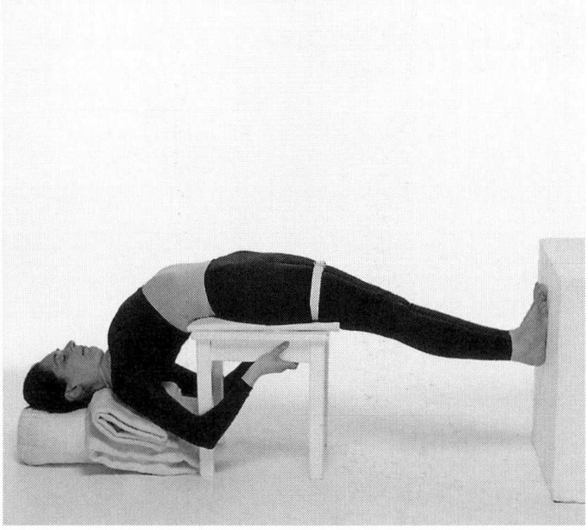

सेतुबन्ध-सर्वाङ्गासन

Setubandha-Sarvāṅgāsana Shoulder Balance Bridge (on bench)

Method

Place a low stool 2 to 2½ feet away from the wall, with a blanket on top for padding. Place a bolster lengthwise in front of it. Place a folded blanket on the bolster. Sit on the stool facing the wall. Tie the mid-thighs together with a belt. Lie back so that the waist curves over the edge of the stool and rest the shoulders on the folded blanket, the head on the bolster. Raise the legs, tighten the knees and press the feet against the wall. Grip the stool firmly, press the shoulders down and move the chest forward. Keep the throat relaxed.

Stay for 5 minutes or longer. Bend the legs and slide backwards off the stool.

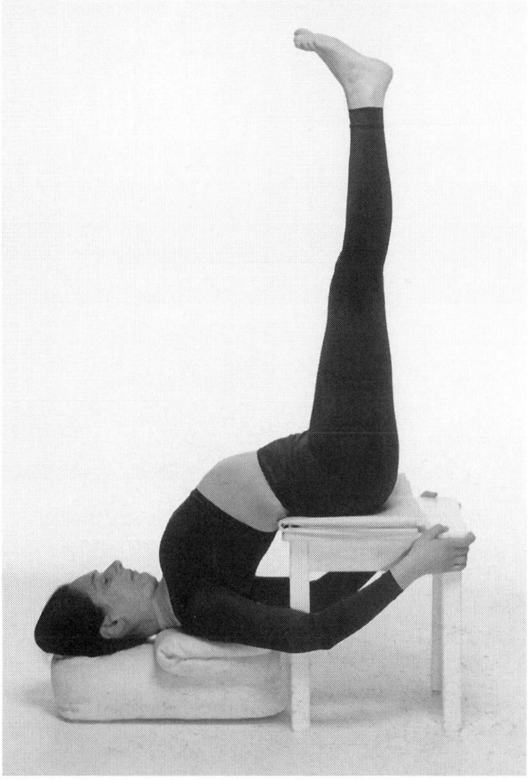

विपरीत-करणी मुद्रा

Viparīta-Karaṇī Mudrā Reverse Action Position

Method

Be in *Setubandha-Sarvāṅgāsana* as above. Bend the legs, raise them over the abdomen and straighten them vertically up. Press the outer hips down, tighten the knees and stretch the feet. Press the shoulders down and open the chest.

Stay for 2–5 minutes. Bend the legs and slide backwards off the stool.

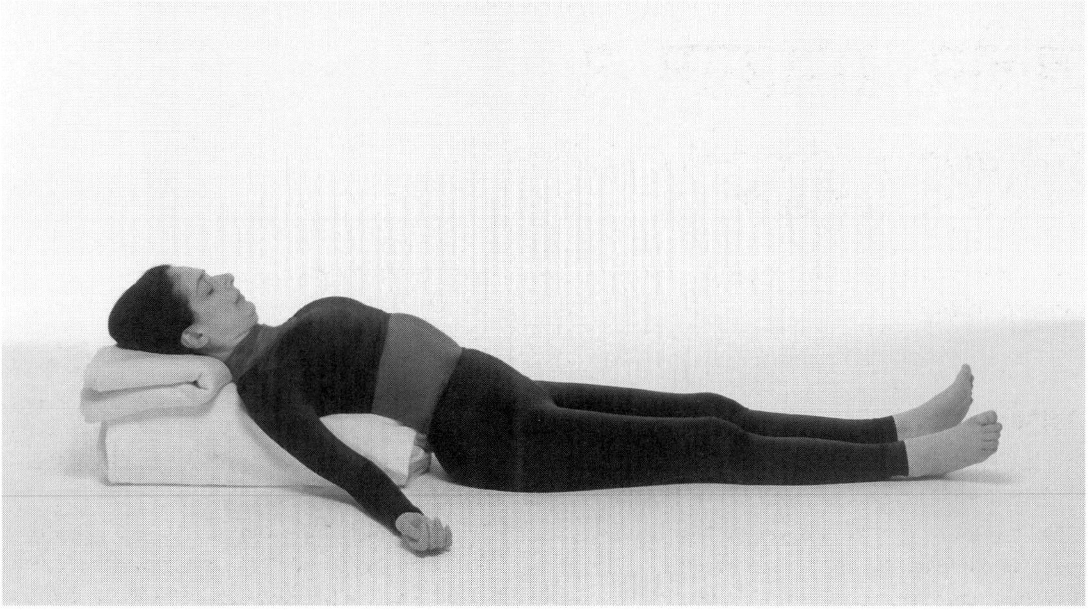

शवासन

Śavāsana Corpse Pose (on bolster)

Method

Follow the method of *Śavāsana* and *Ujjāyi-Prāṇāyāma* given on page 167.

Then continue with the following *prāṇāyāma*:

विलोम-प्राणायाम ९

Ābhyantara-Viloma-Prāṇāyāma
Inhalation in Stages

ābhyantara = internal; viloma = against the grain; prāṇa = breath, life-breath, vital air; āyāma = restraint, control

Method

Exhale completely, to empty the lungs of stale air.

Inhale in three stages as follows:

Inhale partially, pause, inhale partially, pause, complete the inhalation. Make the partial inhalations smooth and unhurried. Start the inhalation mentally from the sides of the pubis and draw the breath smoothly upwards towards the chest. Experience the breath spreading in the lungs during the pauses. During the successive partial inhalations keep the abdomen deflated towards the spine and open the rib cage outwards and upwards. Do not strain. Keep the face, throat and eyes relaxed. After inhaling fully, press the shoulders down and move the shoulder blades in. Bring the chin down.

Maintain the lift of the upper trunk and slowly exhale. Towards the end of the exhalation allow the abdomen to recede further towards the spine. Do not let the sternum collapse.

After the exhalation take two, three or more normal breaths so that the lungs recover.

Repeat from up to 6 times.

Revert to normal breathing and lie quietly. Open the eyes. Turn to the right, coming down off the bolster. Stay on the side, with the blanket still supporting the head. Roll to the other side and get up.

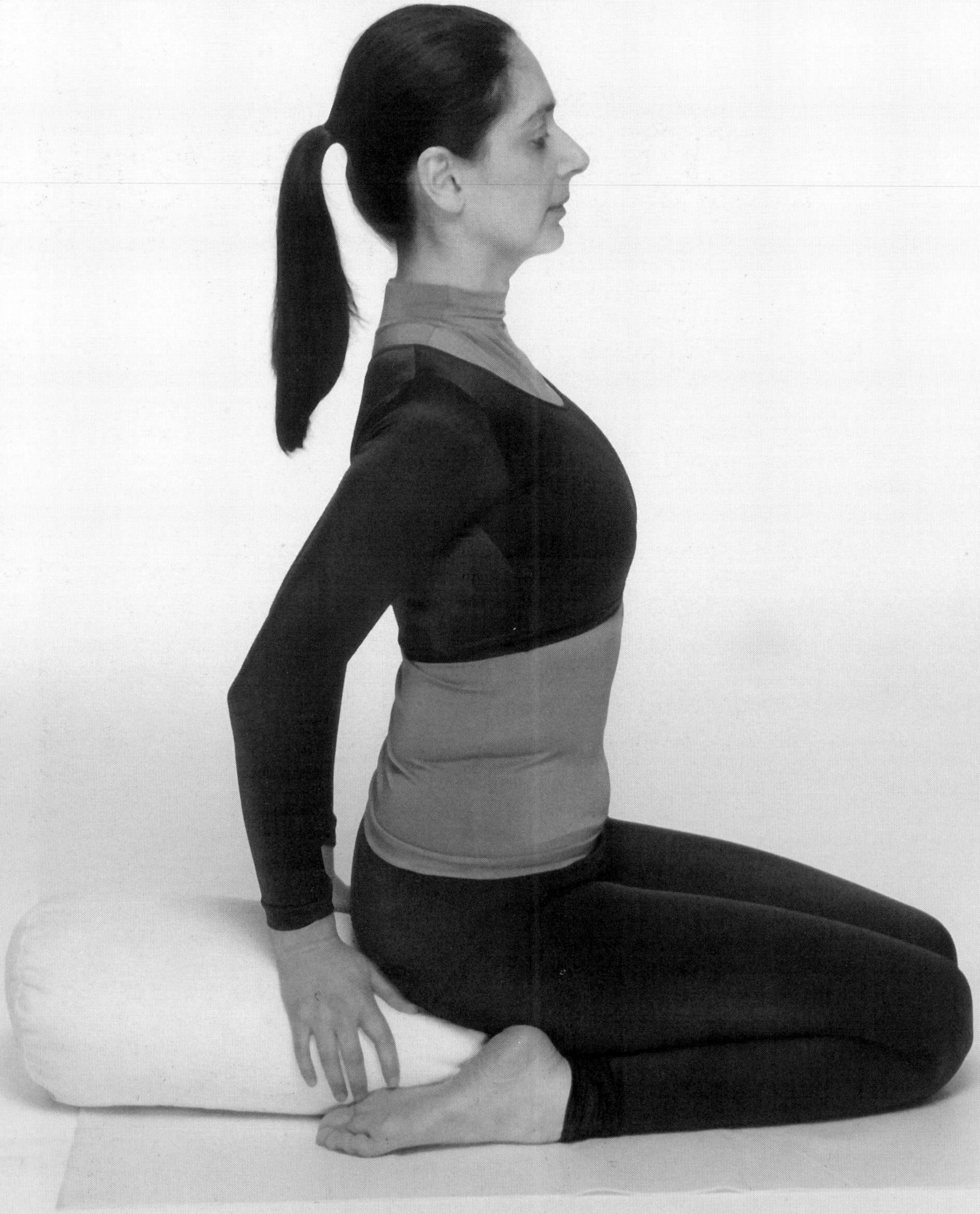

READINGS FOR SERENITY

Gaining knowledge, one soon attains surpassing peace.

(BG 4.39)

Supreme happiness approaches this Yogin
Of serene mind and abated passion.

(BG 6.27)

About the Readings

Originally when planning this section I had envisaged something small, but as I worked on it, it grew and grew, much like Alice after nibbling the cake. Passages cried out for inclusion, either because they illustrated important themes or because of the sheer beauty of their language and imagery, and very often for both reasons. The result is, I hope, an anthology which does justice to the subject, as far as is possible in a book such as this.

In taking up the challenge to do my own translations I came to have immense appreciation for the genius of the authors. In the art of storytelling they are supreme. Take, for example, the conversation of Naciketas with the God of Death in the *Kaṭha Upaniṣad*. The subject, what happens to a person after death, is a grand one, but the poet places it in the mouth of a child. The duologue cleverly reveals character by speech rather than description. Death, the adult who has made a rash promise and regrets it, resorts to pleading and offering numerous temptations to the child Naciketas in order to get out of it. The boy is unimpressed and will not be swayed; the god is forced to keep his word.

Another endearing story, found in both the *Bṛhadāraṇyaka* and *Chāndogya Upaniṣads*, is that of Śvetaketu, a boy who is sent away to school and comes back puffed up with the pride of learning. But what has he learnt? Nothing, it turns out, or at least, nothing worth knowing.

Such gentle satire occurs in many places. A prime example is an audacious metaphor in the *Kaṭha Upaniṣad* likening life to a dish of rice enlivened by the sauce of death.

Other vivid images abound. The *Maitreyānī Upaniṣad* has a host of them: past deeds are compared to the waves of an ocean which cannot be rolled back and the world to an actor changing costume every moment. In the *Bṛhadāraṇyaka Upaniṣad* the human being is likened to a tree, complete with leaves, bark, sap, sapwood and so on. In the *Muṇḍaka Upaniṣad* the multifarious beings of creation are said to spring from the immutable ground of the universe like sparks from a blazing fire. The prolific use of simile and metaphor reflects the teaching skill of the authors in drawing parallels from ordinary experience to illustrate and make comprehensible their teachings.

Another feature of *Upaniṣadic* style is the repetition of phrases and passages almost like a refrain. It is not, however, simple reiteration but a progression of the argument by means of the substitution of key words within a familiar frame. As a teaching technique – drilling without loss of interest – this is highly effective; as a literary device it is superlative. A fine example is a long passage from the *Chāndogya Upaniṣad* which links the following in a series in which the latter is always greater than the earlier: word, speech, will, intelligence, meditation, comprehension, strength, food, water, fire, space, memory, hope and breath.

The Bhagavad-Gītā, from which many passages are taken, needs almost no introduction. Its profound spiritual message, its rhythmic verse and its striking imagery all contribute to make it the well-loved work that it is. It is a first-class example of the difficult art of simplicity. Only a master can achieve the simple presentation of a complex thought, and the author of the *Bhagavad-Gītā* does this time and again. There is inexorable logic in the presentation of the destructive chain beginning with attachment, passing through desire, anger, delusion, confused memory and loss of reason and ending in ruin. As a totally different example, the state of peace is likened to that of the ocean which is continuously filled but remains unmoved. The transcendent form of God is described as a mass of splendour, shining on all sides, with the sun and moon as eyes, pervading the space between heaven and earth and making the three worlds tremble by its awesomeness.

This selection also includes excerpts from the *Yoga Sūtra* of Patañjali and its commentary by

Vyāsa. These are the most difficult of the passages; they represent pure, abstract philosophy with its specialized terminology and method of argumentation. My interest in philosophy was kindled at school, with the Greek and Latin philosophers, and I came to Yoga philosophy much later. But I fell in love with Patañjali's text. It is extremely short, taking up only five or six pages in the original Sanskrit. What a bold and ambitious undertaking: to summarize the essential aspects of a subject in the minimum number of words! His consummate success is proved by the fact that he is still, after two millennia, regarded as the final authority on Yoga. Vyāsa's commentary is extensive, and those of many later commentators voluminous. This gives a more realistic idea of the complexity of the subject. To appreciate Vyāsa needs time and concentration. He both explains the *sūtras* and also gives insights of his own. Consider his detailed elaboration of the causes of pain, which Patañjali merely enumerates as after-effects, anxiety, imprints of experience and the impermanence of everything in nature. To drive his point home, Vyāsa gives a graphic description of the Yogin being like an eyeball – sensitive to the slightest touch, and wishing to avoid all pain.

It has been a great pleasure for me to get to know all these works – the *Upaniṣads*, the *Bhagavad-Gītā* and the Yoga literature – and to read authors who are profound thinkers, broad in their vision of life and at the same time excelling in literary skill. It is my privilege to present their thoughts, and my wish that they afford similar delight to others.

THE SOURCE MATERIAL

These readings have been selected from the major works relevant to Yoga: the *Upaniṣads*, the *Bhagavad-Gītā* and the *Yoga Sūtra* of Patañjali together with its commentary by Vyāsa. All are recognized as classics of world literature as well as important texts on spiritual subjects. (The text of the *Upaniṣads* was checked against the critical edition of the *Upaniṣads* by V.P. Limaye and R.D. Vadekar, *Vaidika Saṃśodhana Maṇḍala*, Pune 1958. The *Yoga Sūtra* and *Bhāṣya* text used was that of the *Ānandāśrama*, Pune 1974.)

THE TRANSLATIONS

The original works are in Sanskrit and are all elegant compositions of verse or prose. Because of the beauty of expression and thought of the ancient sages their words speak directly to the heart and mind. For this reason no attempt has been made to interpose extraneous explanations. For this reason also an attempt has been made in the translations to do justice both to accuracy and to graceful language. Where a construction would be clumsy if translated word for word, a more natural English structure is used, for example, the active voice rather than the passive. Similarly, for the sake of clarity in English, long, complex sentences are broken up into short ones or redundant pronouns omitted. Sometimes a single Sanskrit word repeated in the same passage is rendered by several English synonyms, to bring out the nuances of the original. In the *Bhagavad-Gītā* Arjuna is often addressed by matronyms or patronyms; these have been left untranslated.

THE TOPICS

These readings give a perspective on all aspects of living. They deal with metaphysical issues and the great problems of philosophy: Who am I? What is this world? What is the purpose of life? What is the ultimate reality? They also deal with psychological issues: What is the mind? How can the mind be controlled? Is suffering inevitable? What course of action brings happiness? The ancient answers to these questions, the fruit of profound reflection, are as relevant and gladdening today as when they were formulated.

LIST OF TOPICS

I	LIFE
II	THE HUMAN BEING
III	ULTIMATE REALITY
IV	KNOWLEDGE
V	THE WORLD
VI	EXPERIENCE
VII	THE MIND
VIII	THE CONQUEST OF MIND: YOGA

I Life

Peace of mind, that rare but much sought-after commodity, results from contentment. Contentment is a superior form of happiness based not on the highs of emotion but on approach to life. The quest for contentment as the way to peace of mind thus needs to be informed by a perspective on life.

Pondering over the nature and meaning of life, the ancient Indian thinkers set as a goal the achievement of equanimity in the face of its vicissitudes. In a series of arresting images one *Upaniṣad* captures the essence of the problem and puts forward the solution (*Analogies*).

The embodied soul is involved in an endless chain of lives whose dramas unfold consequent to the actions played out before. The soul's transmigration to different bodies is explained by means of comparisons drawn from the natural world (*Transmigration*). The initiating cause is a forgetting of the true core of being, which is the ultimate reality of the universe (*brahman*).

A mechanistic explanation of the law of *karma* that underpins the cycle of birth, death and rebirth is given in the *Yoga Sūtras* (*Root and Fruit*). Though its approach is stringent philosophical enquiry rather than poetic statement, it also uses picturesque analogies to make its argument clear.

What constitutes the essence of life is another aspect of the large question. It is, asserts an *Upaniṣad*, the life-breath, which is inextricably associated with intelligence and the senses (*Breath and Intelligence*). The departure of these from the body indicates death.

Is there existence after death? The query is put by a child to the God of Death in a famous passage (*A Conversation with Death*). The god would rather bestow untold riches on the boy than reveal his secret, though he does disclose it in the end (it is nothing less than the entire science of Yoga). To be noted here is the priceless value placed on this knowledge.

A similar theme is pursued by a sage's wife (*The Way to Immortality*). Mortal life is contrasted to immortality. The key to the latter is understanding of the self.

Analogies

(MaiU 4.2–3)

Deeds and Death

Like the waves of great rivers, there is no turning back of one's previous deeds;
Like the tide of the ocean, the approach of one's death is hard to avert.

The Embodied Soul

Like the lame, bound by fetters composed of the fruits of good and evil;
Like a prisoner, lacking independence;
Like one in the realm of Death, beset by many fears;
Like one intoxicated with liquor, drunk with the wine of delusion;
Like one possessed by an evil spirit, going astray;
Like one bitten by a huge snake, bitten by the objects of sense;
Like utter darkness, blind with passion.

The World

Like a magic net, consisting of illusion;
Like a dream, false in appearance;
Like the interior of a plantain tree, frail;
Like an actor, changing costume every moment;
Like a painted scene, falsely delighting the mind.

And therefore it is said, "Objects of sound, touch and the like reside in a mortal man like calamities. Through attachment to them, the elemental self does not remember the highest state."

Transmigration

(BU 4.4.3–5)

Just as a leech reaches the end of a blade of grass, draws near another support, crosses onto it and pulls itself along, exactly so does the self drop this body down, render it unconscious, contact another [seat], cross over into it and pull itself along.

Just as a goldsmith takes aside a small quantity of gold and fashions another newer and lovelier form, exactly so does the self drop this body down, render it unconscious, and fashion another newer and lovelier form: that of an ancestral spirit, a heavenly minstrel, a god, a lord of creation, *brahman* or some other beings.

This self, indeed, is *brahman,* this self composed of the intellect, composed of the mind, composed of the life-breath, composed of eyes, composed of ears, composed of earth, composed of water, composed of air, composed of space, composed of fire, composed of what is not fire, composed of desire, composed of the negation of desire, composed of anger, composed of the negation of anger, composed of righteousness, composed of unrighteousness, composed of everything. It is composed of this [the perceivable] and composed of that [the inferable]. As one acts and behaves, so one becomes. One who does good becomes good; one who does evil becomes evil. One becomes virtuous through virtuous acts and evil through evil acts. And so they say, "A person consists only of desire. According to the desire is the intent; what one intends one does, what one does one becomes."

On this there is a verse:

Attached closely to it, he goes together with his deed
To where his mind and subtle body cling.
Reaching the end of whatever deed he has done in this world,
From that world he comes again to this world, to action.

Thus it is for the desiring. For one who has no desires, who is without desire, freed from desire, with fulfilled desires, desiring the Self, his senses do not depart. Being *brahman*, he merges into *brahman*.

On this there is a verse:

When all desires abiding in the heart are shed
Then the mortal becomes immortal and attains brahman in this very life.

Just as the slough of a snake, lifeless and discarded, lies on an anthill, precisely so lies this body. Then this incorporeal and immortal – life-breath is *brahman* itself, light itself.

Root and Fruit

(PYS 2.12–14; VB 2.13)

The deposit of actions rooted in afflictions is experienced in the current or a future birth.
The root surviving, its maturation is species, life span and [worldly] experience.
These fructify in joy and anguish on account of virtue and sin.

COMMENTARY

The deposit of actions begins to mature when the afflictions exist, not when the afflictions are uprooted. Rice is able to sprout when covered with its husk and when its kernel is not roasted, but not when its husk is removed or the kernel is roasted. Similarly, the deposit of actions grows to maturity when covered with the afflictions, but not when the afflictions are removed or when the seed potency of the afflictions is burnt by discriminative knowledge.

The maturation is threefold: species, life span and [worldly] experience. Here the following is to be considered: Is one action the cause of one birth or does one action involve several births? The second consideration is: Do many actions bring about many births or do many actions bring about one birth?

It is not possible that one action is the cause of one birth. Why? Because there would be no rule of succession governing the fruits of actions, the innumerable ones left over from those accumulated from time without beginning and current ones, and as a consequence people would lose faith [in good actions]. This is not acceptable.

Nor is it possible that one action is the cause of many births. Why? Because when there are many actions and one among them would be the cause of many births, there would be no time for the maturation of the remaining ones. This also is not acceptable.

Nor is it possible that many actions are the cause of many births. Why? As those many births cannot occur simultaneously, it must be said [they occur] only in turn. In that case the previous fallacy obtains.

Therefore, the diverse accumulation of virtuous and sinful actions performed between [a given] birth and [the subsequent] death remains dormant in a relation of dominant and subordinate. At death it is activated and, through a single shake-up, it becomes consolidated, brings about death and produces only a single birth. That birth gets its life span from that same action. Within that life-span experience occurs from that same action. This deposit of actions is called "three-fruited" on account of being the cause of birth, life span and experience. Here the deposit of actions is said to be restricted to a single life.

Breath and Intelligence

(KauU 3.3)

One lives when speech has gone, for we see the dumb. One lives when sight has gone, for we see the blind. One lives when hearing has gone, for we see the deaf. One lives when the mind has gone, for we see the simple. One lives when the arms are cut off and when the legs are cut off, for we see such people.

Now, indeed, breath alone is intelligence in essence. Embracing the body, it makes it stand up. Therefore it should be worshipped as the ritual song.

Truly, breath is intelligence and intelligence is breath. For they stay in this body together and leave it together. The perception and understanding of this is in this [fact]: A man who is sound asleep does not see any dreams. Then he becomes unified in the breath itself. Speech together with all names merges into it. Sight together with all forms merges into it. Hearing together with all sounds merges into it. The mind together with all thoughts merges into it. When he wakes, like sparks of a blazing fire flying in all directions, the senses disperse from this self to their respective seats; and from the senses, the gods, and from the gods, the worlds.

The perception and understanding of this is [in] this fact: A man who is sick and about to die becomes weak and drifts into unconsciousness. Then people say, "His consciousness has departed for he does not hear, see, speak with his voice, or think." Then he becomes unified in the breath itself. Speech together with all names merges into it. Sight together with all forms merges into it. Hearing together with all sounds merges into it. The mind together with all thoughts merges into it. When he departs from this body, he departs, indeed, with all these.

A Conversation with Death

(KU 1.1.20–29)

[Nacikatas is given three boons by the God of Death, Yama.]

Naciketas

This doubt there is about a man who is dead:
Some say that he exists, others that he does not.
I wish to know this and you to teach me.
This is the third boon of the three.

Yama

Even the gods of old were unsure of this,
For this doctrine is subtle and hard to know.
Choose another boon, Naciketas,
Do not press me, absolve me from this.

Naciketas

Even the gods of old were unsure of this,
And, O Death, since you say it is hard to know,
And a speaker other than you cannot be found,
No other boon is equal to this.

Yama

Choose sons and grandsons living a hundred years,
Beasts in plenty, elephants, horses, gold!
Choose a great expanse of earth,
And live yourself as many autumns as you wish!

Choose wealth and longevity,
If you think this boon equivalent.
Thrive, Naciketas, on this vast earth,
I will make you enjoy delights at will.

Whatever pleasures are hard to have in the mortal world,
Ask for all pleasures at your will.
These nymphs with chariots and trumpets -
Their like are not attainable by men.
Be waited on by them, a gift from me.
Naciketas, do not ask about death.

Naciketas

O Death, they exist but till tomorrow for a man,
They exhaust the power of all the senses.
Even a whole lifetime is so short.
Keep your mounts, your dances and your songs.

Man cannot be satisfied with wealth.
We shall get wealth since we have seen you.
We live as long as you decree.
The boon I am to choose is still that one.

Coming upon immortals who do not age,
What wise but aging mortal down on earth,
Evaluating beauties, pleasures and delights
Would enjoy too long a life?

O Death, this point of which they are unsure,
Of that great other world, tell me that.
This boon, which is inset deep in mystery,
And no other does Naciketas choose.

The Way to Immortality

(BU 2.4.2–3,5)

[Dialogue between sage Yājñavalkya and his wife Maitreyī]

Maitreyī said, "Well, sir, if this entire earth filled with wealth were mine, would I become immortal through that?" "No," said Yājñavalkya: "Your life would be like the life of the well-to-do. Of immortality, however, there is no hope through wealth."

Then Maitreyī said: "What should I do with something that does not make me immortal? Tell me, sir, what you know [of the way to immortality]."

...

Then he said, "Truly, a husband is not dear for love of the husband but a husband is dear for love of the self. A wife is not dear for love of the wife but a wife is dear for love of the self. Sons are not dear for love of the sons but sons are dear for love of the self. Wealth is not dear for love of wealth but wealth is dear for love of the self. The priest is not dear for love of the priest but the priest is dear for love of the self. The warrior is not dear for love of the warrior but the warrior is dear for love of the self. The worlds are not dear for love of the worlds but the worlds are dear for love of the self. The gods are not dear for love of the gods but the gods are dear for love of the self. Beings are not dear for love of beings but beings are dear for love of the self. Everything is not dear for love of everything but everything is dear for love of the self. Indeed, Maitreyī, the self should be realized, studied from scripture, pondered over and meditated on. Indeed, by realizing, studying, thinking about and understanding the self everything is known."

II The Human Being

The consideration of life leads naturally to the consideration of those who live it: human beings. This anthropocentric view can be justified for the sake of intellectual understanding; it does not diminish the place of other creatures in the scheme of creation.

The central enigma of humankind – the assumption of the mantle of life – is stated by the use of a powerful image (*The Mighty Tree*). While the root of a tree is visibly the cause of its growth, no root can be traced for the emergence of a person.

What constitutes a human being is explained by means of another agricultural metaphor: the field, its knower and its Lord. The body-mind complex, the field, is illumined by its lord, the soul or self (*The Field, its Knower and its Lord*).

There is further probing into the relationship of body and soul. By discarding one after another the externals by which a person relates to the world, the light of the self alone remains (*A Person's Light*).

A different image suggesting this same theme is that of sheaths covering the soul (*The Five Sheaths*). The human being is conceived in the shape of a bird whose soul is encased in layers of increasing subtlety. The outermost is produced by food; within it are those produced by breath, by mind, by determination and by bliss. At the very centre is the blissful core, the self.

The interesting question of the relationship between the soul and its proximate covering, intellect, is discussed in the Yoga literature (*The Soul as the Principle of Consciousness*). The soul as consciousness is said to be neither similar to nor totally dissimilar to the intellect. The intellect in this discussion may be equated with the sheaths of mind and judgement in the *Upaniṣadic* passage introduced above.

The transcendent nature of the soul is affirmed in a verse Upaniṣad of extraordinary lyricism (*The Soul*). Essentially ineffable, it can be described only by negatives and oxymorons. And it can be attained only by the serene and sorrow-free, if the soul itself chooses.

The Mighty Tree

(BU 3.9.28.1–7)

Like a mighty tree, indeed, is a man;
His hairs are the leaves and his skin the outer bark.

From his skin blood flows as sap from the bark;
Therefore it flows from pierced [skin] as sap from a tree that is struck.

His flesh is the sapwood, his sinews are the fibres, undoubtedly;
His bones are the inner wood and his marrow is like the pith.

When a tree is felled it shoots up from its root again with a new form;
From what root does a mortal rise when he is felled by death?

Do not say "from semen", for that is produced from the living.
Like a tree sprouting from a seed, after death it is soon born again.

If a tree is pulled up by its root, it will not sprout again.
From what root does a mortal rise when he is felled by death?

[You say:] Already born, he is not to be born [again],
[I ask:] Who could create him again*?*

The Field, its Knower and its Lord

(BG 13.1,5–6,19–22,31–33)

This body, O Kaunteya,
Is termed the field;
One who knows this the learned
Call the knower of the field.

...

Gross elements, ego principle,
Intellect and the unmanifest,
Ten senses plus one [mind],
Five objects of the senses,

Desire, hatred, pleasure, pain,
Body complex, percipience, grit -
This is the field plus modulations,
In brief narrated.

...

Know that matter and spirit
Are both without beginning;
Attributes and modulations too
Know to be sprung from matter.

When body and organs act,
Matter is said to be the cause;
Of experience of pleasure and pain,
Spirit is said to be the cause.

For spirit, set in matter,
Experiences the attributes of matter born;
Its alliance with the attributes causes
Births in wombs both good and bad.

Observer, approver,
Sustainer, experiencer, great Lord,
The sublime spirit in this body
Is also called the Supreme Self.

...

Devoid of beginning and attributes,
This unchanging Supreme Self,
O Kaunteya, though in the body housed,
Neither acts nor is defiled.

As ubiquitous space is not defiled
By virtue of its intangibility;
So, omnipresent in the body,
The Self is not defiled.

Just as one single sun
Illumines this whole world,
So the Lord of the field
Illumines the whole field, O Bhārata.

A Person's Light

(BU 4.3.2–6)

[Dialogue between sage Yājñavalkya and King Janaka.]

"What light does a person here have?" "He has the light of the sun, Your Majesty," he said, "for with the sun, indeed, as the light, one sits, moves about, does one's work and returns." "Just so, Yājñavalkya."

"When the sun has set, Yājñavalkya, what light does a person here have?" "The moon, indeed, is his light, for with the moon, indeed, as the light, one sits, moves about, does one's work and returns." "Just so, Yājñavalkya."

"When the sun has set, Yājñavalkya, and the moon has set, what light does a person here have?" "Fire, indeed, is his light, for with fire, indeed, as the light, one sits, moves about, does one's work and returns." "Just so, Yājñavalkya."

"When the sun has set, Yājñavalkya, and the moon has set and the fire has died down, what light does a person here have?" "Voice, indeed, is his light, for with voice, indeed, as the light, one sits, moves about, does one's work and returns. Therefore, Your Majesty, even where one's own hand is not discerned, there when voice emerges one reaches there." "Just so, Yājñavalkya."

"When the sun has set, Yājñavalkya, and the moon has set and the fire has died down, and voice is silent, what light does a person here have?" "The self, indeed is his light," said he, "for with the self, indeed, as the light, one sits, moves about, does one's work and returns."

The Five Sheaths

(TU 2.1.1–2.5.1)

The knower of *brahman* attains the highest. On this point it is said:

> *Brahman is truth, knowledge and the infinite.*
> *He who knows [brahman] to be lodged in the cave [of the heart], in the highest heaven*
> *Attains all his desires, together with the wise brahman.*

From that [*brahman*], from this self, space came into being. From space came air; from air, fire; from fire, water; from water, earth; from earth, plants;

from plants, food; from food, man. This man, indeed, is the product of food. This is his head. This is his right wing. This is his left wing. This is his centre. This is his tail, his firm base.

Regarding this there is a verse:

From food, truly, all creatures that dwell on earth are born,
Furthermore, they live by food alone and proceed towards it at the end.
Food is the oldest of beings; therefore it is called the medicine for all.
Those who venerate food as brahman acquire all food.
Food is the oldest of beings; therefore it is called the medicine for all.
From food beings are born, once born they grow by food.
It is eaten, and it eats beings; therefore it is called food and feeder.

Different from this which is the product of food is an inner self consisting of life-breath (*prāṇa*). By that [breath body] is this one [food body] filled. It also has the form of a person. Its man-form corresponds to the man-form of that. The out-breath (*prāṇa*) indeed is its head. The pervading breath (*vyāna*) is its right wing. The down-breath (*apāna*) is the left wing. The space [in the middle] is its centre. The earth is its tail, its firm base.

Regarding this there is a verse:

The gods breathe, and so do men and beasts.
For breath is the life of beings; therefore it is called the life of all.
Those who venerate the breath as brahman live life to its full [span].
For breath is the life of beings; therefore it is called the life of all.

Of the body of that earlier one, this indeed is the self. Different from this which is the product of breath is an inner self consisting of mind. By that [mind body] is this one [breath body] filled. It also has the form of a person. Its man-form corresponds to the man-form of that. The *Yajurveda* [sacrificial hymns] indeed is its head. The *Ṛgveda* [sacred hymns] is its right wing. The *Sāmaveda* [chants] is its left wing. Ritual injunctions are its centre. The *Atharvan* and *Aṅgiras* hymns are its tail, its firm base.

Regarding this there is a verse:

Whence words together with the mind turn back, without attaining it,
One who knows that bliss of brahman never has fear.

Of the body of that earlier one, this indeed is the self. Different from this which is the product of mind is an inner self consisting of determination. By that [determination body] is this one [mind body] filled. It also has the form of a person. Its man-form corresponds to the man-form of that. Faith indeed is its head. Right is its right wing. Truth is its left wing. Yoga [tranquillity] is its centre. Cosmic intelligence is its tail, its firm base.

Regarding this there is a verse:

Determination performs the sacrifice, and also performs acts.
All the gods venerate brahman as the oldest determination.
If one knows brahman as determination and does not mistake this,
Leaving all sins in the body one obtains all one's wishes.

Of the body of that earlier one, this indeed is the self. Different from this which is the product of intelligence is an inner self consisting of bliss. By that [bliss body] is this one [determination body] filled. It also has the form of a person. Its man-form corresponds to the man-form of that. Love, indeed, is its head. Delight is its right wing. Joy is its left wing. Bliss is its centre. *Brahman* is its tail, its firm base.

Regarding this there is a verse:

One becomes non-existent, undoubtedly, if one knows brahman as non-existent;
If one knows brahman exists, then they know one to be existent.

The Soul as the Principle of Consciousness

(PYS 2.20 +VB)

The seer is nothing but the power of consciousness; although pure, it is the witness of ideation.

COMMENTARY

The soul (*puruṣa*) is reflected in the intellect. It is neither similar nor totally dissimilar to the intellect. Firstly it is not similar. Why? Because the intellect is changeable, according as objects are known or unknown to it. Its changeable nature stands proved because its objects – a cow, a pot, and so on – may be known or unknown. In contrast, the constant knowing [by the soul] of its object [the intellect] makes it clear that the soul is immutable in nature. Why? Because the intellect as an object for the soul could not be both comprehended and not comprehended. Thus is proved the soul's eternal consciousness of its object, and hence also its immutability.

Moreover, the intellect serves the purpose of another, as it acts in conjunction [with others]. The soul serves its own purpose. So, because of being the means of apprehension of all objects, the intellect consists of the three strands (*guṇas – sattva, rajas, tamas*) of matter, and because it consists of the three strands of matter, it is unconscious. The soul is an onlooker of the qualities of Nature; hence it is not similar [to the intellect]. Suppose then that it is dissimilar. It is not totally dissimilar either. Why? Because although it is pure it is the witness of ideation. It witnesses the ideation of the intellect, and hence, witnessing that, although it is dissimilar in nature to [the intellect] it appears to be similar to it.

The Soul

(KU 2.18–25)

The sapient one is neither born nor dies,
It came from nowhere and became no thing,
Unborn, eternal, everlasting and primaeval,
It is not slain when the body is slain.

If the slayer thinks he slays,
If the slain thinks that he is slain,
Neither understands:
He does not slay, he is not slain.

Smaller than an atom, greater than the vast,
The Self is set in a living creature's cave [heart].
One without volition and sorrow-free sees
Through tranquillity of the senses, the greatness of the Self.

Sitting, it ranges far;
Lying, it passes everywhere;
Who but me is fit to know
That god of gaiety and gravity?

Realizing the Self, great, all-pervading,
Abiding without a body,
In unabiding bodies,
One who is wise does not grieve.

Not by instruction may this Self be gained,
Nor intellection, nor much erudition,
That one alone gains it whom it chooses,
To whom the Self reveals its own form.

Not one who does not desist from evil ways,
Nor one lacking calm or contemplation,
Nor also one with unquiet mind
May attain it by intelligence.

For it priesthood and power
Are both like a dish of rice
With death as the sauce;
Who, indeed, knows where it is?

III Ultimate Reality

From knowledge of the individual self the enquiry turns to the self writ large: the ultimate essence of the universe, known as *brahman*. They are identical by virtue of being spiritual, as opposed to material, entities.

The connection between them is charmingly explained in a dialogue between a father and son (*The Imperceptible Subtle Essence*). Employing the time-honoured method of introducing the unknown via the familiar, the father demonstrates the unity of existence by means of seeds and salty water. The invisible interior of the seed and the salt permeating the water both exemplify the truth that there is a single substrate for the universe and that "You are that".

Brahman as the all-pervasive substrate of the universe is a major focus of *Upaniṣadic* teaching. Realization of this principle consists not merely of intellectual comprehension but of experience. To this end meditation on it is repeatedly enjoined. One such meditation passage combines a concise portrayal of *brahman* with an emphasis on its deep significance to the individual (*Brahman*).

Because an abstract principle is hard to conceptualize, many different analogies are used as an aid to understanding. In another teacher-pupil dialogue, this time between a husband and wife (met in an earlier section), the great infinite in which all individuality dissolves is likened to the ocean in which all waters merge. Similarly, it is like the heart in which all yearnings meet, or the feet in which all journeys unite, and so on (*The One Rendezvous*).

God is a concretization of this abstract principle. While God is visualized in various ways, the Yoga aphorisms give a particularly clear definition and description (*God*). Beyond afflictions and actions, and transcending time, He is said to be the supreme teacher.

A more personal panegyric represents God as having a superabundance of human attributes: many arms, mouths, eyes. His marvellous form pervades the space between heaven and earth as a mass of splendour (*The Transcendent Form*).

Similar paeans depict *brahman* in its impersonal form, from whom multifarious beings spring forth as sparks from a fire. It abides with all things as their inmost self, in the cave of the heart. By knowledge of *brahman* the knot of ignorance is sundered (*The Sublime Spirit*).

The Imperceptible Subtle Essence

(ChU 6.12.1–3; 6.13.1–3)

"Bring a fruit from that banyan tree." "Here it is, sir." "Break it." "It is broken, sir." "What do you see in it?" "These minute seeds, sir." "Break one of them." "It is broken, sir." "What do you see in it?" "Nothing, sir."

Then he said to him, "My dear, you cannot see that subtle essence at all, but out of that very essence arises this great banyan tree. Believe me, my dear."

"That subtle essence forms the self of this whole world. It is Reality. It is the self (*ātman*). You are that, Śvetaketu." "Teach me once again, sir." "Very well, my dear," he said.

"Put this salt in water and then come to me in the morning." He did so. He said to him, "My son, bring the salt which you put in water last night." He looked for it but could not find it, as it had completely dissolved.

"Take a sip from the [surface] layer, son. What is it like?" he said. "Salty." Take a sip from the middle. What is it like? " "Salty." "Take a sip from the [bottom] layer. What is it like?" "Salty." "Throw it away and then come to me." He did so. "It is there everywhere." Then he said to him, "Truly, my dear, it exists but you do not see it; indeed, it is here.

"That subtle essence forms the self of this whole world. It is Reality. It is the self (*ātman*). You are that, Śvetaketu."

Brahman

(ChU 3.14.1–4)

All this universe, indeed, is *brahman*. It is its origin, dissolution and spirit. One should meditate on that in tranquillity. Now, a person is endowed with resolve, and as is his resolve in this world, so a person becomes on departing from here. Let him make this resolve:

That which consists of mind, whose body is breath, whose form is luminous, whose intention comes true, whose soul is the sky, which [*brahman*] contains all actions, all desires, all smells and all tastes, which overspreads the whole world, which is without speech and without attachment,

That is my Self within the heart. It is smaller than a grain of rice, than a grain of barley, than a mustard seed, than a grain of millet, than the kernel of a grain of millet. This is my self within the heart. It is greater than the earth, greater than the sky, greater than heaven, greater than these worlds.

Containing all actions, all desires, all smells, all tastes, overspreading the whole world, without speech and without attachment, this is my Self within the heart. It is *brahman*. On departing from here I shall become that. One who has this certainty has no doubt.

The One Rendezvous

(BU 2.4.11–12)

[Dialogue between Yājñavalkya and Maitreyī]

As the ocean is the one rendezvous of all waters, so the skin is the one rendezvous of all touches; so the nostrils are the one rendezvous of all smells; so the tongue is the one rendezvous of all tastes; so the eye is the one rendezvous of all forms; so the ear is the one rendezvous of all sounds; so the mind is the one rendezvous of all thoughts; so the heart is the one rendezvous of all yearnings; so the hands are the one rendezvous of all actions; so the sexual organ is the one rendezvous of all pleasures; so the anus is the one rendezvous of all excretions; so the feet is the one rendezvous of all journeys; so speech is the one rendezvous of all Vedas.

As a lump of salt dropped into water dissolves in the water itself and cannot be picked up at all, but wherever one sips, there is salt, so, my dear, this great being is an infinite, limitless mass of intelligence itself. Arising out of these elements it [individuality] perishes along with them. After departing [from them] there is no awareness [of individuality], I say. So said Yājñavalkya.

Maitreyī said, "Here, sir, you have confused me by saying that after departing there is no awareness." He said, "I do not say what is confusing. This is enough for understanding:

When there is duality, as it were, one smells another, one sees another, one hears another, one greets another, one thinks of another, one understands another. But when everything has become the Self, what and with what can one smell, what and with what can one see, what and with what can one hear, what and with what can one greet, what and with what can one think, what and with what can one understand? With what can one understand that [self] by [the existence of which] which everything is understood? With what can one understand the one who understands?"

God

(PYS 1.24–29)

God is a distinct Spiritual Entity untouched by affliction, action, the fruit of action and the deposit of action.

In Him is the seed of omniscience that cannot be exceeded.

He is the mentor of the ancients also, not being limited by time.

OM denotes Him.

Its utterance and contemplation of its meaning [should be made].

Thence comes understanding of the inner self and also the disappearance of obstacles.

The Transcendent Form

(BG 11.16–20)

I see You everywhere, infinite in form,
With many arms, stomachs, mouths, eyes;
I see neither end, nor middle nor yet the
beginning of You,
O Lord of all, Whose form is the universe.

With crown, mace and discus,
Shining on all sides, a mass of splendour,
Immeasurable, bright as the sun and blazing fire,
Hard to behold, I see You all around.

You are indestructible, the transcendent truth to be known,
You are the sublime repose of this world;
You are the immutable guardian of the eternal law,
You are the primaeval spirit, I hold.

Without beginning, middle or end, of infinite might,
With numberless arms, with the sun and moon as eyes;
I see You, with mouth like incandescent fire,
Burning this universe with Your blaze.

This space between heaven and earth,
Is pervaded by You alone, and all directions;
Seeing Your marvellous, fearsome form,
The three worlds tremble, O Majesty.

The Sublime Spirit

(MU 2.1.1–10)

Just as from a blazing fire sparks
By the thousand appear with like form,
So, my dear, from the Immutable multifarious beings
Spring forth, and merge into it alone.

Divine and formless is the spirit,
Without and within, unborn,
Without breath, without mind,
Resplendent, beyond the ultimate imperishable.

From it are born breath, mind
And all the sense organs;
Space, wind, light, water
And earth, the sustainer of all.

Fire is its head, the sun and moon its eyes,
The directions its ears, its speech the Veda revelation;
Air its breath, the world its heart, from its feet the earth;
Indeed, it is the inner self of each and every being.

From it, fire, whose kindling is the sun,
Rain from the moon, plants on earth,
A man pours seed into a woman;
From the spirit a multitude of offspring take their birth.

From it, the verses, chants and formulae [the three Vedas],
Consecration, sacrifice and all rites and sacerdotal fees,
The year, the sacrificer, the worlds
In which the moon and sun give purity.

From it in various ways take birth the gods,
Celestials, people, beasts and birds,
The in-breath and the out-breath, rice and barley,
Austerity, faith, truth, celibate life and sacred laws.

From it the seven breaths arise,
The seven flames, the [seven] kindlings, the seven offerings,
These seven worlds in which the breaths move
Set seven each in the hidden sanctuary.

From it, all the seas and mountains,
From it flow rivers of every kind,
From it, all plants and the sap
By which it abides with elements as their inmost self.

This world is the spirit alone,
Deeds, penance, brahman, the supreme immortal;
One who knows this placed in the cave [of the heart],
Sunders the knot of ignorance, my dear, here on earth.

IV Knowledge

Knowledge is logically tied to its antithesis, ignorance. Being aware of one's ignorance is the first step towards knowledge, and as knowledge increases, ignorance decreases.

An engaging repository of ignorance in the *Upaniṣads* is the boy Śvetaketu (encountered earlier, undergoing instruction from his father). His story serves to illustrate the importance of knowing what to know (*Ignorance*).

Knowledge is differentiated into mundane and spiritual. The latter is ranked higher as it leads to the summum bonum, self-realization (*Two Kinds of Knowledge*).

The acquisition of knowledge, by study and teaching, is enhanced by the cultivation of character and adherence to duty (*The Accessories of Knowledge*). These include uprightness and self-restraint as well as hospitality and the rearing of children.

What does realization consist of? The nature of cognition occurring in this state is explained in the Yoga literature (*Realization*). It is filled with truth and perceives objects directly, without the mediation of reason or the senses.

At this point knowledge becomes infinite, its compass far exceeding the infinitesimal knowable world (*The Firefly in Space*). Appended to this statement, however, is a wry riddle hinting that such a scenario is impossible.

Acquiring knowledge of the ultimate Reality involves understanding a whole series of connected elements (*Comprehension*). In descending order these are comprehension itself, reasoning, faith, devotion, exertion, happiness and the great vastness. It is from the great vastness that the ego principle arises, and from this, the reference to the self. Expanding outwards again, from the self comes everything.

Ignorance

(ChU 6.1.1–7)

There was one Śvetaketu, the grandson of Aruṇa. His father [Āruṇi] said to him, "Śvetaketu, my dear, follow the discipline of sacred knowledge. There is no-one in our family who is not learned and is a brahmin in name only."

Thus he went away at the age of twelve and at the age of twenty-four, having studied all the *Vedas*, he returned, conceited, proud of his erudition and haughty. His father said to him, "Śvetaketu, my dear, here you are, conceited, proud of your erudition and haughty. Did you ask for that instruction..."

Through which what is not heard becomes heard, what is not thought of becomes thought of, what is not understood becomes understood."Sir, what is this instruction like?"

"My dear, just as through a single lump of clay everything made of clay would be understood; modification is a verbal tool, an appellation; clay alone is the reality."

"My dear, just as through a single gold ornament everything made of gold would be understood; modification is a verbal tool, an appellation; gold alone is the reality."

"My dear, just as through a single nail clipper everything made of iron would be understood; modification is a verbal tool, an appellation; iron alone is the reality. My dear, this is the instruction."

"Surely, my revered [teachers] did not know this, for if they knew it, how is it they did not tell me? Sir, explain it to me yourself." "Very well, my dear," he said.

(BU 6.2.1–2; also ChU 5.3.1–3)

Śvetaketu Āruṇi, came to the assembly of the Pañcālas. He approached Pravāhana, the son of Jīvala, as he was being waited on [by attendants]. Seeing him, he addressed him, "Young man!" "Sir?" he responded. "Has your father taught you?" "Yes," he said.

"Do you know how people here, on dying, go in different ways?

"No," he said.

"Do you know how they return to this world?"

"No," he said, simply.

"Do you know how the other world is not filled up by many people dying over and over again?"

"No," he said, simply.

"Do you know the sequence of the sacrificial offering in which, when an offering is made, water becomes a human voice, rises up and speaks?"

"No," he said, simply.

"Do you know the means to the path of the gods or to the ancestors, i.e. by doing what [actions] people reach the path of the gods or the ancestors? For have you not heard the words of the seer:

I have heard of two routes for mortals,
That of the gods and of the ancestors.
Going by these this world unites
That which is between the father and the mother [heaven and earth]."

"I do not know even a single [of these]," he said.

Two Kinds of Knowledge

(MU 1.1.4–7)

There are two kinds of knowledge to be learnt, the higher and the lower, so those who know *brahman* say.

Of these, the lower comprises the *Ṛgveda*, the *Yajurveda*, the *Sāmaveda*, the *Atharvaveda*, phonetics, the code of rituals, grammar, etymology, metrics and astronomy. Then the higher is that by which one realizes the imperishable.

That which is invisible, imperceptible, unclassifiable,
Colourless, without eyes, ears, hands and feet,
Eternal, supreme, ubiquitous, most subtle, undying, the womb of creation,
The wise see all around them.

As a spider spins and draws in [its web],
As plants emerge from the earth,
As the hair of the head and body [grows] from a living man,
So the universe here issues from the imperishable.

The Accessories of Knowledge

(TU 1.9.1)

Right, and study and teaching;
Truth, and study and teaching;
Austerity, and study and teaching;
Self-restraint, and study and teaching;
Serenity, and study and teaching;
The sacred fires, and study and teaching;
The fire sacrifice, and study and teaching;
Guests, and study and teaching;
Humanity, and study and teaching;
Progeny, and study and teaching;
Procreation, and study and teaching;
Propagation of the race, and study and teaching.

Realization

(PYS 1.48–49; also VB 1.48–49)

The cognition in that state is truth-filled.

It has a different [kind of] object from the cognitions of the Holy Word and inference, as its object is the specific.

COMMENTARY

In that state, the cognition which is born of a mind in absorption is termed "truth-filled." This term is in accord with its meaning as it consists of truth exclusively and there is not even a trace of falsity. Thus it is said, " Developing cognition in three ways – through scripture, inference and devotion to the practice of meditation – one gains the highest yoga."

The Holy Word is scripture; it has a generality as its object. For scripture is not able to describe the particular. Why? Because a word does not have a convention with the specific. Similarly, inference has a generality as its sole object. For instance, "Where there is arrival, there is motion; where there is no arrival, there is no motion." Hence it is said that through inference conclusions are drawn concerning generalities. Therefore no specific object can be the object of scripture and inference.

The thing [comprehended in *samādhi*] is subtle, concealed or distant and is not apprehended through ordinary perception. But it is not that the specific, being beyond proof, does not exist. It is to be apprehended exclusively through the cognition in absorption. The specific relates to the subtle elements or to the soul. Therefore it has a different object from the cognition of scripture and inference as its object is the specific.

The Firefly in Space

(PYS 4.31; also VB 4.31)

Then, because of the infiniteness of knowledge, which has been cleared of all obscuring impurities, the knowable world becomes infinitesimal.

COMMENTARY

Knowledge becomes infinite when it is freed from all impurities of afflictions and actions. The illuminating intellect (*sattva*) is overpowered and obscured by darkness (*tamas*). Only sometimes, when impelled and uncovered by energy (*rajas*), does it become capable of comprehension. At the point when it has been cleared of all obscuring impurities it attains infiniteness. As it becomes infinite the knowable world becomes infinitesimal, like a firefly in space.

On this it has been said:

A blind man pieced a pearl;
One without fingers threaded it;
One without a neck wore it;
One without a tongue praised it.

Comprehension

(ChU 7.16.1–26.1)

"Now, one speaks surpassingly when one speaks surpassingly with [awareness of] Reality."

"Sir, I wish to speak surpassingly with [awareness of] Reality."

"Then you must desire to comprehend Reality."

"Sir, I do desire to comprehend Reality."

"Only when one has comprehended does one speak of Reality; without comprehending Reality one does not speak of it. Only after comprehending does one speak of it. So you must desire to comprehend comprehension.

"Sir, I do desire to comprehend comprehension."

"Only when one reasons does one comprehend; without reasoning one does not comprehend. Only after reasoning does one comprehend. So you must desire to comprehend reasoning."

"Sir, I do desire to comprehend reasoning."

"Only when one has faith does one reason; without having faith one does not reason. Only after having faith does one reason. So you must desire to comprehend faith."

"Sir, I do desire to comprehend faith."

"Only when one has devotion does one have faith; without having devotion one does not have faith. Only after having devotion does one have faith. So you must desire to comprehend devotion."

"Sir, I do desire to comprehend devotion."

"Only when one exerts does one have devotion; without exerting one does not have devotion. Only after exerting does one have devotion. So you must desire to comprehend exerting."

"Sir, I do desire to comprehend exerting."

"Only when one gains happiness does one exert; without gaining happiness one does not exert. Only after gaining happiness does one exert. So you must desire to comprehend happiness."

"Sir, I do desire to comprehend happiness."

"Only the great vastness is happiness; smallness is not happiness. Only the great vastness is happiness. So you must desire to understand the great vastness."

"Sir, I do desire to comprehend the great vastness."

"Where one sees nothing else, hears nothing else, comprehends nothing else, that is the great vastness. Where one sees something else, hears something else, comprehends something else, that is the small. Only the great vastness is immortal; what is small is mortal."

"Sir, on what is it founded?"

"On its own greatness; or, perhaps, not on its greatness."

"Here [in ordinary life] cows, horses, elephants, gold, servants, wives, fields, houses are called "greatness". I do not say so. What I say is that they are founded on each other."

"That [great vastness] is below; it is above; it is to the west; it is to the east; it is to the south; it is to the north. Indeed, it is everything. Now, from this alone comes the very reference to the ego principle. 'I am below; I am above; I am to the west; I am to the east; I am to the south; I am to the north. Indeed, I am everything.' "

"Now, from this alone comes the very reference to the Self. 'The Self is below; the Self is above; the Self is to the west; the Self is to the east; the Self is to the south; the Self is to the north. Indeed, it is everything. Seeing in this way, reflecting in this way, understanding in this way, delighting in the Self, playing with the Self, uniting with the Self, finding bliss in the Self, one becomes one's own lord and roams all the worlds at will. But those who understand otherwise are ruled by others and exist in perishable worlds. They cannot roam the worlds at will.

When one sees in this way, reflects in this way, comprehends in this way, it is thus: from the Self comes the life-breath; from the Self comes hope; from the Self comes memory; from the Self comes space; from the Self comes fire; from the Self comes water; from the Self comes appearance and disappearance; from the Self comes food; from the Self comes strength; from the Self comes intelligence; from the Self comes meditation; from the Self comes consciousness; from the Self comes will; from the Self comes the mind; from the Self comes speech; from the Self comes Word; from the Self come prayers (*mantra*); from the Self come rites; from the Self, indeed, comes this everything."

V The World

In contrast to the world of the spirit, consisting of the individual self and the all-pervading *brahman*, is the world of matter. Living creatures and inanimate objects alike are part of nature and subject to its laws. An understanding of the world adds a necessary dimension to the spiritual quest by demarcating its boundaries.

The view of the self as the source of the world is expanded in several creation myths. More than just stories, they have a psychological import. For example, it is said that from one arise many, but from solitude arise ego, fear and uneasiness (*Animate Creation*).

The interconnectedness of the universe, the macrocosm, and the human being, the microcosm, is another characteristic teaching. In the regulated order of creation, speech is linked to fire, the life-breath to air, sight to the sun, hearing to the directions, and so on. At the bidding of the creator self they arise in a newly created man and, in a mirror-image concept, they also enter him (*Macrocosm and Microcosm*).

The duality of experience is the subject of another allegory featuring gods and demons. The sense organs and the mind are tainted by the demons and as a result perceive good as well as evil. Only the life-breath itself, which nourishes and supports these organs, is untainted and unassailable (*Good and Evil*).

The diversity of the world is noted and analysed. The different qualities observed in objects are traced to three fundamental elements of nature: fire, water and earth. At a superficial level all objects have a distinct identity; at a deep level they reduce to these three elements. Individual identity is thus a function of nomenclature and is not a reality (*Fire, Water, Earth*).

Nature itself is constituted of three intertwining and inseparable qualities: light, energy and darkness/inertia. These strands run through both the objective and the mental world. Mind, being other than spirit, is considered to be part of matter. In psychological terms light is illumination, energy is activity and emotion, and darkness/ inertia is ignorance and dullness. This provides a rationale for judgements about human personalities and endeavours (*The Three Strands of Matter*).

For a statement about the world in a nutshell one must turn to the Yoga literature (*The Constituents and Purpose of the World*). Characterised by the three stands of nature, it consists of elements and senses. It serves the purposes of the embodied soul by facilitating two kinds of knowledge: that of experience and that of spiritual emancipation.

Animate Creation

(BU 1.4.1–4,8)

In the beginning this world was only the Self in the form of a person. Looking around, he saw nothing other than himself. He first said, "I am." From that he came to have the name "I". Therefore, even today one who is addressed says first, "This is I" and then tells whatever other name he may have...

He was afraid. Therefore one who is alone is afraid. Then he thought to himself, "Since there is nothing other than myself, what should I fear." Thereupon, indeed, his fear went away, for, what could he have feared? It is, after all, because of another that there is fear.

He had no ease at all. Therefore one who is alone has no ease. He wished to have a second. He became as large as a man and woman in close embrace. He caused himself to fall into two. From that arose husband and wife. Therefore ... this (body) is like half of a pea. Therefore this vacuum is filled by a wife. He united with her. From that human beings were produced.

She thought, "How can he unite with me after procreating me from his own self? Well, let me hide!" She became a cow. The other became a bull and did, indeed, unite with her. From that cows [and] bulls were born. The one became a mare, the other a stallion. The one became a female ass, the other a male ass. He did, indeed, unite with her. From that one-hoofed animals were born. The one became a she-goat, the other a he-goat. The one became a ewe, the other a ram. He did, indeed, unite with her. From that goats and sheep were born. In this way he created everything that exists in pairs, right down to ants.

Macrocosm and Microcosm

(AU 1.1.1–4; 1.2.1–4)

In the beginning this world was the one self alone. There was nothing else whatsoever that blinked. He thought, "Let me create the worlds."

He created these worlds: fluidity, the motes of light, the mortal and the waters. Up beyond heaven is fluidity; the firmament is its support. The motes of light are the middle space. The mortal world is the earth. What is below are the waters.

He thought, "These are the worlds; let me now create the protectors of the worlds." From the water itself he pulled out and solidified a man.

He incubated him, and in this incubated [man], a mouth cracked open, like an egg. From the mouth came speech, and from speech, fire.

Two nostrils cracked open; from the nostrils came the life-breath, and from the life-breath, air.

Two eyes cracked open; from the eyes came sight, and from sight, the sun.

Two ears cracked open; from the ears came hearing, and from hearing, the directions.

A skin cracked open; from the skin came hairs, and from the hairs, plants and trees.

A heart cracked open; from the heart came the mind, and from the mind, the moon.

A navel cracked open; from the navel came the downward wind (*apāna*), and from the downward wind, death.

A penis cracked open; from the penis came semen, and from semen, water.

These deities that had been created fell into this vast ocean [of transmigratory life]. He [the self] subjected him [the man] to hunger and thirst. They said to him, "Provide an abode for us in which we can be established and eat food."

He brought a bull to them. They said, "This is not enough for us at all." He brought a horse to them. They said, "This is not enough for us at all."

He brought a man to them. They said, "This one is well fashioned. "Man is indeed well fashioned." He said to them, "Enter into your respective abodes."

Becoming speech, fire entered the mouth; becoming the life-breath, air entered the nostrils; becoming sight, the sun entered the eyes; becoming hearing, the directions entered the ears; becoming hairs, plants and trees entered the skin; becoming the mind the moon entered the heart; becoming the downward breath, death entered the navel; becoming semen, water entered the penis.

Good and Evil

(ChU 1.2.1–9)

There was a time when the gods and demons, both descendents of Prajāpati [the Creator], engaged in a fight. Then the gods invoked *OM* (the symbol of the highest principle), saying, "With this we shall defeat them."

They worshipped the life-breath (*prāṇa*) in the nose as *OM*. The demons stabbed it with evil. Therefore, with it one smells both the fragrant and the foul, for it has been stabbed with evil.

Then they worshipped speech as *OM*. The demons stabbed it with evil. Therefore, with it one speaks both truth and falsehood, for it has been stabbed with evil.

Then they worshipped the eye as *OM*. The demons stabbed it with evil. Therefore, with it one sees both the attractive and the unsightly, for it has been stabbed with evil.

Then they worshipped the ear as *OM*. The demons stabbed it with evil. Therefore, with it one hears both the pleasant and what is unpleasant, for it has been stabbed with evil.

Then they worshipped the mind as *OM*. They stabbed it with evil. Therefore, with it one thinks both good thoughts and bad thoughts, for it has been stabbed with evil.

Then they worshipped the life-breath (*prāṇa*) in the mouth itself as *OM*. The demons attacked it and were smashed, just as [a clod of earth] strikes a hard rock and is shattered.

Thus, anyone who wishes evil on or who injures one who knows this is smashed just as [a clod] striking a hard rock disintegrates. He is like a hard rock.

With this life-breath (*prāṇa*) one perceives neither fragrance nor foul smell, for it is free from evil. Whatever one eats or drinks, with that one protects the other vital breaths. Failing to find it at the end, one departs; and, indeed, at the time of death one opens [one's mouth].

Fire, Water, Earth

(ChU 6.3.2–6.6.6)

That same deity willed,"Let me enter these three deities (fire, water, earth) along with the soul of a living being and differentiate it in name and form."

"Let me make each one of these tripartite." So saying, that deity entered the three deities along with the soul of each living being and differentiated it in name and form.

It made each of them tripartite. Learn from me, my dear, in what manner each of these three deities becomes threefold.

In a fire, the red colour is the form of fire, the white that of water and the black that of earth. [Thus] the identity of the fire vanishes; the modification is an appellation, a mere name. The reality is in fact the three (constituting) forms.

In the sun, the red colour is the form of fire, the white that of water and the black that of earth. [Thus] the identity of the sun vanishes; the modification is an appellation, a mere name. The reality is in fact the three forms.

In the moon, the red colour is the form of fire, the white that of water and the black that of earth. (Thus) the identity of the moon vanishes; the modification is an appellation, a mere name. The reality is in fact the three forms.

In lightning, the red colour is the form of fire, the white that of water and the black that of earth. (Thus) the identity of lightning vanishes; the modification is an appellation, a mere name. The reality is in fact the three forms.

It was, indeed, knowing this that the great householders and great scholars of old, said: "Now no one shall tell us anything unheard of, unthought of or unknown." For from that they knew [all].

They knew that whatever appeared red was the form of heat; they knew that whatever appeared white was the form of water; they knew that whatever appeared black was the form of earth.

They knew that whatever seemed to be unknown was the combination of these same deities. Now, my dear, know from me the manner in which these three deities each becomes tripartite on entering a person.

Food, once eaten, is divided into three parts. The grossest constituent becomes faeces, the medium, flesh and the subtlest, the mind.

Water, once drunk, is divided into three parts. The grossest constituent becomes urine, the medium, blood and the subtlest, breath.

Fire, once ingested, is divided into three parts. The grossest constituent becomes bone, the medium, marrow and the subtlest, the voice.

For, my dear, the mind consists of food, breath consists of water and speech of fire.

"Sir, teach me once again." "Very well, my dear," he said.

When curd is churned, my dear, the finest part rises upwards and it becomes butter.

Likewise when food is eaten, my dear, the finest part rises upwards and it becomes the mind.

When water is drunk, my dear, the finest part rises upwards and it becomes breath.

When fire is ingested, my dear, the finest part rises upwards and it becomes speech.

For, my dear, the mind consists of food, breath consists of water and speech of fire.

"Sir, teach me once again." "Very well, my dear," he said.

The Three Strands of Matter

(BG 14.5–8; 17.2–22)

[Kṛṣṇa instructs Arjuna.]

Sattva, rajas, tamas,
The attributes innate in matter,
Bind to the body, O Strong-Armed One,
The imperishable bodiless one.

Of these, sattva*, being stainless,*
Illuminates and is harmless;
It binds by attachment to pleasure,
O Sinless One, and by attachment to
knowledge.

Know that rajas has the nature of passion,
Arising from desire and attachment;
It binds the embodied one, O Kaunteya,
By attachment to action.

Know that tamas *born of the ignorance*
Deludes all embodied beings;
It binds, O Bhārata,
By negligence, indolence and sleep.
...

Of three kinds is faith
Inborn in embodied souls,
Sattvic, rajasic
And tamasic*; listen!*

Faith, O Bhārata, is in accord
With the mindset of each one.
A man is made of faith;
As his faith is, so is he.

The sattvic *worship gods,*
The rajasic, jinn *and demons;*
The rest, tamasic *folk, worship*
Spirits and the hordes of ghosts.

Men who practise awful penances,
Unsanctioned by holy writ,
Who are full of hypocrisy and ego,
As well as driving lust and passion,

Indiscreet, torturing the insentient
Set of elements in the body,
And thus Myself, dwelling in the body,
Know them to have devilish intent.

Now, the food favoured by all
Is also of three kinds,
And so is sacrifice, austerity and gift;
Hear of their divisions.

Enhancing life, goodness, strength, health,
Happiness and pleasure,
Succulent, oily, substantial and agreeable,
Are the foods liked by the sattvic.

Pungent, sour, salty, over-hot,
Sharp, dry and burning
Are the foods desired by the rajasic*;*
They cause pain, grief and sickness.

Undercooked, insipid,
Putrid, stale,
Leftover and unfit for sacred use,
Is the food liked by the tamasic.

Sacrifice offered as prescribed,
By those not yearning for its fruit,
Thinking only, with resolved mind,
That sacrifice must be done, is sattvic.

But that which is offered, O Great Bhārata,
With the objective of its fruit
And motivated by hypocrisy,
Know that sacrifice to be rajasic.

If not ordained, with food omitted,
Without prayers and the priest's fee,
Devoid of faith, a sacrifice
Is considered as tamasic.

The gods, the twice-born, mentors and the wise –
Worship of these, purity, rectitude,
Celibacy and non-violence
Are called austerity of body.

Words that do not cause distress,
Are truthful, pleasant and of help,
And iteration of the sacred texts
Are called austerity of speech.

Serenity, gentleness,
Silence, self-control,
Purity of intention, all these,
Are called austerity of mind.

This threefold austerity,
Practised with utmost faith by men
Not coveting the fruit, but disciplined,
Is considered to be sattvic.

Austerity hypocritically performed
For esteem, prestige and adulation
Is proclaimed here to be rajasic,
Fickle and ephemeral.

Austerity performed as torture of oneself,
With a deluded understanding,
Or with the aim of ruining another
Is declared to be tamasic.

A gift given because it should be given,
To one to whom no debt is owed,
To a fit recipient, at fit place and time,

That gift is recognized as sattvic.
But that given for a favour in return,
Or else motivated by the fruit,
And with vexation,
Is recognized as rajasic.

A gift given out of place and time
And to the undeserving,
With disrespect and scornfully,
Is declared to be tamasic.

The Constituents and Purpose of the World

(PYS 2.18 + VB)

The perceivable [world] is characterized by illumination, activity and inertia. It consists of the elements and the senses, and serves the purpose of [worldly] experience and [spiritual] emancipation.

COMMENTARY

Light is the character of *sattva*; activity is the character of *rajas*; inertia is the character of *tamas*. These strands of matter (*guṇas*) are distinct but affect one another. They mutate, conjoin and separate. Their forms are acquired by taking the support of one another. Although they are mutually dependent each has a distinct power and the proportions of their powers vary vis-à-vis like and unlike products. When one is predominant the other strands exhibit themselves as subsidiary, but although they are subsidiary their presence is inferred solely by their functions. Their power is employed in serving the purpose of the soul (*puruṣa*). They serve it merely by proximity, enabled in the manner of a magnet. They follow, without an external cause, the mode of one amongst them. They are called by the term "primordial". This is said to be the objective [world]. This it is which consists of the elements and the senses. It evolves in the form of the elements, earth, etc. in their gross and subtle aspects. Similarly, it evolves in the form of the senses, the ear, etc. in their gross and subtle aspects.

This is not without a purpose. It operates on the basis of a purpose. For the perceivable world has as its objectives [worldly] experience and emancipation of the soul (*puruṣa*). Of these, experience is the ascertainment of the characters of the strands of matter (*guṇas*) as welcome and unwelcome, when not distinguished [from the soul]. Emancipation is the ascertainment of the essential nature of the experiencer. There is no other form of knowledge besides these two.

VI Experience

Life is a ceaseless pageant of experiences. The messages they hold can be discarded or analysed and reflected on for their meaning. In this way wisdom accumulates. Actions performed on the basis of properly digested experience are likely to be right ones, for they build constructively on the past towards the future good.

Quotidian experiences occur in two states: waking and dreaming. The dream state is said to be the junction between this world and the next. In it a person fabricates an idiosyncratic world based on portions of this world and roams in it like an immortal god (*Waking and Dreaming*).

An object of experience is set within time. The reality of time, existing in the forms of past, present and future, underpins the schedule of manifestation of attributes of objects from genesis to extinction. If this were not so, cause and effect would have no temporal basis. This in turn would negate the logic for doing good actions (*The Reality of Time*).

Discriminating between good and pleasant experiences is important for the higher goal of life. The wise person chooses the good, for spiritual welfare, rather than the pleasant, which brings only temporary enjoyment (*Choices*).

Since pleasure is ephemeral it is regarded as pain, for its termination engenders mental suffering in the form of frustration, regret or anger. The pursuit of pleasure, being dependent on external objects, is ridden with anxiety and may involve harm to others. It breeds attachment and insatiable appetite. Wishing to avoid all these painful experiences, which are ultimately rooted in ignorance, the wise person (the Yogin) seeks eternal bliss through true knowledge (*Pleasure and Pain*).

The truth of a life is revealed at the time of death. What other recourse is there at this moment than to review one's actions and pray for a good outcome for oneself? An exquisite hymn to the Sun resonates with this urgent beseeching (*The Moment of Truth*).

What is to be learnt from the experiences of life? It is not knowledge of objects but knowledge of the being who experiences these objects, who speaks, who sees, who feels, who thinks (*The Point of Experience*).

Waking and Dreaming

(BU 4.3.8–14)

A person (*puruṣa*), on being born and attaining a body, is connected with evils [the body and organs], and on dying and leaving the body, discards those evils.

That person has only two abodes, this world and the next. The dream state, which is the third, is at their junction. Standing at that junction, he sees the two abodes, this world and the next. Then, according to his course [of life] he is at a location of the other world, and, stepping on that platform, he sees both evils and joys. When he dreams, he takes a portion of this entire world, demolishes [his gross body] himself and re-creates [a subtle body] himself. He dreams by his own light, by his own lustre. In that place the person becomes his own light.

There are no carriages, no yoke-animals and no roads there; but he creates carriages, yoke-animals and roads. There are no pleasures, no delights and no joys there, but he creates pleasures, delights and joys. There are no pools, no lakes and no rivers there, but he creates pools, lakes and rivers. For he is the fabricator.

On this point there are some verses:

When the body is overcome with sleep,
The waking one witnesses the sleeping senses.
Taking their pure form, he returns to the [waking] state,
The golden person, the unique gliding swan.

Preserving by breath the lowly nest,
The immortal roams outside the nest.
The immortal goes wherever he likes,
The golden person, the unique gliding swan.

In the dream, wandering high and low,
The god fashions many forms.
Now as if enjoying himself with women,
Now as if laughing, or seeing dreadful things.

All see his pleasure, but none sees him...

The Reality of Time

(PYS 4.12; VB 4.12)

What has passed and what is to come exist in their own essence because attributes of objects differ in appearance in the course of time.

COMMENTARY

What is to come means what manifests in the future. What has passed means what was manifested in the past. The present is what is engaged in an operation. This threefold aspect of knowledge is to be noted. If the [attributes] did not exist in their own essence this [fact of] knowledge being devoid of content and would not have arisen. Therefore a past and a future [object] does exist in essence. Moreover, if the due fruit of actions geared to enjoyment and that geared to emancipation is [regarded] as imaginary, then the performance of right actions in that regard, i.e. with that motive would not stand to reason. A cause has the power to actualize in the present a result that exists, not to produce one that does not pre-exist. An already existing cause makes perceptible an effect in its specificity; it does not produce something not previously there.

An object has many attributes. The attributes stand separately by virtue of their different schedules. While a present [object], having arrived at a specific manifestation, exists in a substance, the past and the future do not. How, then? A future [object] exists as if in its own unmanifest form, a past [object] exists in its own experienced form of manifestation. Only a present [object] has a manifestation of its form. [Objects in] the past and the future do not have it. At the time of the journey of one, the other two exist merged in the object. [Thus] the three times [i.e. the objects in them] do not exist without having existed before.

Choices

(KU 2.1–2)

The good is one thing, and the pleasant quite another;
They both, with different object, bind a man.
Of these, good ensues for one who takes the good;
One who selects the pleasant misses the goal.

Good and pleasant both approach a man;
Considering the two, the wise discriminate.
A wise man selects the good above the pleasant.
A fool selects the pleasant, for worldly weal.

Pleasure and Pain

(PYS 2.15 + VB)

On account of the pains of after-effects, anxiety and imprinted experience, and of the antithetical modes of the strands of matter, everything is pain alone to the discriminating.

COMMENTARY

For everyone this experience of pleasure, depending on animate and inanimate instruments, is permeated with attachment. Hence there must be a deposit of actions produced by attachment. Similarly, one hates the instruments of pain and suffers bewilderment and hence there must also be a deposit of actions produced by hatred and delusion. And so it is said: "Enjoyment does not occur without harming creatures. Hence there is also a deposit of actions relating to the physical which is produced by violence."

It has [already] been said that pleasure in sensory objects is [rooted in] ignorance (*avidyā*). Pleasure is the appeasement of the senses resulting from their gratification in enjoyments. Pain is non-appeasement [of the senses] due to dissatisfaction. It is not possible to make the senses free from craving by means of continued enjoyments, because both attachments and the aptitude of the senses increase with continued enjoyment. Therefore continued enjoyment is not the means to happiness. Indeed, a person seeking pleasure is like one who, afraid of a scorpion's sting, is bitten by a snake. Addicted to sensory objects, he is sunk in a great quagmire of pain.

This is called the pain of after-effects. Being [ultimately] unfavourable, it only torments a yogin even during the state of happiness.

Now, what is the pain of anxiety? The experience of anxiety depends on animate and inanimate instruments and is permeated with aversion. As a result there is a deposit of actions produced by aversion. Someone who seeks instruments of pleasure acts in body, speech and mind and either favours or hurts others. From favouring and oppressing others merit and sin pile up, and there is a deposit of actions rooted in greed and delusion. This is called the pain of anxiety.

To proceed: what is the pain of the imprints of experience? From the experience of pleasure there is a deposit of the imprints of pleasure. From the experience of pain there is a deposit of the imprints of pain. Thus when pleasure or pain is experienced as the maturation of actions, the deposit of actions increases further. Thus this beginningless, over-flooding stream of pain distresses the yogin alone on account of its [ultimately] unfavourable nature. Why? Because a wise man is like an eyeball. Just as a woollen thread fallen on the eyeball hurts it by its touch, but not [if it falls on] any other part of the body, so these pains afflict the yogin only, being like an eyeball, and not anyone else who experiences them.

However, the tripartite pain, rooted in both external and internal causes, pursues the other [i.e. the non-yogin] again and again from the moment of birth. He sheds the pain brought by his own actions as he receives it again and again, and shedding it, receives it again and again. He is wholly permeated, as it were, by ignorance housed in the mind and variegated with beginningless instincts. He holds fast to the concepts of "I" and "mine," which should in fact be cast off. Thus the yogin, seeing himself and the host of living beings being carried away by a stream of pain without beginning, takes refuge in right knowledge, which eliminates all pain.

And also on account of the antithetical modes of the strands of matter everything is sheer pain to the discriminating. The strands of the intellect take the form of light, activity and inactivity. Being mutually dependent, they initiate experiences composed of the three strands, peaceful, vehement or deluded. The modes of the strands are ever-moving; hence the mind is said to be quick-changing. Specific attitudes [piety, impiety, etc.] and specific states [pleasure, pain, etc.] conflict with each other, but general ones operate with specific ones. Thus these qualities [in their general characters], by supporting each other, cause the experiences of pleasure, pain and delusion. All of them exist in all forms and hence they partake of the character of each other. Their specificity is produced by [their] subordination to or predominance over [each other]. Therefore everything is pain alone to the discriminating.

Ignorance is the generating seed of this great aggregate of pain, and the cause of its annihilation is right knowledge.

The Moment of Truth

(ĪU 15.18; also BU 5.15.1)

The face of truth is hidden by a golden bowl;
O Sun, reveal it, that I, dutiful to truth, may see it!

O Nourisher, Sole Seer, Death, Sun, Son of Creation's Lord,
Disperse your rays! Gather up your shine
So that I see your most blessed form.
That which is that spirit, that am I.

Let the breath of the immortal "I" merge in wind;
Let this body end in ashes.
OM; O Resolve, recall your deeds, remember!
O Resolve, recall your deeds, remember!

O Fire, lead us on good paths to prosperity,
O God who know all avenues.
Remove the crooked sin in us!
With repeated orisons we bow to you.

The Point of Experience

(KauU 3.8)

One should not seek to understand speech; one should know the one who speaks. One should not seek to understand smell; one should know the one who smells. One should not seek to understand form; one should know the one who sees form. One should not seek to understand sound; one should know the one who hears. One should not seek to understand the taste of food; one should know the one who perceives the taste of food. One should not seek to understand action; one should know the one who acts. One should not seek to understand joy and sorrow; one should know the one who perceives joy and sorrow. One should not seek to understand bliss, love or procreation; one should know the one who perceives bliss, love and procreation. One should not seek to understand going; one should know the one who goes. One should not seek to understand the mind; one should know the one who thinks.

VII The Mind

The mind is the interface between the soul and the world. To know the soul it is necessary to have sovereignty over the mind. Then it can be turned away from engagement with the external world towards the inner reality.

The role of the mind as intermediary between the soul, on the one hand, and the body, senses and sense objects, on the other, is explained by way of a metaphor. The soul is the owner of a chariot, the body is the chariot, the intellect is the charioteer and the mind the reins. The senses are the horses and sense objects their coursing ground. Like ungovernable horses the senses can run wild and lead all astray, or they can be reined in by the mind in order to reach the desired destination (*Chariot and Horses*).

As the instrument of cognition the mind performs a number of functions. It moves between five basic states, much as a radio tunes in to different stations. These five are right cognition, erroneous cognition, language-dependent cognition and the cognitions of sleep and memory (*The Modes of the Mind*).

The mind operates according to a blueprint that predisposes it to experience worldly life and suffering. The root of the problem is failure to recognize the spiritual core of being. From this arise the sense of identity, feelings of attachment and aversion, and the tenacious will to live (*The Blueprint of the Mind*).

The will to live is the force that drives the individual through life after life. In each, the imprints of experiences are laid down in the subconscious mind, becoming memories and instincts. Memories and instincts are triggered by circumstances, and circumstances occur in accordance with the cause-effect law of karma. They surface in the mind despite temporal or spatial discontinuity of lives, and also despite disparity of species. It is said that a Yogin can transcend this otherwise inexorable law, because his actions are divested of motivation (*Memory, Experience and Instinct*).

In contrast to the extroverted, transmigratory mind is the introverted mind that aids meditation and the experience of the spirit. The mind is likened to a crystal. Transparent itself, the crystal takes on the hue of whatever it rests on. Similarly the mind, neutral by nature, is coloured by whatever object it lights on. Focused on external objects, it possesses them and assumes their form. Focused on the self, it assumes the character of the self (*The Crystal*).

To make this inward journey requires a perspective encompassing both the outer and the inner worlds. If it is not to be a random roaming there must be a starting point and a well-defined route to the destination. The mind must expand from narrow horizons to cosmic vistas. In a breathtaking passage teaching of "the shore beyond sorrow", facets of mental involvement with the world are graded on a scale of greatness. Starting with word, we are taken through speech, the mind, will, intelligence, meditation, comprehension, strength, food, water, fire, space, memory and hope to reach, finally, breath, which is the hub of all beings (*A Perspective*).

Chariot and Horses

(KU 3.3–9)

Know the Self as the chariot's owner
And the body as the chariot itself,
Know the intellect as the charioteer
And the mind as the reins.

The senses are the horses, they say;
Sense objects, their pastures;
With body, senses and mind conjoined
It is the enjoyer, the wise declare.

An ignoramus,
Ever undisciplined in mind,
Has senses that cannot be controlled,
Like a charioteer's rogue steeds.

But a sagacious man,
Ever disciplined in mind,
Has senses that can be controlled,
Like a charioteer's good steeds.

An ignoramus,
Unmindful and ever impure,
Does not reach that [highest] state
But returns to the round of life.

But a sagacious man,
Mindful and ever pure,
Attains that place
From which he is not born again.

With understanding as charioteer,
And with his mind as reins, a man
Reaches the journey's end
That is Viṣṇu's supreme abode.

The Modes of the Mind

(PYS 1.5–11)

The modes of the mind are five, arising from sufferings and devoid of them.

[They are] right cognition, wrong cognition, verbal cognition, sleep and memory.

Right cognition consists of perception, inference and scripture.

Wrong cognition is false knowledge founded on the appearance of a thing other than what it is.

Verbal cognition is knowledge involving words without objective reality.

Sleep is the mode of mind which takes as its object the cognition of the absence [of the waking state and dream].

Memory is the non-relinquishing of objects experienced.

The Blueprint of the Mind

(PYS 2.3–9; VB 2.6,9)

Ignorance, sense of identity ('I-am-ness'), attachment, aversion and the will to live are the afflictions.

Ignorance is the seedbed of the subsequent ones, which are dormant, reduced, interrupted or active.

Considering as permanent, pure, pleasing and the Self [what is in fact] transient, impure, painful and the non-Self is ignorance.

The powers of cognition and of the means of cognition seeming identical is the sense of identity ("I-am-ness").

Attachment is the concomitant of pleasure.

Aversion is the concomitant of pain.

The will to live flows from natural instinct and is deep set even in the wise.

COMMENTARY

The Self is the power of cognition. The intellect is the power of the means of cognition. The apparent conflation of these two into one is known as the affliction of the sense of identity. When the powers of the experiencer and the experienced appear non-distinct, despite being totally different and totally exclusive, [worldly] experience ensues. But on retrieving their true natures the Self stands absolutely alone. Where then is experience? Thus it is said: *Not seeing that the Self is beyond the intellect on account of its nature, character, consciousness and so on, through delusion one considers the intellect the Self.*

Every living creature has this constant yearning for itself, "Let me not cease to exist! Let me exist!" One who has not experienced death cannot have such a yearning for itself. The experience of a previous birth is concluded from this. And this will to live is an affliction that flows from natural instinct, right from birth, even for worms. The dread of death, consisting of the vision of extinction, is not derived through direct perception, inference and traditional lore. This leads to the inference of the death agony experienced in a previous life. Just as this affliction is seen in the grossly ignorant so also it is deep set in the learned who understand the starting point [transmigratory life] and the final state [liberation]. Why? Because the expert and the untutored alike have the same instinct on account of the experience of the death agony.

Memory, Experience and Instinct

(PYS 4.7–10; VB 4.7–9)

A Yogin's action is neither white nor black; that of others is of three kinds.

Thence [comes] the manifestation only of such instincts as are congruent with its maturation.

Despite the intervention of [other] species, place and time, they [instincts] are sequential because memory and imprints of experience (*saṁskāra*) are identical.

And they are beginningless owing to the perpetuation of the desire to live

COMMENTARY

There are four classes of actions (*karma*): black, white-and-black, white and neither-white-nor-black. Of these, the evil-minded have the black. The white-and-black is achieved through external means. Basically, the deposit of actions accumulates through the oppression and advantaging of others. Those who engage in austerities, scriptural study and meditation have the white. As it is restricted solely to the mind it is not dependent upon external instruments, [and does] not [result from] causing harm to others. Renunciates with attenuated afflictions, who are in their last bodies, have the neither-white-nor-black. In this context, the not-white variety pertains to the Yogin only, as he has renounced their fruit, and [also] the not-black as he does not perform [black actions]. But other beings have the three kinds mentioned before.

In the maturation of a particular kind of action, instincts consistent with it accompany the maturation of the action. They alone manifest. For when an action in the life of a god is fructifying it does not cause the manifestation of hellish, animal or human instincts. On the contrary, only instincts appropriate to the divine are manifested. The reasoning is the same in respect of hellish, animal and human [actions].

The occurrence of fruition [of action] in a cat [-birth] manifests through an appropriate manifesting power. Even if a hundred births or distant lands or a hundred aeons intervene, because the appropriate drive for manifestation arises instantaneously, it would emerge again, prompted by the appropriate drive, and take on the instincts imprinted during the fruition of a previous experience as a cat. Why? Because despite the intervening factors these instincts are sequential because a similar action becomes the cause of their manifestation. Again, how is that? Because memory and the imprints of experience must be identical. As are experiences, so are the imprints of experiences, and they accord with instincts relating to action. As are instincts, so is memory. Thus, memory comes from the imprints of experience, albeit interrupted by species, place and time. Imprints of experience in their turn arise from memory. Thus memory and imprints of experience are manifested by virtue of the operation of the deposit of actions. Hence it is established that because of the certainty of the relation of cause and effect, [instincts] are proved to be sequential, howsoever separated they may be.

The Crystal

(PYS 1.41; VB 1.41)

When the modes of the mind are enfeebled and when it dwells on an object – perceiver, instrument of perception and object of perception – and, like a fine crystal, is suffused with it, that is absorption.

COMMENTARY

"Modes enfeebled" means the cessation of intellection. "Like a fine crystal" is given as an illustration. A crystal, on account of the difference of its supporting bases is imbued with various colours, and appears to have the same colour as its base. Similarly, the mind is coloured by its supporting object, and, possessed of that object, appears to have the same character as it.

[To explain:] Suffused with a subtle element, it is possessed of that subtle element and becomes illumined by the form of that subtle element. Similarly, suffused with a gross supporting object, it is possessed of that gross object, and becomes illumined by the form of that gross object. Similarly, suffused with the different objects in the universe, it is possessed of the different objects in the universe and becomes illumined by the form of the universe. The same is to be seen in the case of the instruments of perception, the sense organs. Suffused with an instrument of perception as its support, it is possessed of that instrument of perception and shines with its aspects in the form of that instrument of perception. Similarly, suffused with the soul, the perceiver, as its support, it is possessed of the soul, the perceiver, and shines with the aspects of the perceiving soul. Similarly, suffused with a liberated soul as its support, it is possessed of the liberated soul and shines with the aspects of the liberated soul. Thus, the mind, resembling a fine crystal, rests on and is suffused with an object - perceiver, instrument of perception, object of perception, [i.e. in this case] soul, senses, elements - and is firm in it and takes on its forms. That is called absorption.

A Perspective

(ChU 7.1–15)

[Sanatkumāra instructs Nārada.]

"Teach me, Sir," Nārada approached Sanatkumāra. He replied, "Come to me with what you know. What is beyond that I shall explain." He said:

"Sir, I know the *Ṛgveda*, the *Yajurveda*, the *Sāmaveda*, the *Atharvaveda* as the fourth, history and legend as the fifth [*Veda*], the *Veda* of the *Vedas* [grammar], ancestral rites, mathematics, divination, the science of treasures, logic, ethics, etymology, the *Vedic* sciences, exorcism, the science of weaponry, astronomy, snake-lore and divine arts. This, sir, I know."

"Sir, I am merely a connoisseur of texts; I am ignorant of the Self. I have heard from respected people like yourself that one who knows the Self passes beyond sorrow. Sir, I am full of sorrow. Sir, take me across to the shore beyond sorrow." He replied, "Whatever you have studied is but word."

"Word, indeed, is the *Ṛgveda*, the *Yajurveda*, the *Sāmaveda*, the *Atharvaveda* as the fourth, history and legend as the fifth [*Veda*], the *Veda* of the *Vedas* [grammar], ancestral rites, mathematics, divination, the science of treasures, logic, ethics, etymology, the *Vedic* sciences, exorcism, the science of weaponry, astronomy, snake-lore and divine arts. This is but word. Worship the word."

"One who worships word as *brahman* goes wherever one wishes as far as word reaches, one who worships word as *brahman*." "Is there, Sir, anything greater than word?"

"Certainly, there is something greater than word." "Sir, please tell me it."

"Speech, certainly, is greater than word. Speech makes us understand the *Ṛgveda*, the *Yajurveda*, the *Sāmaveda*, the *Atharvaveda* as the fourth, history and legend as the fifth [*Veda*], the *Veda* of the *Vedas* [grammar], ancestral rites, mathematics, divination, the science of treasures, logic, ethics, etymology, the *Vedic* sciences, exorcism, the science of weaponry, astronomy, snake-lore and divine arts; and also heaven and earth, air and space, water and fire, gods and men, beasts and birds, grasses, trees, animals right down to worms, insects and ants, right and wrong, truth and falsehood, good and bad, pleasant and unpleasant. If speech did not exist, right and wrong would not exist, nor truth and falsehood, nor good and bad, nor pleasant and unpleasant. Speech alone makes all this known. Worship speech."

One who worships speech as *brahman* goes wherever one wishes as far as speech reaches, one who worships speech as *brahman*. "Is there, Sir, anything greater than speech?"

"Certainly, there is something greater than speech." "Sir, please tell me it."

"The mind, certainly, is greater than speech. Just as a fist encompasses two myrobalan fruits or two kola berries or two dice, so the mind encompasses speech and word. When one formulates the thought with the mind that 'I should learn the texts,' one learns them; that 'I should perform actions,' one does so; that 'I should desire sons and cattle,' one so desires; that 'I should desire this world and the next,' one so desires. For mind is the Self, mind is the world, mind is *brahman*. Worship the mind."

One who worships the mind as *brahman* goes wherever one wishes as far as the mind reaches, one who worships the mind as *brahman*. "Is there, Sir, anything greater than the mind?"

"Certainly, there is something greater than the mind." "Sir, please tell me it."

"Will, certainly, is greater than the mind. When one wills then one formulates thought, then utters speech, and utters it in a word. Sacred recitations become consolidated with the word, and rites with the sacred recitations."

All these, indeed, have will as their single abode. They have will as their essence and will as their firm base. Heaven and earth willed, air and space willed, water and fire willed. By their will, rain wills [is effective]; by the will of rain, food wills; by the will of food, the vital breaths will; by the will of the vital breaths, the sacred recitations will; by the will of the sacred recitations, the rites will; by the will of the rites, the world wills; by the will of the world, everything wills. This is will. Worship will."

"One who worships will as *brahman* attains the worlds willed by him: one who is constant, constant worlds, one who is firmly based, firmly based worlds, one who is untroubled, untroubled worlds. One goes wherever one wishes as far as will reaches, one who worships will as *brahman*." "Is there, Sir, anything greater than will?"

"Certainly, there is something greater than will." "Sir, please tell me it."

"Intelligence, certainly, is greater than will. When one reasons, then one wills then one formulates thought, then utters speech, and utters it in a word. The sacred recitations become one with the word, and the rites with the sacred recitations."

"All these, indeed, have intelligence as their single abode. They have intelligence as their essence and intelligence as their firm base. Therefore even if someone is very learned but is without intelligence, people say of him, "He is not this [learned]. If he knew, if he were learned, he would not lack intelligence in this way." If someone has little learning but has intelligence, people wish to listen to him alone. For intelligence is their single abode. Intelligence is their essence and intelligence is their firm base. Worship intelligence."

"One who worships intelligence as *brahman* attains the worlds of intelligence: one who is constant, constant worlds, one who is firmly based, firmly based worlds, one who is untroubled, untroubled worlds. One goes wherever one wishes as far as intelligence reaches, one who worships intelligence as *brahman*." "Is there, Sir, anything greater than intelligence?" "Certainly, there is something greater than intelligence." "Sir, please tell me it."

"Meditation, certainly, is greater than intelligence. The earth meditates, as it were. The sky meditates, as it were. Heaven meditates, as it were. The waters meditate, as it were. The mountains meditate, as it were. Gods and men meditate, as it were. Therefore those who attain greatness here among men indeed share, as it were, in the reward of meditation. Those who are petty are quarrelsome, malicious and censorious. But those who are high-minded indeed share, as it were, in the reward of meditation. Worship meditation."

"One who worships meditation as *brahman* goes wherever one wishes as far as meditation reaches, one who worships meditation as *brahman*." "Is there, Sir, anything greater than meditation?" "Certainly, there is something greater than meditation." "Sir, please tell me it."

"Comprehension, certainly, is greater than meditation. By comprehension, indeed, one understands the *Ṛgveda*, the *Yajurveda*, the *Sāmaveda*, the *Atharvaveda* as the fourth, history and legend as the fifth [*Veda*], the *Veda* of the *Vedas* [grammar], ancestral rites, mathematics, divination, the science of treasures, logic, ethics etymology, the *Vedi*c sciences, exorcism, the science of weaponry, astronomy, snake-lore and divine arts; and also heaven and earth, air and space, water and fire, gods and men, beasts and birds, grasses, trees, animals right down to worms, insects and ants, right and wrong, truth and falsehood, good and bad, pleasant and unpleasant, food and drink, this world and the next. By comprehension alone one understands. Worship comprehension."

"One who worships comprehension as *brahman* attains worlds full of comprehension and knowledge. One goes wherever one wishes as far as comprehension reaches, one who worships comprehension as *brahman*." "Is there, Sir, anything greater than comprehension?" "Certainly, there is something greater than comprehension." "Sir, please tell me it."

"Strength, certainly, is greater than comprehension. A single strong man makes a hundred men of understanding tremble. When one becomes strong, then one rises. Rising, serves; serving, one comes close [to a teacher]; coming close, one sees, hears, thinks, reasons, acts and understands. By strength, indeed, the earth stands; by strength, the sky; by strength, the heaven; by strength, the mountains; by strength, gods and men; by strength, beasts and birds; by strength, grasses and trees; by strength, animals right down to worms, insects and ants. By strength, the world stands. Worship strength."

"One who worships strength as *brahman* goes wherever one wishes as far as strength reaches, one who worships strength as *brahman*. "Is there, Sir, anything greater than strength?" "Certainly, there is something greater than strength." "Sir, please tell me it."

"Food, certainly, is greater than strength. Therefore, if one did not eat for even ten days and yet lived, one would not see, hear, think, reason, act and understand. But with the coming of food one sees, hears, thinks, reasons, acts and understands. Worship food."

"One who worships food as *brahman* attains worlds full of food and drink. One goes wherever one wishes as far as food reaches, one who worships food as *brahman*." "Is there, Sir, anything greater than food?" "Certainly, there is something greater than food." "Sir, please tell me it."

"Water, certainly, is greater than food." Therefore when there is no rain life is blighted, for 'Food will be scarce.' But when there is good rain life becomes joyful, for 'Food will be plentiful.' Water, indeed, incarnate, has become these beings: this earth, the sky, heaven, mountains, gods and men, beasts and birds, grasses, trees, animals right down to worms, insects and ants. Water, indeed, incarnate is these beings. Worship water."

"One who worships water as *brahman* obtains all desires and becomes satisfied. One goes wherever one wishes as far as water reaches, one who worships water as *brahman*." "Is there, Sir, anything greater than water?" "Certainly, there is something greater than water." "Sir, please tell me it."

"Fire, certainly, is greater than water. For seizing the wind, it heats space. Then people say, 'It is sweltering, it is scorching, it is going to rain.' Thus fire shows this as precursor, then creates water. Then, with upward and criss-cross lightning, come thunder rolls, and so they say, 'There is lightning, there is thunder, it is going to rain.' Thus fire shows this as precursor, then creates water. Worship fire."

"One who worships fire/heat as *brahman*, as a radiant being attains worlds full of radiance and lustre, with darkness quelled. One goes wherever one wishes as far as fire reaches, one who worships fire as *brahman*." "Is there, Sir, anything greater than fire." "Certainly, there is something greater than fire." "Sir, please tell me it."

"Space, certainly, is greater than fire. For in space are both sun and moon, and lightning, stars and fire. One calls out across space, one hears across space, one replies across space. One enjoys oneself in space. One does not enjoy oneself in space. One is born in space. One grows in space. Worship space."

"One who worships space as *brahman* attains worlds full of space and light, unobstructed and wide in compass. One goes wherever one wishes as far as space reaches, one who worships space as *brahman*." "Is there, Sir, anything greater than space?" "Certainly, there is something greater than space." "Sir, please tell me it."

"Memory, certainly, is greater than space. Therefore even if there were many people, without remembering they would not hear anything, they would not think, they would not understand. When, however, they remembered, then they would hear, then they would think, then they would understand. Through memory one knows one's sons, and through memory, one's cattle. Worship memory.

"One who worships memory as *brahman* goes wherever one wishes as far as memory reaches, one who worships memory as *brahman*." "Is there, Sir, anything greater than memory?" "Certainly, there is something greater than memory." "Sir, please tell me it."

"Hope, certainly, is greater than memory. For memory lit with hope learns sacred texts, performs rites, desires sons and cattle, and desires this world and the next. Worship hope."

"One who worships hope as *brahman* has all desires fulfilled through hope. One's prayers are effective. One goes wherever one wishes as far as hope reaches, one who worships hope as *brahman*." "Is there, Sir, anything greater than hope." "Certainly, there is something greater than hope." "Sir, please tell me it."

"Breath, certainly, is greater than hope. Just as spokes are set on a hub so is everything mounted on this breath. Breath moves by breath. Breath gives breath. It gives to breath. The father is breath. The mother is breath. The brother is breath. The sister is breath. The teacher is breath. The *brahman* is breath."

If one retorts harshly to one's father or mother, to one's brother or sister, to one's teacher or a *brahmin*, people say, "Shame on you! You are a father-killer! You are a mother-killer! You are a brother-killer! You are a sister-killer! You are a teacher-killer! You are a brahmin-killer!"

Now if their breath has departed and one were to cremate them, piled up together with a poker, people would not say, "You are a father-killer! You are a mother-killer! You are a brother-killer! You are a sister-killer! You are a teacher-killer! You are a brahmin-killer!"

For breath alone is all these beings. One who sees, thinks and understands in this manner becomes a surpassing speaker.

VIII The Conquest of Mind: Yoga

The outward-ranging powers of the mind need to be harnessed in order to make the inward journey to the source of being. This is achieved through the discipline of Yoga. As the mind participates in all aspects of activity – moral, behavioural, physical, physiological, sensory and intellectual – all these are addressed in Yoga. As a result of the conquest of the mind a tranquil, pellucid state of being is attained that reflects truth, bliss and infinity.

The method of entering this state is to sit erect and motionless, restraining the breath and mind. Various apparitions arise that presage success, such as mist, smoke, fire and crystal. The establishment of the Yogic state brings visible changes in the Yogin, including lightness, health, absence of greed and a melodious voice (*The Procedure of Yoga*).

Yoga is defined as the control of the modes of the mind. The mind has levels of concentration: unstable, dull, restricted to pleasure, one-pointed and controlled. It is only at the last two levels that Yogic meditation and absorption are possible. These levels are created by the preponderance of one of the three strands of nature, illumination, activity and inertia (*sattva*, *rajas*, *tamas*). When every speck of the last two is removed, the illuminative quality of mind alone remains. Discarding that also leads to the highest Yogic state of absorption that is beyond mental involvement (*The Yogic Mind*).

The action part of Yoga, as opposed to the moral, disciplinary (relating to body, breath and senses) and meditative, has three components. These are the practice of austerity, the study of scripture and surrender to God. They stabilize the Yogic state of absorption and weaken the root afflictions that set the mind up for worldly life (*The Stepping Stones of Yoga*). Without these actions there can be no progress.

Yoga practice is divided into eight parts, corresponding to the various spheres of human activity. These are ethical vows, observances, posture, breath control, sensory control, concentration, meditation and absorption (*The Eight Limbs of Yoga*). They are also known as limbs, suggesting their role within an organic whole.

The stability of mind envisioned by Yoga results from deliberate acts to that end. Pre-eminent is the cultivation of positive and non-emotive attitudes. Other methods include the practice of breath control or concentration on sublime objects. Examples of these are preternatural sense perceptions, engrossment in the awareness of the existence of the self, reflection on a saintly character and knowledge arising from deep sleep (*Attaining Stability of Mind*).

The conduct of someone who has attained stability of mind is described; it is that of a Yogin. Such a person is not distressed by woes, does not crave sensual pleasures, and is fearless, free of anger and disciplined in mind and senses. Breaking the chain which begins with attachment, moves through desire, anger, delusion, confused memory and loss of reason, and ends with ruin, the Yogin secures the ultimate serenity: the beatitude of *brahman* (*The Sage Yogin*).

The Procedure of Yoga

(ŚU 2.8–14)

Holding the body erect its three parts [chest, neck, head] aligned,
Fixing senses and mind in the heart,
The wise man should cross by the boat of brahman
All rivers generating fear.

Suppressing his breaths here, his movement restrained,
With attenuated breath he should breathe through the nose;
Like a carriage yoked to vicious horses
The wise man should alertly hold his mind in check.

In a level, clean [place], free of pebbles, fire and sand,
Through such things as sounds, water and abodes
Agreeable to the mind, but not offensive to the eye,

In a secure refuge without wind, should he practice.

Mist, smoke, sun, wind, fire,
Fireflies, lightning, crystal, moon,
These forms are the precursors
Bringing the revelation of brahman *in Yoga.*

When earth, water, fire, wind and space are refined
And the fivefold quality of Yoga [subtle smell, etc] sets in,
There is no disease, old age or pain for one
Who has gained a body made of the fire of Yoga.

Lightness, health, absence of greed,
Clear complexion and melodious voice,
Sweet smell, slight urine and stool,
Is the first setting in of Yoga, they say.

As a mirror besmeared with grime
Shines brightly when it is cleaned,
So the embodied one, seeing the soul's real nature
Becomes single, with aim fulfilled, and sorrow-free.

The Yogic Mind

(PYS 1.1–4; VB 1.1–2)

Now the instruction on Yoga.

Yoga is the control of the modes of the mind.

Then the self abides in its own form.

At other times it is identified with the modes [of the mind].

COMMENTARY

Yoga is absorption. It is [not] a feature of the mind at all levels. The levels of the mind are (i) unstable, (ii) dull, (iii) restricted [to pleasure], (iv) one-pointed and (v) controlled. Here, perfect absorption in the [pleasure-]fixed mind does not belong to Yoga as it is connected with [pleasure] fixation. But in the one-pointed mind that which illumines an object as it really is, diminishes the afflictions, loosens the bonds of action and inclines it towards control, that is known as absorption (*samādhi*) with awareness of other elements. It is [fourfold, being] accompanied by deliberation, judgement, bliss and [pure] existence. When all the modes are controlled it is absorption (*samādhi*) without awareness of other elements.

The mind is composed of the three strands [of matter] as it has the character of illumination, activity and inertia (*sattva*, *rajas*, *tamas*). The illuminative faculty of mind, when contaminated by activity and inertia, becomes fond of [Yogic] powers and sensory objects. When permeated by inertia it tends towards wrongdoing, ignorance, lack of detachment and disability. When it shines on all sides and the veil of delusion has been destroyed, and it is tainted with an iota of activity, it tends towards righteousness, knowledge, detachment, and [Yogic] powers. When the taint of even the smallest element of *rajas* is removed it stands in its own character and remains as nothing but the distinction between the mind and the self. It [then] tends to the meditation known as "cloud of righteousness." Meditators describe this as the supreme mediation. The power of consciousness is [by nature] unchanging. It does not move [to objects]. Objects are reflected into it. It is pure and infinite. In contradistinction to it is this differentiating knowledge, which is composed of the strand of illumination (*sattva*). The mind, free from attachment to that [differentiating knowledge], halts even that knowledge. That state retains only memory imprints (*saṁskāras*); it is seedless absorption. In it nothing is cognized; hence it is called "without awareness [of other elements]." This twofold Yoga is comprised in the control of the modes of the mind.

The Stepping Stones of Yoga

(PYS 2.1–2 + VB)

Austerity, study of scriptures and dedication to God are the action part of Yoga.

Its objectives are to stabilize absorption [*samādhi*] and to enfeeble the afflictions.

COMMENTARY

Yoga does not succeed when one does not practise self-mortification. Impurity, (i) diversified by beginningless actions, instincts and afflictions and

(ii) comprising the net of sense objects, cannot be eliminated except by mortification. Hence mortification is mentioned. And [the author] implies that it should be practised so as not to disturb the serenity of mind.

The study of scriptures is the recitation of *OM* and other holy [utterances], or the study of the treatises on liberation.

Dedication to God is the offering of all actions to the Supreme Teacher, or the renunciation of their fruit.

[The action part of Yoga] when assiduously performed stabilizes *samādhi* and enfeebles the afflictions such that, through the fire of meditation, the enfeebled afflictions are made sterile like roasted seeds. Because of the enfeeblement of the afflictions the subtle insight which discriminates between the mind and the Self will not be affected by them again. Its [subtle insight's] purpose fulfilled, it will be due for dissolution.

The Eight Limbs of Yoga

(PYS 2.29, 30, 32, 46, 48, 54 & 3.1–3; VB 2.30, 32, 46, 49, 54 & 3.1–3)

Ethical vows, observances, posture, breath control, withdrawal of senses, concentration, meditation and absorption are the eight limbs of Yoga.

Non-injury, truthfulness, non-stealing, celibacy and non-acquisition are the vows of abstention.

Cleanliness, contentment, ascetic discipline, study of scriptures and dedication to God are the observances.

Posture is what is stable and comfortable.

When it [posture] is there, the regulation of the flow of inhalation and exhalation is breath control.

When disjoined from their objects, the senses seeming to imitate the state of the mind is sensory withdrawal.

Focusing consciousness on a locus is concentration.

The continuity of attention thereon is meditation.

Meditation with the appearance of the object alone, seemingly devoid of its own form [as cognition], is absorption (*samādhi*).

COMMENTARY

Of these non-injury is the complete absence of cruelty towards living beings at all times. The subsequent forbearances and observances stem from this and are performed purely in order to accomplish it and bring it to perfection. And so it is said, "As this *brahman* purposefully undertakes many vows progressively, he avoids occasions for cruelty created by carelessness and refines non-injury."

Truthfulness is when speech and mind are in accord with fact. As it is seen and inferred, so should be speech and thought. Speech is uttered in order to communicate one's understanding to another in such a way that it is not misleading, ambiguous or conveying no sense at all. It is employed for the benefit of all creatures and not to do them harm. If, despite this, an utterance were to harm a living being, that would not be truth but in fact sin. Through this apparent virtue, which is the opposite of virtue, one would attain the miserable darkness [of hell]. Therefore, one should, after close consideration, speak the truth for the good of all creatures.

Theft is the unauthorized appropriation of others' goods. Abstention from theft is its contrary and consists of the absence of desire.

Celibacy is the control of the sex organ with the other organs [also] guarded.

Non-acquisition is non-appropriation springing from the awareness of the demerits of objects: earning, keeping, loss, attachment and hurt.

Of these [observances], cleanliness produced by earth, water and so on, and by taking in pure substances is external. Internally it is washing away the impurities of the mind.

Contentment is not wishing to acquire more than that which serves one's immediate needs.

Ascetic discipline is the endurance of opposites. The opposites are hunger and thirst, heat and cold, standing and sitting, and log-like silence and cessation of gestures. It includes vows as appropriate: bodily mortification, the lunar fast and the austere fast.

Study of scriptures is the study of the treatises on liberation or the repetition of *OM*.

Dedication to God is the surrender of all actions to that supreme teacher.

[Postures:] These are as follows: the lotus pose, the hero pose, the blessed pose, the cross, the staff pose, the supported [pose], the couch, the heron seat, the elephant seat, the camel seat, the symmetrical placement, the easily stable, the comfortable, and so on.

After posture has been mastered [breath control comes]. The in-breath is the intake of external air and the out-breath is the expulsion of abdominal air. The interruption of the flow of both is breath control.

When the mind is controlled the senses, like the mind, are controlled. They do not need any independent effort as in the case of the other [non-Yogic] subjugation of the senses. Just as bees follow the flight of the leader bee and alight when it alights, so the senses are controlled when the mind is controlled. This is the withdrawal of the senses.

Concentration is the fixing of the mind only by [mechanical] attention on the navel plexus, the lotus of the heart, the head, light, the top of the nose, the tip of the tongue, or other loci or external objects.

Meditation is the unidirectional flow of attention towards the object of meditation in that locus, undisturbed by any other cognition.

When meditation with exclusive illumination of its object becomes devoid, as it were, of its own [cognitive] nature because it has merged with the nature of the object, it is said to be absorption (*samādhi*).

Ways of Attaining Stability of Mind

(PYS 1.33–39 + VB)

Serenity of mind comes by the cultivation of goodwill, compassion, joy and impassivity towards the happy, the suffering, the virtuous and the wicked.

Or by the expulsion and retention of breath.

Alternatively the apperception arisen with respect to a sense object holds the mind steady.

Or the sorrow-free, Luminous state.

Or the mind having a dispassionate person as its object.

Or having the support of knowledge from a dream or sleep.

Or through meditation on what holds the mind.

COMMENTARY

Of these [attitudes], one should feel goodwill towards all creatures experiencing happiness, compassion towards the wretched, joy for the virtuous-minded and impassivity towards the evil-minded. In one exercising these feelings "white" merit (cf. PYS 4.7) is engendered. Thereby the mind is purified and, when purified, attains the serene, one-pointed state of steadiness.

Expulsion is the ejection of abdominal air through the nasal apertures with special effort. Retention is *prāṇāyāma*. Alternatively through these one attains steadiness of mind.

For one who concentrates on the top of the nose, the perception of smell is the awareness of divine smell; on the tip of the tongue, the awareness of divine taste; on the palate, the awareness of [divine] colour; on the middle of the tongue, awareness of [divine] touch, on the root of the tongue, awareness of [divine] sound. When these perceptions have arisen they hold the mind steady, dispel doubts and become the doorway to the insight of *samādhi*. A perception arising in regard to the moon, sun, a planet, a gem, a light, a treasure should also be regarded as object-based.

The truth of a thing understood through scripture, inference or the instruction of a teacher is no doubt its reality, because they [scripture etc.] are able to explain the thing precisely as it is. However, as long as even any one aspect is not known by one's own senses the whole is, as it were, indirectly known, and this does not bring about the unshakeable understanding of subtle objects such as liberation. Therefore, in order to reinforce scripture, inference and the instruction of teachers it is imperative that some specific object should be directly perceived. When there is direct perception of an aspect which has been taught, faith is created in all subtle objects, right up to liberation. For this very reason the purification of the mind is advised. The [second] reason is with regard to uncontrolled mental operations; when consciousness of mastery over those [chosen] objects arises, the mind is capable of directly perceiving each object. When this occurs, faith, dynamism, memory and absorption [*samādhi*] arise in it unhindered.

The *sattva* strand of the mind is luminous and like space. Through undiluted concentration on the consciousness of the mind focusing on the lotus of the heart, a mode of the mind assumes the effulgent forms of the sun, moon, a planet or a gem. Similarly, the mind engrossed in the awareness of the existence of the self is like a sea without waves, peaceful, limitless, consisting only of the awareness of the existence of the self. On this point it is said, "Discovering the atomic Self, one is conscious only of the sense of 'I am.' This twofold, sorrow-free perception is object-based, while [the other], consisting of the mere sense of "I am", is said to be Luminous. Through these the Yogin's mind attains a state of steadiness.

Alternatively, the Yogin's mind, imbued with the thought of some dispassionate person, attains steadiness.

Alternatively, the Yogin's mind, resting on knowledge from dreams or knowledge from deep sleep, and taking its shape, attains steadiness.

One should meditate on whatever holds the mind. Gaining steadiness there, one gains steadiness elsewhere also.

The Sage Yogin

(BG 2.55–72)

When one renounces all desires
Set within the mind, O Pārtha,
Content just with the Self and in the Self,
Then one is called a steadfast seer.

One who is not distressed by woes,
Is without the wish for pleasures,
Free of passion, fear and anger,
Is called a contemplative, firm in thought.

One who is unattached in every way,
And meeting the auspicious or inauspicious,
Neither rejoices nor abhors it,
Has stability of intellect.

And when such a one retracts
From all sides, like a tortoise its limbs,
The senses from their sense objects,
He has stability of intellect.

Objects of sense retreat
From the embodied soul who fasts;
Except for taste; taste too retreats
From him, on seeing the Supreme.

Even for one who strives, O Kaunteya,
For a man of learning
The tormenting senses
Forcibly abduct the mind.

Holding all those in check,
Composed, he should stay engrossed in Me.
For one whose senses are subdued
Has stability of intellect.

In a man brooding on sense objects,
Attachment to them is born;
From attachment springs desire,
From desire anger springs.

From anger comes delusion,
From delusion, confused memory;
From confused memory, loss of reason
From loss of reason, one is ruined.

One free from love and hate
Among sense objects moving
With organs mind-controlled, controlled in mind,
Attains serenity.

In serenity there comes surcease
Of all one's sufferings,
For in the tranquil-minded
The intellect stays firm.

For the undisciplined there is
Neither judgement nor meditation;
For the non-contemplative, no peace;
For the non-peaceful, where is happiness?

When the mind is ruled
By the roving senses
It bears away one's wisdom
As the wind a ship on water.

Therefore, O Strong-Armed One,
One whose senses are held back
On all sides from sense objects,
Has stability of intellect.

The ascetic stays awake
In what is all creatures' night,

When creatures are awake,
That is, for the seer, night.

As waters enter the ocean,
And it is filled yet stays unmoved,
Likewise one in whom all desires enter
Finds peace, not one seized with desire.

The man who discards all desires
Moves about free from wants;
Free from the sense of "mine" and "I",
He secures peace.

This, O Pārtha, is the Absolute state;
Attaining it, there is no delusion.
Abiding there, even if at the time of death,
One gains the beatitude of brahman.

A Note on the Source Texts

Imagine a teacher surrounded by pupils. The teacher has planned the main topics for the term, but in individual classes digresses from it in response to students' questions, expatiating on details or on other branches of the science. From time to time the need arises for recapitulation or for a restatement of important basic principles. By the end of the course the smooth, linked flow of exposition has been interrupted, even subverted, though the original scheme is still recognizable.

The classical texts on Āyurveda suggest just such an exposition based on the oral transmission of knowledge. Information relating to a single subject may be found in various parts of the works. This makes the navigation of these works a formidable task.

In writing about Āyurveda I have drawn heavily on the source texts. My purpose in doing so has been to present the subject as faithfully as possible, and to give the reader direct access to the ancient way of thought, as far as possible without obtruding myself as interpreter and intermediary. Many of the paragraphs are virtual translations. I have attempted below to chart the topics, and in so doing to provide a summary of the material presented. The passages referred to are key ones, though not necessarily the only ones, dealing with a particular topic.

Introducing Āyurveda

Life

Regarding life, the main work used has been the *Caraka Saṁhitā* and to a minor extent *Vāgbhaṭa's Aṣṭāngahṛdaya*. The Section on Principles (*Sūtrasthāna*) gives the definition of life (CS-Sū 1.42; CS-Sū 30.22) and states the importance of health as the sustainer of achievements and aims (VA-Sū 1.2; CS-Sū 1.15; CS-Sū 11.3–4). It notes disease as an obstacle to achievement (CS-Sū 1.16) and Āyurveda as the subject that deals with the science of life (CS-Sū 1.14). It considers types of life, listing the characteristics of happy, unhappy, good and bad lives (CS-Sū 30.24). Other Sections, on the Body (*Śārīrasthāna*), on Portents and Prodromes (*Indriyasthāna*) and on Measures (*Vimānasthāna*), discuss life span, giving indications of longevity and imminent death (CS-Śā 8.51; CS-In), the ways of determining life span (CS-Vi 8.96–99) and the factors affecting it (CS-Vi 3.38).

The Conceptual Framework of Āyurveda

To understand the conceptual framework of Āyurveda, all three of the great classics have been consulted, primarily from their Sections on Principles (*Sūtrasthāna*) and on the Body (*Śārīrasthāna*). These texts discuss the important doctrine of the five elements (*Pañca Mahābhūta Siddhānta*), explaining what they are (SS-Śā 1.4 & 19; VA-Sū 9.1–2; CS-Sā 4.12) and their properties (CS-Śā 1.27). They state the characteristics of substances according to predominance of element and relevance to the body (VA-Sū 9.5–9) and the role of the elements in body parts and functions (CS-Śā 4.12; VA-Śā 3.3). They further give the correlation between *doṣas* and elements (SS-Sū 42.5) and between senses and elements (CS-Sū 8.14).

Information on the properties and tastes occurring in substances is again found in the Section on Principles of all the works. Lists are given of the twenty properties (SS-Sū 46. 513–523) and the six tastes (VA-Sū 1.14). Post-digestion taste (VA-Sū 9.20) is discussed, as well as potency (CS-Sū 26. 64–65) and special property (CS-Sū 26.67).

The theory of similarity and dissimilarity (*sāmānya viśeṣa siddhānta*) is found in Caraka's Section on the Body (*Śārīrasthāna*). It explains this principle in relation to the maintenance of the body (CS-Śā 1.44) and its three types (CS-Śā 6.9–10).

The theory of the correspondence between the human being and the universe (*loka puruṣa sāmya siddhānta)* is also expounded in the same section.

It discusses the microcosm and macrocosm (CS-Śā 4.13; 5.3-6), the main correspondences between them (CS-Śā 5.5) and the value of understanding their relationship (CS-Śā 5.7).

The Body

Information on the body is drawn from the Section on Principles (*Sūtrasthāna*) and the Section on the Body *(Śārīrasthāna)* of all three authorities, and, with respect to digestion, from Caraka's Section on Treatment (*Cikitsāsthāna*). The body is defined (CS-Śā 6.4; SS-Śā 1).

The constituents of the body are enumerated: *doṣas*, tissues (*dhātus*) and waste products (*mala*) (VA-Sū 11.1). To understand the *doṣas* it is necessary to know the overall role of each *doṣa* (SS-Sū 21.5), its area of operation (VA-Sū 1.7; VA-Sū 11.26) and its sites and detailed functions (VA-Sū 11–12).

The body tissues form the base of the body (VA-Sū 1.13 commentary; VA-Sū 11.35; VA-Sū 1.7) and have various functions (VA-Sū 11.4; SS-Sū 15.7). Their quintessence, *ojas*, is the strength of the body (SS-Sū 15.23; VA-Sū 11.37–40).

The waste products of the body also have a function (VA-Sū 11.5). As well as the main waste products subsidiary ones are noted (SS-Sū 46.527).

The action of the digestive and metabolic fire (*agni*) is considered crucial in Āyurveda. There is discussion of its function and location (CS-Ci 15.40) and of the consequences of its impairment (CS-Vi 6.12; VA-Sū 1.8; VA-Sū 13.25). On it depends the process of digestion (CS-Ci 15.6–14) and the formation of body tissues (CS-Ci 15.15–16).

Āyurveda recognizes the role of constitution (*prakṛti*) in health. Different constitutional types are noted (VA-Sū 1. 9–10) and their characteristics enumerated (VA-Śā 3.85–103). Psychological traits are correlated with the *guṇas* of Nature (SS-Śā 1.18), which in their turn also have a correlation with *doṣas* (SS-Ni 1.8). The characteristics of the various psychological types are listed (CS-Śā 4.36–39).

Āyurveda discusses the soul and mind. In order to do so it posits two eternal principles, spirit and matter or Nature (SS-Śā 1.9). It outlines the process of evolution (SS-Śā 1.4) and the correlation between the elements and the *guṇas* (SS-Sū 42.5). It discusses the nature of the soul (CS-Śā 1.53–54) and of true knowledge, which is knowledge of the soul (CS-Śā 1.54–55). It traces emotions to faulty understanding (CS-Śā 1.53), resulting in the cycle of birth and death (CS-Śā 1.67–69). It lists the signs of the soul in the body (CS-Śā 1.70–74).

The relationship between the soul and the mind is considered (CS-Śā 1.75). Probing into the mind, it discusses knowledge and the mind (CS-Śā 1.18–19), the actions of the mind (CS-Sū 8.4, 7) and the objects of the mind (CS-Śā 1.20–21).

Finally, in respect of anatomy, Āyurveda identifies the most vulnerable sites of the body (*marmasthānas*) (SS-Śā 6; VA-Śā 4).

Health

The topic of health (*svāsthya*) is covered in the Section on Principles (*Sūtrasthāna*) of all three works, although some information on food is also found in Caraka's Section on Measures (*Vimānasthāna*) and on the causes of disease in his Section on the Body (*Śārīrasthāna*). Suṣruta's Section on Treatment (*Cikitsāsthāna*) discusses exercise. As a preliminary, statements are made regarding the concept of health (CS-Sū 5.13 Commentary), its definition (SS-Sū 15.45), and regarding the twofold objective of Āyurveda (CS-Sū 30–26) of prophylaxis and cure.

There are three types of guidelines for the maintenance of health (*Svasthavṛtta*): daily regimen, seasonal regimen and safeguards against disease. Details of a health-promoting daily regimen are given (VA-Sū 2). This includes diet, sleep, exercise and good conduct.

There is detailed discussion on the importance of food (CS-Sū 27.349–350), on how to gain the optimum benefit from food (CS-Vi 1.21–24) and on conditions detrimental to digestion (CS-Vi 2.9). Wholesome foods suitable for all constitutional types (SS-Sū 20.5; VA-Sū 6.62,65) and for individual constitutions (CS-Vi 1.6) are listed.

The vital role of sleep is recognized (CS-Sū 21.59, 36) and the optimum time for sleeping and rising is given (CS-Sū 21.35). There is a discussion on sleep and the *doṣas* (CS-Sū 21.44, 50).

The texts give a definition of exercise

(CS-Sū 7.31) and what it comprises and excludes (CS-Sū 7.31 commentary). They discuss the benefits of exercise (VA-Sū 2.10; CS-Sū 7.32; SS-Ci 24.39, 41–44) and when and how much to exercise (SS-Ci 24.45, 48; VA-Sū 2.11). Importantly, they note the signs of over-exercising (CS-Sū 7.33[1]; SS-Ci 24.46) and the dangers resulting from it (CS-Sū 7.33). They indicate the people who should avoid exercise (CS-Sū 7.35[1]).

Good conduct (*sadvṛtta*) is said to consist of positive acts (CS-Sū 8.18), ethical behaviour (CS-Sū 8.19) and actions to be avoided (CS-Sū 8.19–29).

Following a seasonal health regimen (*ṛtucarya*) involves understanding the relationship between the seasons and the body (CS-Sū 11.42) and the qualities of the seasons (CS-Sū 6.6) with their accumulation of specific *doṣas* (VA-Sū 12.24). Recommended regimens are given for each season (CS-Sū 6).

Emphasis is placed on safeguarding against disease (VA-Sū 4). Disease is defined (CS-Sū 9.4) and classified into types (CS-Sū 10.45; SS-Sū 24.4). Its causes are analysed. They are said to be the wrong use of the senses (CS-Śā 1.118–126; CS-Sū 11.37), wrong actions (CS-Sū 11. 37–39) and unseasonable climate (CS-Sū 11.42). The root cause of disease is traced to the failure of intellect (CS-Śā I.102; CS-Sū. 7–51). Disease can be prevented by the non-suppression of the physical urges (VA-Sū 4.1) and the suppression of undesirable impulses of mind, speech and body (CS-Sū 7.27, 28, 29). Safeguarding against diseases impinging from outside is achieved by the exercise of intellect (CS-Śā 1.147). Finally, there are purificatory treatments (VA-Sū I.34) to remove toxins and thus maintain the body's health.

Understanding Yoga through Āyurveda

Anatomy and Physiology

In applying the principles of Āyurveda to Yoga practice, it is necessary to refer to traditional Yoga manuals, of which the most pre-eminent is the *Haṭha Yoga Pradīpikā*. This does not, however, provide a guide to many of the aspects which have been considered here. For example, the vital sites of the body (*marmasthānas*) identified by Āyurveda (SS-Śā 6; VA-Śā 4) are not discussed in Yoga texts, though they are helpful in understanding the dynamics of *āsanas*.

Physiology: *Asanas* and *Doṣas*

The physiological benefits of some *āsanas* are recorded (HYP 1.26–32ff). An explanation of these benefits can be found in the Āyurvedic view that the imbalance of *doṣas* leads to disease. Various symptoms indicate the increase and decrease of *doṣas* (VA-Sū 11). On the basis of this it is possible to correlate *āsanas* with *doṣas*, relating actions of the former to effects on the latter, and to use *āsanas* for *doṣa* management.

Āyurveda classifies each *doṣa* into five subsidiary ones, based on precise location and function (VA-Sū 12.4–18). This facilitates a detailed understanding of *āsana* dynamics with respect to different parts of the body.

Psychology: *Doṣas* and *Prāṇayāma*

The benefits of *prāṇāyāma* are also recorded (HYP 2.48–158ff), as well as a caution regarding premature practice (HYP 2.15–17). *Prāṇayāma* involves respiration and so is related to *vāta doṣa*, which it controls partly by means of certain locking actions. However, it primarily concerns *prāṇa*, the life-force, and is thus connected with the cosmic *guṇas* and the mind. Mind and breath have an intimate, invariable connection (HYP 4.22–25).

Energy Management

Āyurveda delineates the influence of various factors such as constitution, age, state of health, time of day, climate, season and diet on day-to-day living. It also distinguishes between right use, overuse, under-use and misuse of the senses (CS-Śā 1.118–126; CS-Sū 11.37), and between right and wrong actions (CS-Sū 11. 37–39). All this information can be used as a tool for the management of energy throughout life. Importantly, it provides a guide to Yoga practice. By following the rules for health, Yoga can ultimately enhance and transcend it.

It is possible to maintain constitutional balance by *āsana* practice.

Āyurveda notes the various stages of life

(VA-Sū 1.8). While these should be taken into account, it is certainly the case that Yoga practice is suitable for all (HYP 1.64).

Āyurveda treats illness, stress and trauma in two stages (CS-Ci 1.4): remedy and restoration of strength. Yoga therapy follows the same approach.

Āyurveda notes that the day consists of periodic cycles of *kapha, pitta* and *vāta* (VA-Sū 1.8), each with its own quality. The time and content of Yoga practice should vary accordingly. The time of *prāṇāyāma* practice is more restricted (HYP 2.11).

Similarly, climates and seasons are characterized by different *doṣas*, and different regimens are recommended for each (CS-Sū 6). On the same lines, Yoga practice should be adapted to suit these variations.

Āyurveda stresses the importance of diet in health and gives guidelines on food (CS-Vi 1.21, VA-Sū 8.46). For Yoga practitioners certain foods are advised or forbidden (HYP 1.58–63; 2.14) on the basis of their effect on body and mind. These accord with Āyurvedic classifications. The practice of *āsanas and prāṇāyāma* enhances digestion and sensitivity to what is consumed.

Pain Management

Āyurveda theory is helpful in understanding the development of pain. It outlines the general pattern of disease (SS-Sū 21.36), and this can be used as a paradigm for the process of pain. It also identifies different types of pain (various references). On the basis of this knowledge the management of pain through Yoga can be better understood: the recognition of pain due to wrong movements, the alleviation of pain and the significance of inflammation and itching. Mental pain can be understood on the analogy of physical pain.

Cleansing Treatments

Āyurveda has a system of cleansing treatments *(pañcakarma)* for maintaining the health of the body by eliminating excess *doṣas* (VA-Sū 1.25; 14.5). Each is preceded by pre-operative procedures (VA-Sū 16.36), particularly oleation and sudation (VA-Sū 16.13). The principal cleansing treatments are emesis (*vamana*) (VA-Sū 18.1; 13.30); purgation (*virecana*) (VA-Sū 18.1), enema (*basti*) (VA-Sū 1.19), nasal medication (*nasya*) (VA-Sū 20.1) and bloodletting (*rakta mokṣa*) (SS-Sū 13.4). These are followed by post-operative procedures (VA-Sū 16.29) which ease the transition to normal diet and activity.

These cleansing treatments have an equivalent in Yoga (HYP 2.21–38). In particular, the regular practice of *āsanas and prāṇāyāma* promotes internal purification.

The effects of other treatments in Āyurveda such as massage (*abhyaṅga*) (VA-Sū 2.8), the streaming of oil onto the head (*śirodhāra*) (VA-Sū 22.23) and sudation (*svedana*) can also be obtained through Yoga practice. Yoga practice also includes post-operative procedures.

Other Specializations

Some of the specialized branches of Āyurveda (CS-Sū 30.28; VA-Sū 1.5) also provide information that is useful for understanding Yoga practice. Specializations include psychiatry, paediatrics, women's health, aphrodisiacs and reproductive disorders, and rejuvenation.

Diseases of the mind are classified according to cause and type (VA-Ut 6). This is helpful when using Yoga therapy to treat mental disorders. Its rationale conforms to Āyurvedic guidelines.

In the Āyurvedic view of children, account is taken of the predominant *doṣa* in each stage of life (VA-Sū 1.8). The Yogic approach to children is consonant with the fact that childhood is the stage of *kapha*-predominance.

With regard to women, Āyurveda classifies the physiological changes in a woman's life. It delineates the menstrual cycle (VA-Śā 1.26) and advises a quiet mode of living during menstruation (VA-Śā 1.24). The Yogic approach accords with this, recommending a special regime of *āsanas* during menstruation and other phases of womanhood.

A special branch of Āyurveda deals with aphrodisiacs and reproductive diseases (*vājīkarañā*), recognizing the importance of sex in life (CS-Ci 2; CS-Sū 11.35). Yoga, in contrast, primarily advocates celibacy, which is said (almost paradoxically) to increase virility and desirability (HYP 2.54–55). Yoga practice improves the health of the pelvic organs and can help to overcome infertility.

Another important branch of Āyurveda concerns rejuvenation (*rasāyana*) of the body tissues. Rejuvenation therapy is defined and its aim stated (CS-Ci 1.1. 7–8). The causes of degeneration are identified (CS-Ci 1.2.3), and the process of degeneration and regeneration is explained (VA-Sū 11.34–35). The benefits of rejuvenation therapy are enumerated (CS-Ci 1.7). Yoga similarly can be considered a rejuvenation therapy (HYP 2.78), and a comparison drawn between Āyurvedic *rasāyana* and Yogic *āsanas* and *prāṇāyāma*.

An integral part of rejuvenation therapy is ethical conduct and the observation of life disciplines (CS-Ci 1 2.30-36). These have their parallel in Yoga (PYS 2.30-32).

Āyurveda's objective of promoting longevity is echoed in Yoga (HYP 2.3). Yoga techniques as aids to longevity are noted (HYP 3.57–58, 61, 65, 70–71); these have their equivalents also in *āsanas*. However, certain Yoga practices seek to go beyond longevity, to immortality (HYP 3.105–108; 1.9).

Guide to Sanskrit Pronunciation

The spelling of Sanskrit words in this book follows the international convention of transliteration. A guide to pronunciation is as follows:

Vowels

There are long and short vowels. A bar sign over a vowel indicates that it is long.

Pure vowels

a as in *a*bout; **ā** as in *a*rm; **i** as in *i*t; **ī** as in *e*at; **u** as in p*u*ll; **ū** as in pool

Diphthongs

e as in eight; **ai** as in *eye*; **o** as in *o*re; **au** as in *ow*l

Vocalic r

ṛ as ri or ru (approximate equivalents)

Nasalised vowel

ṁ or **ṃ** the nasal is modified by the following consonant: **sāṁkhya** as saankhya

Aspiration

ḥ indicates the breathy repetition of the preceding vowel: **aḥ** as aha; **iḥ** as ihi; **uḥ** as uhu (approximate equivalents)

Consonants

These are grouped according to the place of articulation. Many have both an unvoiced and voiced, and unaspirated and aspirated form. There is a nasal in most groups.

These are grouped according to the place of articulation.

Guttural

k as in *k*ind; **kh** as in bac*k h*and; **g** as in **g**ive; **gh** as in a*gh*ast; **ṅ** as in si*n*k and si*ng*

Palatal

c as in *c*hin; **ch** as in *ch*urch hall; **j** as in *j*am; **jh** as in he*dge*hog; **ñ** as in i*n*ch and e*n*gine

Retroflex

ṭ ṭh ḍ ḍh ṇ: the tongue curls back and hits the upper palate.

Dental

t th d dh n: the tip of the tongue touches the back of the upper teeth (not the alveolar ridge, as in English).

th as in ou*th*ouse; **dh** as in chil*dh*ood

Labial

p ph b bh m

ph as in ha*ph*azard **bh** as in a*bh*or

Semi-vowels

y r l v

Sibilant

ś ṣ s

ś: palatal sh as in *sh*eet; **ṣ:** retroflex sh as in pu*sh*

Aspirate

h

Summary

A bar sign over a vowel indicates that the vowel is long.

An accent on s makes the pronunciation sh.

A dot under r makes the sound vocalic.

A dot under t, d or n makes it retroflex.

A dot above n makes it guttural.

A tilde above n makes it palatal.

A dot above or under m modifies it according to the following consonant.

Abbreviations

Authors and works are abbreviated by their initials; sections or works with identical initials by their first syllable.

Āyurveda Texts	
Caraka Saṁhitā	CS
Suśruta Saṁhitā	SS
Vāgbhaṭa Aṣṭāṅgahṛdaya	VA
Section Headings	
Cikitsāsthāna (Section on Treatment)	Ci
Indriyasthāna (Section on Portents and Prodromes)	In
Nidānasthāna (Section on Diagnosis)	Ni
Sūtrasthāna (Section on Principles)	Sū
Śārīrasthāna (Section on the Body)	Śā
Uttarasthāna (Section on Remaining Topics)	Ut
Vimānasthāna (Section on Measures)	Vi
Philosophy Texts	
Aitareya Upaniṣad	AU
Bṛhadāraṇyaka Upaniṣad	BU
Chāndogya Upaniṣad	ChU
Īśa Upaniṣad	ĪU
Kaṭha Upaniṣad	KU
Kauṣītaki Upaniṣad	KauU
Muṇḍaka Upaniṣad	MU
Maitrāyanī Upaniṣad	MaiU
Śvetāśvatara Upaniṣad	ŚU
Taittirīya Upaniṣad	TU
Bhagavad-Gītā	BG
Yoga Texts	
Pātañjala Yoga Sūtra	PYS
Vyāsa Bhāṣya (Commentary on PYS)	VB
Haṭha Yoga Pradīpikā	HYP

Index